Clinical
Echocardiography

Springer
London
Berlin
Heidelberg
New York
Hong Kong
Milan
Paris
Tokyo

Michael Y. Henein
Mary Sheppard
John Pepper
Michael Rigby

Clinical Echocardiography

With 357 Figures, 255 in Full Color

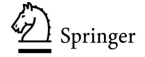 Springer

Michael Y. Henein, MSc, PhD
Senior Lecturer and Hon. Consultant in
 Cardiology/Echocardiography
Royal Brompton Hospital
Imperial College
London, UK

Mary Sheppard, MD, FRCPath
Consultant in Histopathology
Royal Brompton Hospital
London, UK

John Pepper, M.Chir, FRCS
Professor of Cardiothoracic Surgery
Royal Brompton Hospital
Imperial College
London, UK

Michael Rigby, MD, FRCP
Consultant Paediatric Cardiologist
Royal Brompton Hospital
London, UK

British Library Cataloguing in Publication Data
Clinical echocardiography
 1. Echocardiography
 I. Henein, Michael
 616.1′207543

ISBN 1852337737

Library of Congress Cataloging-in-Publication Data
Clinical echocardiography / Michael Henein ... [et al.].
    p. ; cm.
 Includes bibliographical references and index.
 ISBN 1-85233-773-7 (alk. paper)
  1. Echocardiography. I. Henein, Michael, 1959–
  [DNLM: 1. Echocardiography—methods. WG 141.5.E2 C6412 2004]
 RC683.5.U5C566 2004
 616.1′207543—dc22   2003067390

ISBN 1-85233-773-7 Springer-Verlag London Berlin Heidelberg
Springer-Verlag is part of Springer Science+Business Media
Springeronline.com

Typeset by EXPO Holdings, Malaysia
Printed and bound at Kyodo Printing Company, Singapore
28/3830-543210 Printed on acid-free paper SPIN 10917428

To Dr. Derek Gibson

Contents

Mitral Valve

ANATOMY

The mitral valve is composed of two leaflets, an annulus, chordae tendineae, and two papillary muscles. The anterior (aortic) leaflet is attached to the root of the aorta in direct continuity with the aortic valve and the membranous septum, and has a rectangular shape involving one-third of the circumference of the annulus. The posterior leaflet is continuous with the posterior wall of the left atrium and is longer than the anterior leaflet, occupying two-thirds of the circumference of the mitral annulus. The posterior leaflet is generally divided into three scallops, but this may vary. Chordae arise from the ventricular margin of the two leaflets and are inserted into the papillary muscles, which are placed one anteromedially and the other posterolaterally in the wall of the left ventricle. Papillary muscles themselves are continuous with the trabeculae and subendocardial layer of the ventricular wall.

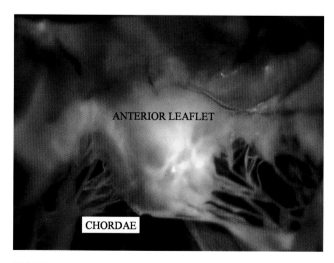

FIGURE 1.1. Normal mitral valve with large, "apron" like anterior leaflet in direct continuity with the aortic valve and posterior leaflet. Note attached chordae and papillary muscles.

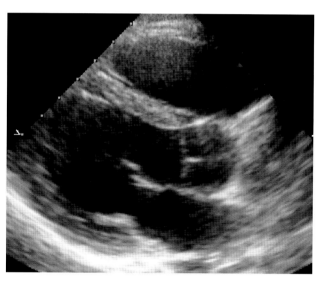

FIGURE 1.2. Parasternal two-dimensional long-axis view showing anterior (extending from the posterior aortic wall) and posterior (extending from the left atrial posterior wall) mitral valve leaflets.

PHYSIOLOGY

The mitral valve orifice cross-sectional area is approximately 5.0 cm^2, allowing left ventricular filling to occur predominantly in early diastole (approximately two-thirds of stroke volume) at a peak rate of 500- to 1000 mL/s. The remaining one-third of the stroke volume passes through the mitral valve during atrial systole. During diastasis, ventricular volume remains unchanged.[1] With exercise and increase in heart rate, diastasis shortens and the early and late filling components approximate until they summate and become indistinguishable.[2] With age the filling pattern reverses so that dominant left ventricular filling occurs in late diastole.[3]

1

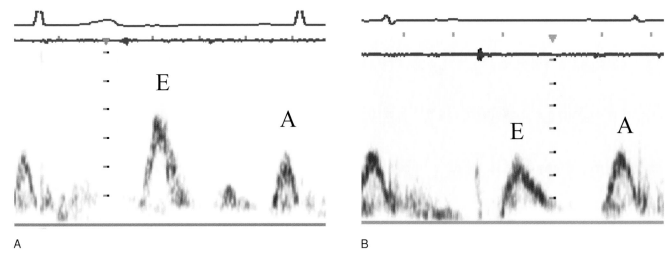

A   B

FIGURE 1.3. Transmitral Doppler flow velocities from (A) young subject showing dominant early diastolic component and (B) an elderly subject showing dominant late diastolic component.

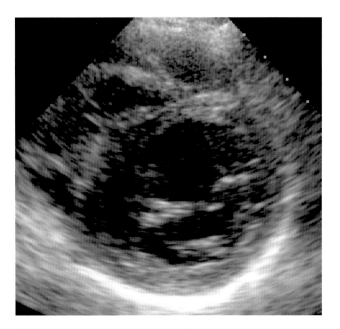

FIGURE 1.4. Minor axis view of the left ventricle and mitral valve showing the anterior and posterior leaflets.

MITRAL STENOSIS

Congenital mitral stenosis is a relatively rare group of anomalies with considerable variations in the morphologic features. Normally included in this diagnosis is cor triatriatum and supra-valvar mitral membrane, which can be identified by four-chamber and long-axis sections. Characteristically, color flow Doppler reveals acceleration proximal to the mitral valve leaflets. It is not unusual, however, for supra-valvar mitral stenosis to be associated with thickened mitral valve leaflets and chordal abnormalities as well. It is unusual to find isolated mitral valve stenosis. In addition to thickened and dysplastic leaflets, anomalies of the cords and of the papillary muscles may be detected. In the classical parachute mitral valve all the chords insert into a single papillary muscle.

Rheumatic Mitral Stenosis

Rheumatic mitral stenosis affects 10/100,000, predominantly in the Middle East, India, and the Far East. Mitral stenosis develops progressively after the occurrence of rheumatic fever in childhood.[4] It results in fusion of the commissures, thickened leaflets and eventually fibrosis. In the early stages, the anterior mitral leaflet is pliable, showing a doming motion in diastole and possibly a degree of leaflet prolapse in systole. The posterior leaflet is always stiff due to the commissural fusion. Thickening of the valve affects predominantly the tips and the leaflet body but tends to spare the base.[5] The subvalvular apparatus may also be involved. The chordae are thickened and fused, and the papillary muscles are scarred as a result of spread of fibrosis into the inferobasal

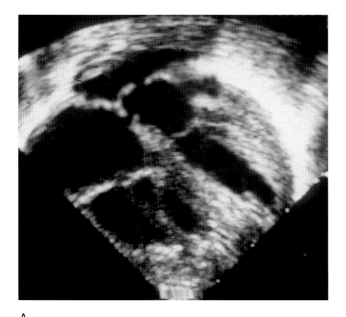

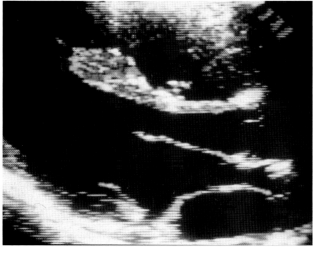

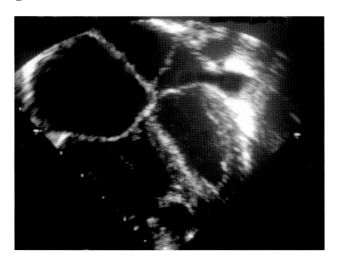

A

B

C

FIGURE 1.5. (A) Subcostal view and (B) Parasternal section from two patients with Cor triatriatum. (C) Subcostal view from a patient with supravalvar membrane.

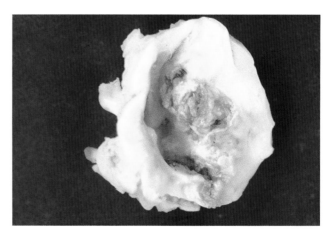

FIGURE 1.6. Pathology section from rheumatic mitral valve disease. Section shows the stenotic orifice with fish-mouth appearance. Note commissural fusion and leaflet calcification. View from the left atrium.

myocardium. Eventually, the mitral ring and leaflets may calcify.[6] Long-standing mitral stenosis may be complicated by dilatation of the left atrium, atrial fibrillation, and development of mural thrombus. Mitral stenosis may also result in pulmonary venous congestion, pulmonary hypertension, right ventricular hypertrophy and dilatation and functional tricuspid regurgitation.

Pathophysiology

As the disease progresses, the leaflets thicken, the commissures fuse, and the mitral valve area falls. With an area of 2.5 cm², symptoms start to appear as transmitral pressure drop becomes influenced by valve area, rhythm, duration of diastasis, and ventricular diastolic function. With a valve area of 2.5 cm², peak left ventricular filling rate falls and diastasis is lost. This is of no physiologic consequence at rest, but with exercise left ventricular filling is only maintained by a significant rise in left atrial pressure and, consequently, pressure drop between the left atrium and left ventricle. As the valve area becomes progressively smaller, a pressure drop develops at rest. This is usually associated with a fall in cardiac output and increase in pulmonary vascular resistance. Subvalvular apparatus involvement with fibrosis may contribute to the stenosis.[7]

To gain a flow-independent measure of the degree of narrowing, the mitral valve area is frequently calculated. A number of methods have been proposed for this, but none is entirely satisfactory. There is no agreed gold standard against which noninvasive measures can be calibrated, and when compared with one another, correlation coefficients are usually too low to be applicable in individual patients. Furthermore, it is questionable whether the complex hemodynamic disturbance to atrioventricular flow can be summed up in a simple statement of area.

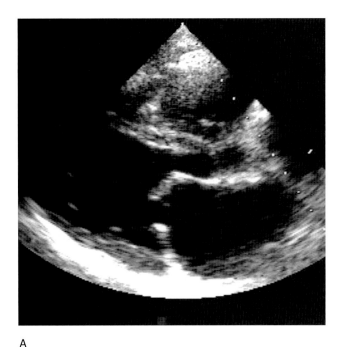

A

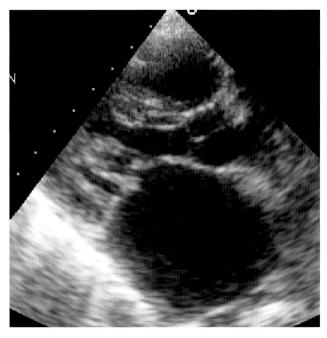

B

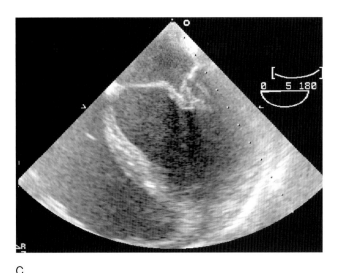

C

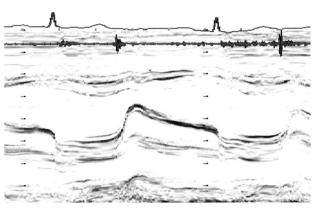

FIGURE 1.8. Mitral valve M-mode echogram from the same patient. Note the characteristic pattern of stiff rheumatic anterior leaflet in diastole and the anterior movement of the posterior leaflet.

FIGURE 1.7. (A) Two-dimensional parasternal long-axis view showing rheumatic mitral valve leaflets. Note the thickening and bowing of the anterior leaflet in diastole. (B) Similar view from a patient with fibrosed subvalvar apparatus causing subvalvar stenosis. (C) Transaesophageal echo showing Rheumatic mitral valve leaflets and fibrosed subvalvar apparatus.

Assessment of Severity of Mitral Stenosis

A number of methods have been used with varying accuracy.

- *Planimetry technique:* This involves tracing the inner border of the mitral valve opening in diastole. This has been shown to correlate with valve area measured by catheterization. It has its limitations particularly in the presence of significant leaflet tip calcification, poor border detection, and varying degrees of opening time due to atrial fibrillation.

- *Color flow Doppler:* The width of color flow jet in two orthogonal planes correlates with planimetry estimated values of mitral valve area.[9]

- *Flow convergence method (proximal isovelocity area-PISA):* Blood flow through a narrowed orifice con-

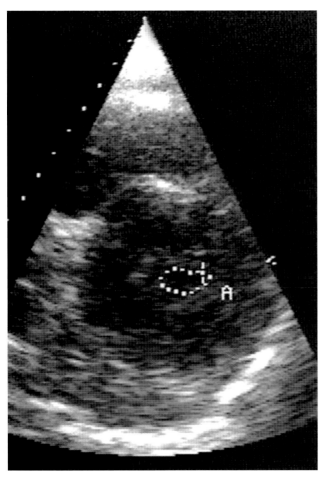

FIGURE 1.9. Parasternal short-axis view of a rheumatic mitral valve showing a traced valve area of 1.0 cm².

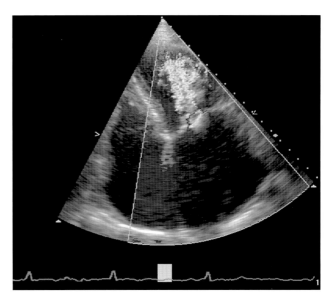

FIGURE 1.10. Transmitral flow convergence velocities from a patient with mitral stenosis. Note the change in velocity before the stenotic orifice.

change in color at the aliasing boundary. The narrowed orifice area can be calculated by dividing peak flow rate by maximal velocity through the orifice (obtained from the continuous wave Doppler). Mitral valve area calculated by this method has been shown to correlate with that obtained by conventional catheterization. However, the flow convergence method is subject to geometric complexities of the mitral valve orifice.[10]

- **Transmitral pressure drop:** Using the modified Bernoulli equation ($4V^2$) peak and minimum mitral pressure drop can be measured and mean value calculated.[11]

- **Pressure half time:** This is the time taken by the early diastolic transmitral pressure to drop to half its peak value (or the time taken for initial velocity divided by square root of 2, which is 1.4). The mitral area is then calculated as a constant (220) divided by pressure half time.

verges in a series of proximal isovelocity hemispheres (isovelocity surface area). In mitral stenosis it can be demonstrated by mosaic color Doppler on the atrial side in diastole. The flow rate is calculated by $2\pi r^2 v$, where r is the distance to a contour of velocity v, defined by the

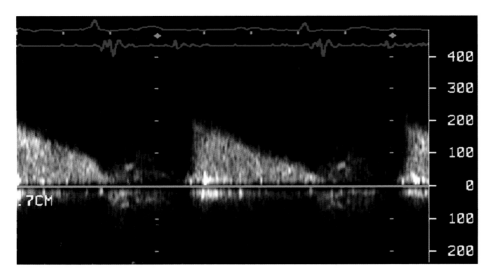

FIGURE 1.11. Left ventricular filling velocities by continuous-wave Doppler, showing raised early diastolic pressure drop component, giving a mean of 8 mmHg.

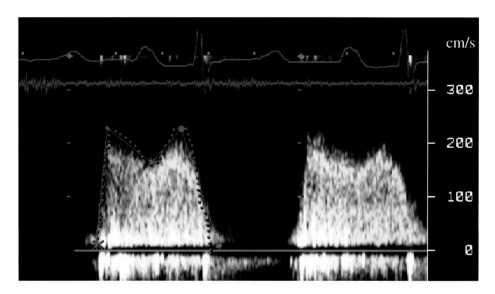

FIGURE 1.12. Transmitral Doppler flow velocities from a patient with mitral stenosis showing pressure decline during diastole (the basis for pressure half time measurements).

Although mitral pressure half time has been found to correlate with invasively measured mitral valve area, it too has major limitations, particularly in patients with atrial fibrillation and fast heart rate. Moreover, pressure half time depends on the left ventricular inflow resistance due to the funnel shape of the mitral apparatus, including both the orifice and the subvalvar component. More resistance at the subvalvar apparatus may slow the pressure decline across the inflow tract, so that pressure half time is usually smaller than that obtained from two-dimensional planimetry. The opposite is seen in patients with concomitant aortic regurgitation or left ventricular hypertrophy, when pressure half time overestimates the degree of mitral stenosis. It may therefore provide unreliable values after mitral valvuloplasty. The main reason for underestimating the accuracy of this method is the fact that it relies on the pressure fall, which is frequently not exponential.[12,13]

• *Continuity equation:* The continuity equation is based on the principle of mass and energy conservation. The flow at all points along a tube is constant and equals the product of mean velocity and the cross-sectional area. The mitral valve area is calculated as the product of aortic or pulmonary annular cross-sectional area and the ratio of the respective valve velocity time integral to that of the mitral stenotic continuous wave velocity. Although a more complex approach, this method is preferable in patients with additional significant aortic regurgitation in whom pressure half time overestimates mitral valve area.[14]

A mitral valve area of more than 1.5 cm² is usually considered mild stenosis, between 1.0 and 1.5 cm² is viewed as moderate, and an area of less than 1 cm² is considered to reveal severe stenosis.

Clinical Picture and Disturbed Physiology

Symptoms can develop at any time after the onset of acute rheumatic fever. The commonest manifestation is breathlessness, reduction of exercise tolerance, or palpitation, usually the result of increased left atrial pressure and atrial fibrillation. Hemoptysis and paroxysmal nocturnal dyspnoea may be related to pulmonary venous congestion. Systemic embolic disease, fluid retention, and symptoms of right-sided congestion are common in untreated cases. Venous pressure is raised if there is tricuspid regurgitation, organic involvement of the tricuspid valve, or pulmonary hypertension. The characteristic opening snap is heard when the leaflets are still pliable, but it disappears as the leaflets calcify with reduced mobility. A loud first heart sound is heard preceded by presystolic murmur if the patient is in sinus rhythm or mid-diastolic murmur.

Complications

• *Leaflet thickening and fibrosis:* With progressive rheumatic disease, chronic leaflet deformation occurs in the form of fibrosis and stiffness, particularly of the posterior leaflet. Fibrosis and calcification of the anterior leaflet may also occur.

• *Valve stenosis* results in progressive dilatation of the left atrium until blood stagnates in it. This results in slow atrial circulation, swirling of blood (spontaneous contrast or smoke), and increased risk of clot formation. The common site for clot location is either the free wall or the left atrial appendage. Since transthoracic echo cannot reliably visualize the left atrial appendage, transesophageal echo has become the technique of choice in confirming the presence of left atrial clot.[15,16]

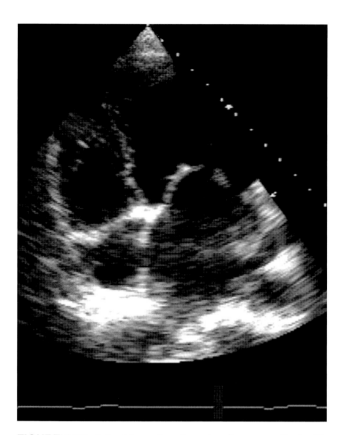

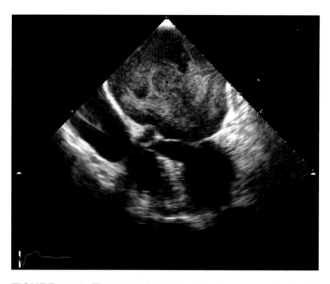

FIGURE 1.14. Transesophageal echo from a patient with rheumatic mitral valve stenosis showing a large left atrium with spontaneous echo contrast.

FIGURE 1.13. Apical four-chamber view from a patient with rheumatic mitral valve. Note the extent of leaflet thickening and fibrosis.

- *Left ventricular function* is often impaired in rheumatic mitral stenosis. In addition to the characteristic M-mode picture of a slow-filling ventricle, posterobasal segmental hypokinesia is commonly seen. This either may be due to primary rheumatic myocardial involvement or may be secondary to the significant fall of the posterior leaflet excursion and hence its corresponding myocardial segment. Ventricular dysfunction may result in significantly low stroke volume, high peripheral resistance, and development of pulmonary hypertension.[17,18]

- *Pulmonary hypertension:* Chronic significant mitral stenosis and increases in left atrial pressure and pulmonary venous pressure can lead to pulmonary arterial hypertension. Pulmonary hypertension is demonstrated as dilated right heart and significant increase in right ventricular-to-right atrial pressure drop. This may be underestimated as the right atrial pressure rises. Systolic right ventricular pressure may significantly fall after successful mitral valvotomy or valvuloplasty.[19,20]

- *Tricuspid regurgitation:* Even in the absence of organic tricuspid leaflet disease, functional tricuspid regurgitation may be present. This varies in its severity from mild to moderate as the tricuspid ring dilates, particularly as pulmonary hypertension develops. Severe tricuspid regurgitation has been reported to develop years after

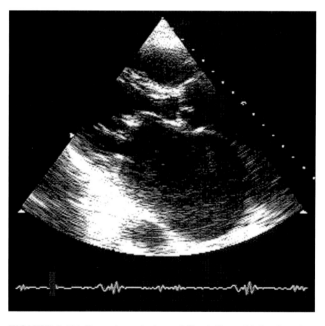

FIGURE 1.15. Parasternal view of the left ventricle showing dilated cavity.

mitral valve replacement, which significantly limits exercise tolerance in individual patients. Recently, some of this tricuspid regurgitation has been shown to be organic in origin, with the leaflets demonstrating signs of disease with fibrosis, calcification, prolapse, and tethering. In contrast to functional regurgitation, severe organic disease results in severe tricuspid annular dilatation, right heart failure, morbid liver complications, and early mortality.[21]

- *Aortic valve disease:* Although the mitral valve is most commonly affected by rheumatic disease, aortic regurgitation may also appear early in life during the sub-

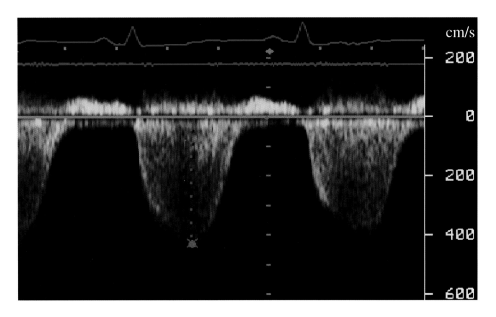

FIGURE 1.16. Continuous-wave Doppler demonstrating raised right ventricular–right atrial pressure drop–70 mmHg, from a patient with pulmonary hypertension (PHT) complicating mitral stenosis.

acute phase. Aortic stenosis tends to develop later. Its severity may be significantly underestimated as long as mitral valve stenosis is present. If missed before correction of mitral stenosis, it usually devalues the success of the procedure.

- **Tricuspid valve stenosis:** Organic tricuspid stenosis is not seen in the absence of mitral stenosis. When it occurs, physical signs are usually mild and overshadowed by those of mitral stenosis. Physiologically significant pressure drops are much less than across the mitral valve (2- to 3 mmHg). Tricuspid stenosis must be recognized by echocardiography before correction of mitral stenosis because, if left, it results in fluid retention. Tricuspid stenosis is often missed at cardiac catheterization and, when confirmed, always requires an open procedure. Thus it is an absolute contraindication to balloon mitral valvuloplasty. Finally, tricuspid stenosis may develop late after mitral valve surgery for mitral stenosis.[22]

Treatment

Valvuloplasty

Valvuloplasty uses a percutaneous catheter double balloon or Inoue balloon valvuloplasty. It is only recommended when mitral valve leaflets are pliable and there is no valve calcification, including the subvalvar apparatus. Left atrial clot should be excluded by transesophageal echo. The increase in mitral valve area occurs along the plan of commissures and results in an increased opening angle, provided there is no calcification. An echocardiographic (Abascal) score is used to assess morphologically mitral valve structure and function.[23–25] Assigning a score ranging from 0- to 4 to each of mitral leaflet mobility, thickening, calcification, and subvalvar thickening provides a numerical assessment of overall valve function. The higher the score, the more anatomically deformed and functionally

abnormal is the valve, and thus the likelihood of poor outcome after balloon valvuloplasty. Mid- and long-term results of the procedure in well-selected cases are promising. A successful procedure is judged by a more than 50% increase in mitral valve area. This can be underestimated early after procedure because of the iatrogenically created left-to-right shunt across the atrial septum. The latter results from the guidewire insertion through the atrial septum. This shunt has been reported to disappear within 6 months after the procedure. Significant mitral regurgitation may occur in more than 30% of patients after balloon valvuloplasty. It is usually more severe when the procedure is complicated by a tear in one of the two leaflets. Transesophageal echocardiography is of particular importance before and during this procedure in order to:

Assess valve structure and calcification before procedure.

Exclude left atrial appendage or free wall thrombus.

Guide the way during septal puncture.

Ascertain balloon position across the valve orifice.

Assess pressure drop and mitral valve area after each inflation.

Detect early complication (i.e., leaflet tear, ruptured chordae, or mitral regurgitation that needs urgent intervention).

Confirm any perforation of left atrial free wall.

Assess left to right shunt.

Surgery

For symptomatic cases not suitable for valvuloplasty, surgery is the only alternative.

- **Closed mitral valvotomy:** This is appropriate for young patients who are in sinus rhythm, with no other

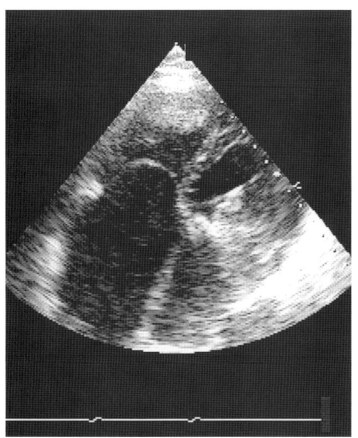

A

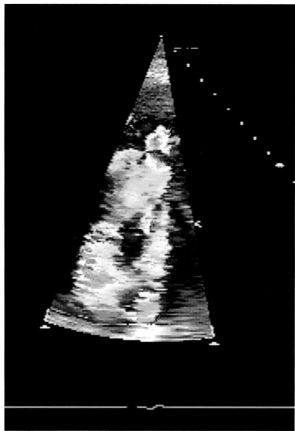

B

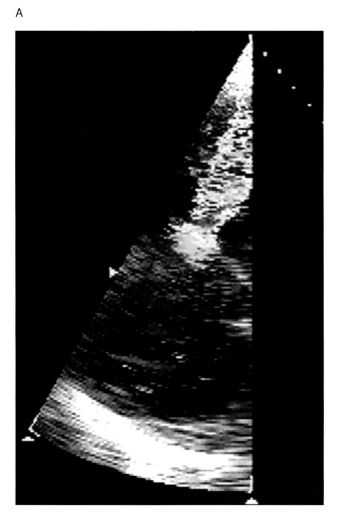

C

FIGURE 1.17(A,B,C). Apical four-chamber views from a patient with rheumatic heart disease involving mitral, aortic, and tricuspid valves. Note the bowing of the tricuspid valve leaflets in diastole, tricuspid regurgitation and the high forward velocity consistent with organic leaflet involvement.

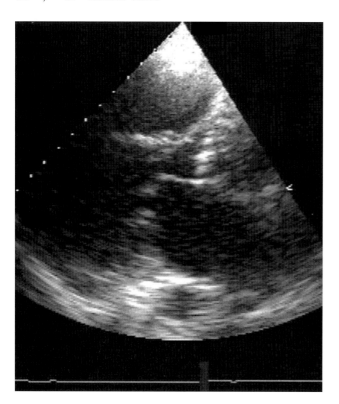

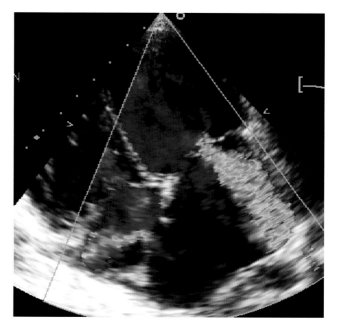

FIGURE 1.19. Apical views from a patient with rheumatic mitral valve leaflets after balloon valvuloplasty demonstrating significant regurgitation and atrial shunt across the mid septum.

FIGURE 1.18. Parasternal long-axis view from a patient with rheumatic heart disease involving mitral and aortic valves. Note the classical picture of mitral leaflet involvement and thickening of the aortic cusps.

valve disease, in whom mitral valve leaflets are mobile and not calcified. This is an underrated operation, and up to 40 year follow up results are exceptionally good.

● *Open valvotomy:* This procedure allows an anatomical repair of the mitral valve under direct vision. Correction of associated rheumatic mitral regurgitation in some cases has been recently undertaken. Open valvotomy requires the use of cardiopulmonary bypass, but can be performed either via a sternotomy or smaller incisions such as a right anterior thoracotomy or with computerised robotic technology via 3 to 4 ports in the chest wall.

● *Mitral valve replacement:* This is required in pure mitral stenosis when the valve is heavily calcified. Valve substitutes are either a bioprosthesis, a single leaflet valve (e.g., Medtronic) or a bileaflet valve (e.g., St. Jude

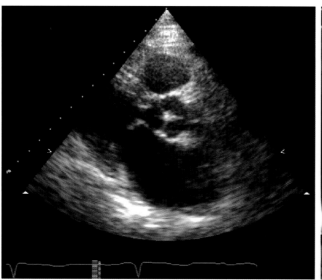

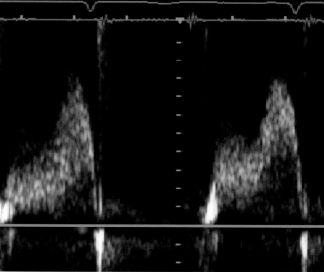

FIGURE 1.20. Parasternal long-axis view from a patient with rheumatic mitral valve disease and flow velocities after valvotomy.

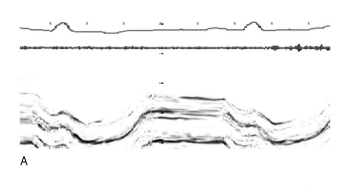

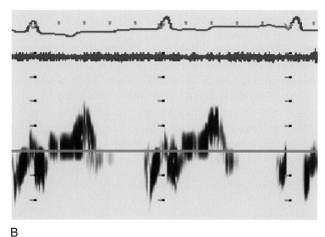

FIGURE 1.21. Long-axis recording from left ventricular free wall of a patient after mitral valve replacement and cutting of papillary muscles. Note the marked incoordinate behavior and the extent of shortening that takes place in diastole rather than systole.

Medical). Traditionally, replacement of the mitral valve required cutting the heads of the papillary muscles to prevent entanglement of chordal in the cage of a Starr-Edwards valve. This resulted in significant incoordination of the left ventricle, particularly the long axis when its main shortening phase occurs in diastole rather than in systole. The loss of longitudinal function renders the ventricle more spherical in diastole and hence has adverse implications on filling pattern and symptoms. The current surgical approach is to preserve the subvalvar apparatus as much as possible. This change in procedural plan has resulted in maintained long axis function and improvement of ventricular hemodynamics and symptoms after surgery.

The Role of Echocardiography in Patient Selection for Surgery

Assessing Ventricular Function: In addition to valve assessment, transthoracic echo provides an exceptional means for quantifying ventricular function in these patients. Symptoms may result from poor ventricular function, whether as part of the rheumatic cardiac disease or from an additional etiology (e.g., coronary artery disease). Raised end-diastolic pressure results in accentuated left ventricular filling velocities, which is complicated by pulmonary venous congestion and hence development of dyspnoea. Additional atrial fibrillation usually worsens the situation by losing the atrial filling component and compromises the stroke volume, particularly when fast. Such severely disturbed physiology should be excluded before signifying mitral valve stenosis as the main cause of symptoms. Furthermore, ignoring such abnormalities before surgery may result in peri- or early post-operative complications with increased mortality.

Degree of Valve Calcification: Transesophageal echo provides additional details on the mitral valve and subvalvar apparatus that may influence decision making. Pliable leaflets with mild calcification suggest valvotomy, whereas extensive calcification requires valve replacement. Subvalvar stenosis by fibrosed chordae and papillary muscles also favors valve replacement. Any evidence for additional endocarditis or possible complications such as "shunt formation" can be dealt with at the time of surgery.

Atrial Fibrillation: Patients with atrial fibrillation and a modestly dilated left atrium may be recommended for elective ablation of the pulmonary venous orifice at the time of mitral valve surgery. When such procedure is performed under transesophageal echo guidance, it may add to its rate of success. Left atrial thrombus, whether mural or in the atrial appendage, can also be decorticated during the procedure.

Other Valve Disease: Transthoracic echo provides quantitative assessment of aortic and tricuspid valve involvement, when combined with pulsed and continuous-wave Doppler. If found, a balanced physiology should be considered when assessing more than one diseased valve (i.e., tricuspid stenosis tends to underestimate mitral stenosis, and mitral stenosis underestimates aortic stenosis). Transesophageal echo may add more clarity in assessing tricuspid valve anatomy in this condition.

MITRAL ANNULAR CALCIFICATION

Mitral annular calcification is usually a disease of the elderly,[26] predominantly females.[27] It is also present in other conditions, such as hypertension and/or aortic stenosis.[28] Calcification affects the heart either in a patchy manner or uniformly. It usually involves the mitral annulus but can extend into the basal septum, the aortic root and cusps, or rarely, the whole of the ventricular basal region. However, if the calcification encroaches on the basal part of the mitral leaflets, it may result in increased filling velocities. It can be associated with mild mitral regurgitation, but more commonly, conduction disturbances occur in approximately 50% of patients. When affecting the mitral annulus, the leaflets themselves are usually spared, and the valve does not become stenotic.

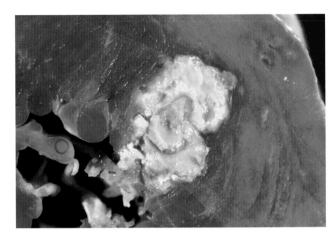

FIGURE 1.22. Pathologic picture showing extensive nodular calcification of the mitral annulus that extends deeply into the myocardium. Note sparing of most of the leaflet apart from base.

Management

In the absence of significant mitral stenosis, valve replacement is not indicated. When involving the aortic root and cusps leading to stenosis, aortic valve and root replacement is usually successful. Calcification of the mitral annulus is not superficial, but it invades deeply into the myocardium. During surgery, decalcifying the mitral

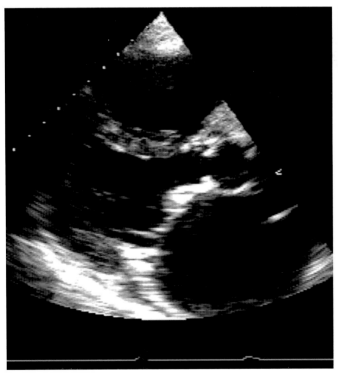
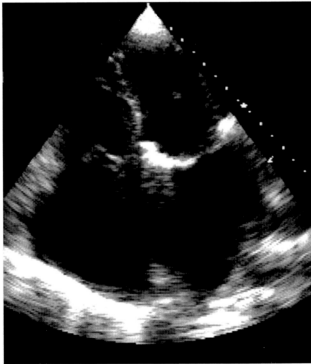

FIGURE 1.23. Parasternal long-axis and four-chamber views of the left heart showing a heavily calcified mitral annulus and normal leaflets.

ring for valve replacement may result in myocardial perforation. Mitral valve replacement, therefore, should never be performed for pure mitral ring calcification.

MITRAL REGURGITATION

Mitral regurgitation results from abnormalities affecting components of the mitral valve–leaflets, annulus, chordae, or papillary muscles. The causes are multiple in comparison to mitral stenosis. Myocardial disease when affecting particularly the basal part of the ventricle may result in some degree of mitral regurgitation.

Common Causes of Mitral Regurgitation

Myxomatous Degeneration

Myxomatous degeneration is the most common cause of isolated mitral regurgitation. It is also called degenerative mitral valve disease of the elderly or floppy valve. The disease involves progressive myxomatous degeneration of the mitral leaflets and may range from stretched, "normal" appearing leaflet to the full-blown thickened myxomatous ballooned leaflet. The terms *prolapse, floppy, redundant, myxomatous,* and *flail* have all been applied to this entity. The classic valve leaflets are thickened, redundant, and increased in area, and prolapse into the left atrium in systole. This process could affect either of the two cusps, most commonly the mid-third of the posterior leaflet. The chordae may become elongated, thinned, and tortuous, predisposing to rupture and acute mitral valve prolapse. In the elderly, it is usually asymptomatic. Echocardiographically, mid-late systolic buckling of the leaflets of more than 2- or 3-mm posterior displacement to the mitral closure point is taken as a clear demonstration of the leaflet prolapse. Myxomatous degeneration, particularly when involving the leaflet tips, may be difficult to differentiate from vegetation caused by endocarditis. The diagnosis of mitral prolapse should be made from the left parasternal view, since the combination of the shape change of the mitral valve ring in systole and the valve closure may appear to represent prolapse in other views.[29] In Marfan's syndrome, the myxomatous degeneration tends to involve commonly the leaflet tips, particularly the anterior leaflet. This does not always result in significant mitral regurgitation but may remain static and asymptomatic for years. Loss of systolic coaption and prolapse of one of the two leaflets into the left atrium constitute a highly sensitive and specific sign of a flail leaflet irrespective of its etiology. Transesophageal echo usually provides clearer images for the leaflets and the degree of loss of coaption. The degree of mitral regurgitation with pure leaflet prolapse may be insignificant, and clinical examination may reveal a mid-systolic click or late-systolic murmur. Mitral prolapse may predispose to infective endocarditis, and pro-

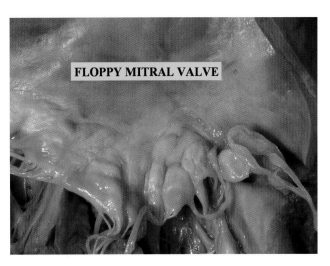

FIGURE 1.24. Pathology section from myxomatous mitral valve leaflets showing the thickened leaflet with ballooning between the chordae.

phylactic antibiotics are recommended. Over the long term, simple mitral prolapse may progress to severe mitral regurgitation that requires surgical repair.

The most common form of so-called congenital mitral regurgitation is that found in association with a primum atrial septal defect or other form of atrioventricular septal defect. In general, it is better to describe the systemic atrioventricular valve in this group of anomalies as the left atrioventricular valve rather than the mitral valve. Another important cause of congenital mitral regurgitation is the so-called isolated cleft of the anterior leaflet of the mitral valve. In essence the valve appears to have three leaflets. The importance of this diagnosis is that in almost every case it is possible to perform a surgical repair by patching anterior leaflet of the mitral valve, thus avoiding the need for mitral replacement.

Infective Endocarditis

Infective endocarditis is a major cause of symptomatic mitral regurgitation.[30] Vegetations develop on the cusp and vary from small nodules along the line of apposition to large friable masses up to 10 mm in diameter or more, especially with fungal infection. Lesions on the anterior (aortic) cusp of the mitral valve may occur in association with aortic valve endocarditis, usually involving the right coronary cusp. Infection with rupture and perforation may occur. These jet lesions vary from localized aneurysms to complete cusp perforation, resulting in severe mitral regurgitation that requires valve replacement. Endocarditis may affect normal valves, particularly in the elderly, but more commonly, valves with minor congenital abnormality or floppy valve.

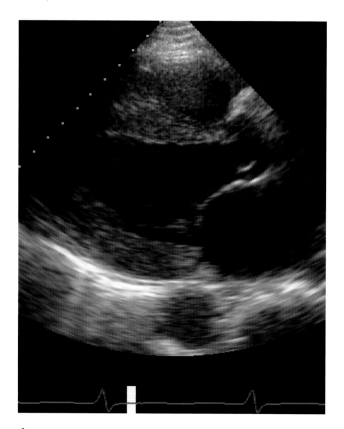

A

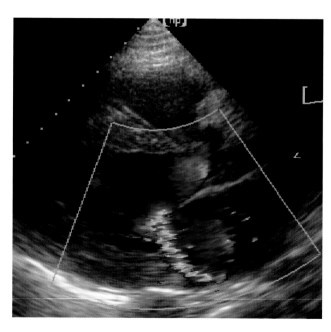

B

FIGURE 1.25. Parasternal long-axis two-dimensional image of the left ventricle and mitral valve. Note the mild prolapse of the anterior leaflet (left) and the resulting mild mitral regurgitation as shown by color Doppler (right).

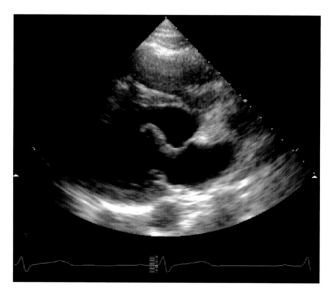

FIGURE 1.26. Flail anterior mitral valve leaflet from a patient with Marfan's syndrome.

Pathophysiology of Mitral Regurgitation

Pure mitral regurgitation is associated with a large increase in left ventricular output.[7] The total stroke volume may be increased up to three or four times the normal. At the time of aortic valve opening, more than a quarter of the stroke volume may have already entered the left atrium. This results in a V wave, which may be as high as 50 to 60 mmHg. This volume of blood re-enters the ventricle in early diastole, thus shortening the isovolumic relaxation time and increasing early diastolic filling velocities, resulting in a third heart sound. When mitral regurgitation is very severe, left ventricular and left atrial pressures may equalize at mid-ejection or even earlier. This occurs particularly with ruptured papillary muscle. At first, left ventricular end-diastolic volume does not significantly increase, whereas end-systolic is greatly reduced. This results in a significant fall in forward cardiac output that can only be maintained by sinus tachycardia.

Assessing Severity of Mitral Regurgitation

The major determinant of mitral regurgitation severity is the effective regurgitant area, which may be fixed in rheumatic mitral valve disease, bacterial endocarditis, and mitral prolapse. A regurgitant volume of 40 mL signifies a regurgitant fraction (volume of blood regurgitated into the left atrium) of 40% and regurgitant area (mitral valve incompetent area in systole) of 40 mm^2.[31]

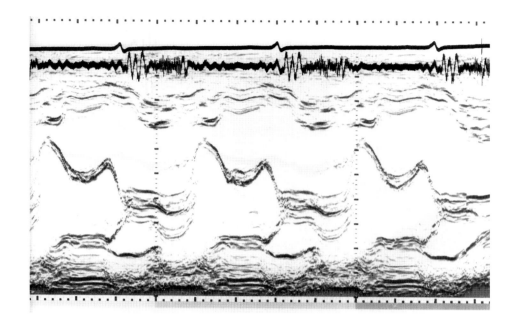

FIGURE 1.27. M-mode echogram of the mitral valve leaflets from a patient showing mid-systolic backward movement of the mitral leaflet coinciding with the click (on the phonocardiogram, top) and late systolic mitral prolapse.

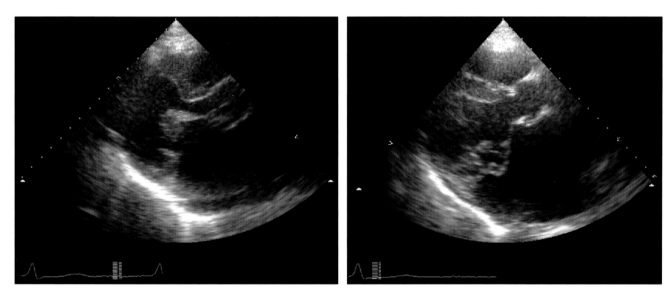

FIGURE 1.28. Parasternal two-dimensional long-axis view from an elderly patient with myxomatous anterior MV leaflet tip. Note the way it prolapses into the left atrium in systole.

Large LV Stroke Volume An increase in left ventricular end-diastolic dimension and fall of end-systolic dimension over time suggests an overloaded ventricle and significant mitral regurgitation.[17,32] In this condition, fractional shortening and calculated ejection fraction should not be taken as measures of ventricular function. Absolute end-systolic diameter or volume may be considered as more accurate markers of ventricular disease. An end-systolic diameter of more than 40 mm suggests independent left ventricular disease, the reversibility of which cannot be confirmed.[33]

Color flow area is the most widely used technique. Maximum jet areas traced in different views correlate with severity of mitral regurgitation assessed by left ventricu-

lography. A regurgitant area of more than 8 cm^2 or a relative area more than 40% that of the left atrium suggests severe regurgitation, whereas a jet area of less than 4 cm^2 or a relative area less than 20% identifies mild mitral regurgitation. This method relies on the clear display of a uniform regurgitant jet. If used alone, it may over or underestimate the regurgitation severity, particularly when the valve leaflets are flail and the jet uniformity is disrupted. Jet areas studied by transesophageal technique also tend to overestimate valve regurgitation.[34–36]

Proximal Isovelocity Surface Area (PISA) As discussed in mitral stenosis, the regurgitant orifice area can be calculated by dividing peak flow rate by maximal velocity through the orifice (obtained from the continu-

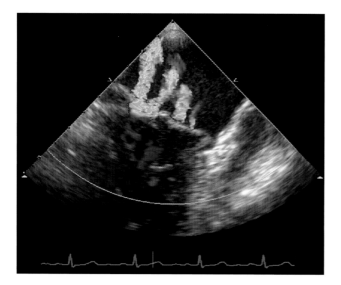

FIGURE 1.29. Transesophageal echo from a patient with myxomatous MV leaflets showing multiple regurgitation jets.

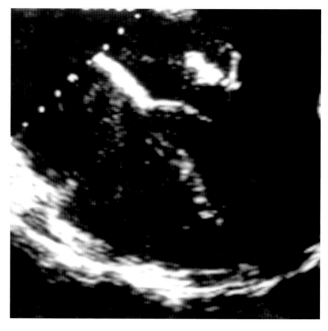

FIGURE 1.30. Transesophageal echo from a patient with bacterial endocarditis and a vegetation attached to the anterior mitral valve leaflet.

ous-wave Doppler). A regurgitant orifice of more than 0.5 cm² corresponds to a regurgitant fraction of more than 50% and thus signifies severe mitral regurgitation that needs surgery. Accurate measurements of flow convergence seem more reliable than color flow area mapping. However, flow convergence method is subject to geometric complexities of the regurgitant orifice that requires correction factors, as in eccentric jets commonly seen in mitral valve prolapse.

Vena Contracta is the narrowest cross-sectional area of the jet that immediately exists at the regurgitant orifice. The width of vena contracta has been found to correlate with the regurgitant volume; a width of 5 mm with a

regurgitant volume of 60 mL suggests severe regurgitation and a width less than 3 mm is consistent with mild mitral regurgitation. Vena contracta has been suggested to be independent of hemodynamic variables, orifice geometry, and instrument setting and is associated with a low interobserver variability.[40]

Systolic flow reversal in pulmonary veins is a sign that is helpful in determining regurgitant severity only when the jet is not eccentric. It is not of great use in patients with severe left ventricular disease in whom the

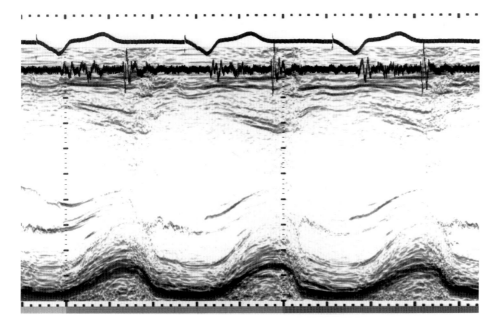

FIGURE 1.31. M-mode of the left ventricular minor axis from a patient with severe mitral regurgitation. Note the relative difference between end-diastolic and end-systolic measurements and the rapid increase in early diastolic dimension due to severe mitral regurgitation.

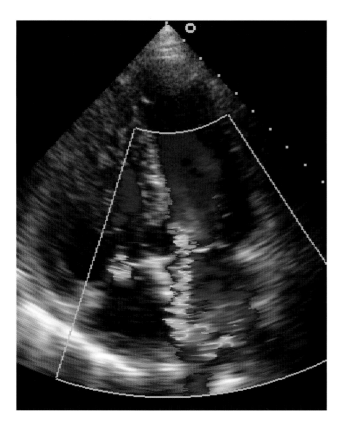

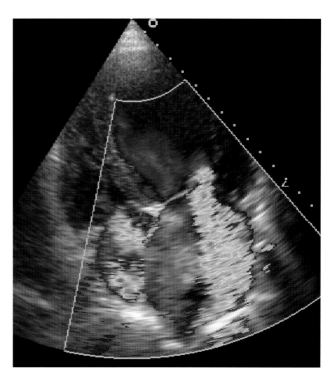

A   B

FIGURE 1.32. Apical four-chamber view from a patient with mild and another with severe mitral regurgitation on color Doppler. Note the absolute and relative difference in the regurgitant area with respect to that of the left atrium.

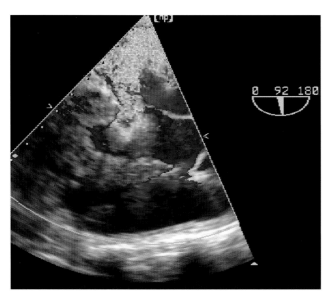

FIGURE 1.33. Color flow Doppler from a patient with severe mitral regurgitation from a transesophageal picture. Note the aliasing velocities proximal to the valve orifice (on the ventricular side).

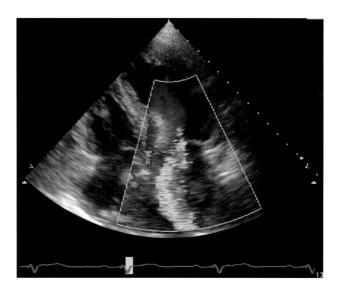

FIGURE 1.34. Apical four-chamber view from a patient with moderate mitral regurgitation showing vena contracta of 4 mm.

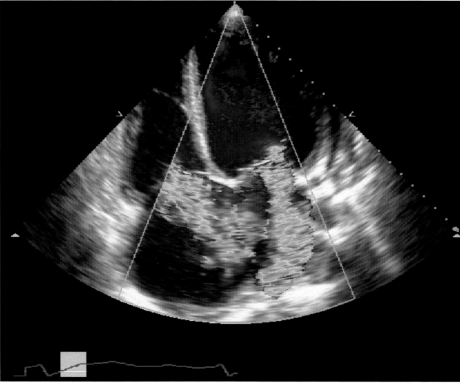

A

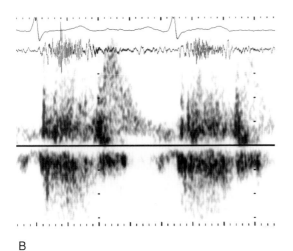

B

FIGURE 1.35. Apical four-chamber view from a patient with severe mitral regurgitation with the jet approaching the orifice of the pulmonary veins (top). Pulsed-wave velocity of the pulmonary venous flow from the same patient showing systolic flow reversal in the veins (bottom).

systolic component of pulmonary venous flow is already poor and those with eccentric mitral regurgitation jet. Moreover, systolic flow in pulmonary veins is affected by left atrial compliance, age, rhythm, and eccentric jets.[41]

Continuous-Wave Doppler Mild mitral regurgitation usually stops well beyond (>80 ms) end-ejection, corresponding to the left ventricular pressure decline during the isovolumic relaxation period.[42] A short deceleration limb of the retrograde transmitral signal suggests significant regurgitation. As left atrial pressure increases, the retrograde pressure drop across the mitral valve also falls and no longer represents left ventricular systolic pressure. Left atrial pressure can be estimated as the transmitral retrograde pressure drop deducted from systolic blood pressure, particularly when it is low.

Left atrial emptying volume is estimated as end-systolic volume–end diastolic volume. A value of more than 40 mL identifies patients with severe mitral regurgitation.[43]

Continuity Equation Relative aortic and mitral stroke volumes using the continuity equation, as previously discussed, determine regurgitation severity.[37]

Three-Dimensional Color Doppler The advent of real-time three-dimensional color Doppler now allows us to quantify the regurgitant volume.

Clinical Picture and Course of the Disease

The clinical picture and course of the disease differ according to the underlying etiology.

Ruptured Chordae Tendineae

Ruptured chordae tendineae often result from the myxomatous degeneration process that occurs with age. The development of significant mitral regurgitation is usually gradual. In some cases it takes an acute onset,

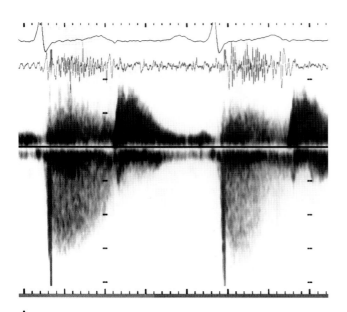

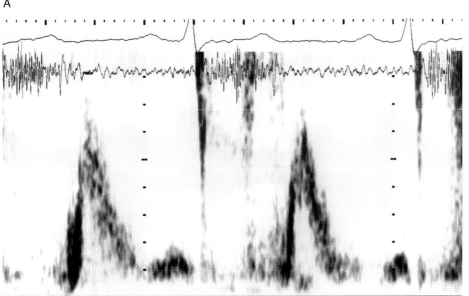

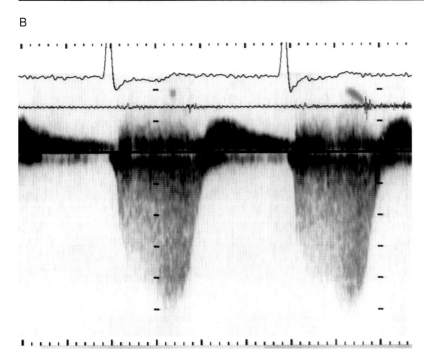

FIGURE 1.36. (A) Continuous-wave Doppler recording of severe mitral regurgitation and (B) left ventricular filling. Note the equalization of left atrial and left ventricular pressures in early diastole, ending retrograde flow at A2, short isovolumic relaxation time, high left ventricular filling velocities in early diastole, and third heart sound. (C) Continuous-wave Doppler from a patient with moderate MR, ending shortly beyond A2.

A

B

C

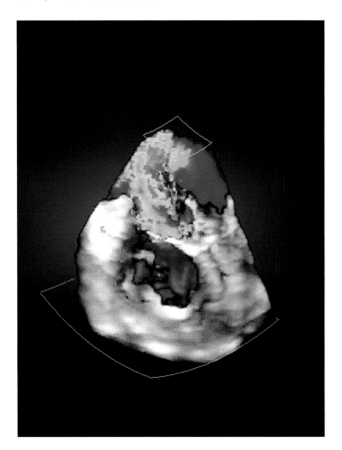

FIGURE 1.37. Three-dimensional reconstruction of color Doppler mitral regurgitation.

improve over the course of the following weeks, by which time the ventricle adapts itself to the volume load. Patients may present in intractable pulmonary edema in severe cases. This can be explained on the basis of long-standing mitral regurgitation, leading to a dilated and diseased ventricle. The combination of raised ventricular diastolic pressures and filling pressures worsen the condition and reduce the probability of a successful repair.[44,45]

Ruptured Papillary Muscles

Ruptured papillary muscles constitute a major complication of myocardial infarction. They occur 2 to 5 days after the onset of the infarct. The prognosis is very poor without prompt surgical repair. Incomplete rupture, usually of only one head of the papillary muscle, occurs 4 to 5 days after the infarct, with gradual deterioration of mitral regurgitation. This increases pre-existing left ventricular dysfunction.

Functional Mitral Regurgitation

The normally functioning mitral valve depends on the leaflets; ring; subvalvar apparatus, including chordae; papillary muscle fibers; and the circumferential muscle layer supporting the mitral ring. Each of these components plays an important role in maintaining the competence of the mitral valve. With papillary muscle dysfunction due to ischemia or other etiologies, cusp closure is not complete, thus resulting in some degree of mitral regurgitation.[46,47] This is usually mild in severity but may be relatively long in duration, enough to compromise filling time and hence cardiac output. With severe left ventricle deterioration of function, particularly

particularly when it is not a complication of myxomatous degeneration but is due simply to chordal rupture. The ventricle does not dilate acutely. The main symptoms are palpitations and dyspnoea. Symptoms tend to

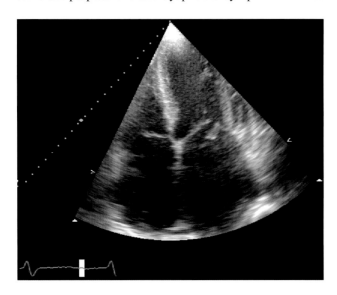

A

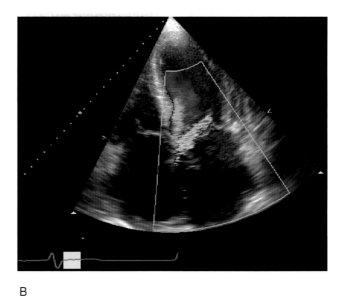

B

FIGURE 1.38. Left: Apical four-chamber view from a patient with ruptured chordae resulting in posterior MV leaflet prolapse. Right: Color flow Doppler showing mitral regurgitation.

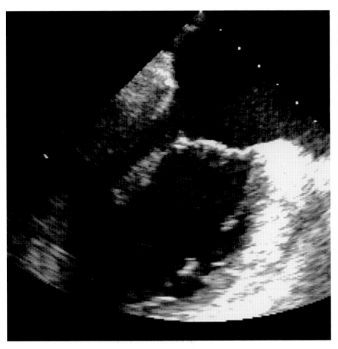
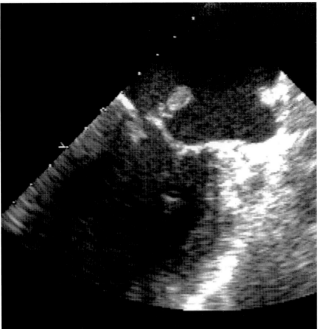

A

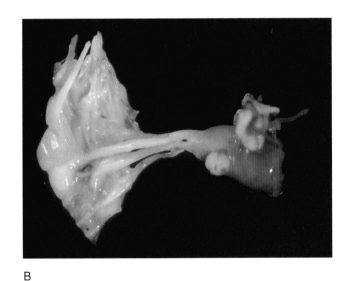

B

FIGURE 1.39. (A) Transesophageal pictures from a patient with ruptured posteromedial papillary muscle. Note bouncing of the detached segment into the left atrium in systole. (B) Part of mitral valve leaflet with attached chordae and infarcted papillary muscle that has ruptured.

at the basal segment and as the ventricle progressively dilates, mitral ring diameter increases. This adds to the degree of regurgitation. Thus, although functional in origin, mitral regurgitation may be hemodynamically significant either in terms of duration with respect to the cardiac cycle length or in terms of volume. Color flow Doppler may overestimate the degree of regurgitation. In some patients with dilated cardiomyopathy, severe regurgitation at rest may become mild with stress, particularly those with enough viable myocardium that reduces basal ventricular dimensions and hence ring diameter. In these patients, achieving satisfactory revascularization of the ventricular base tends to revive its systolic function and reduce the mitral regurgitation.

Endomyocardial Fibrosis

Endomyocardial fibrosis is a fibrotic process that involves the subendocardium and underlying myocardial layer. When it affects the right ventricle, it involves predominantly the apex, then progresses toward the tricuspid valve, but spares the outflow tract. In the left ventricle, the inflow tract, apex, and outflow tract are all involved. As the fibrosis affects the papillary muscle it results in mitral and tricuspid valve regurgitation that can be severe enough to warrant valve replacement. This disease is common in the eastern part of Africa, southern India, and Brazil, and rarely affects Europeans. It is usually linked to hyperesinophilia due to helminthic infection.

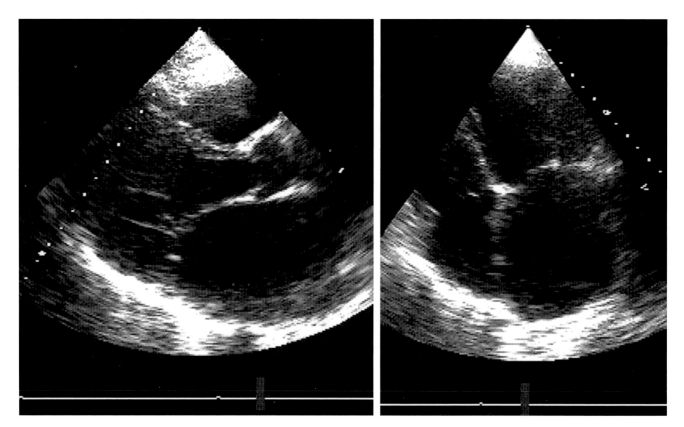

FIGURE 1.40. Parasternal and apical views from a patient with functional mitral regurgitation caused by ischemic left ventricular disease. Note the dilated ventricle, the normal morphology of the mitral valve, and the dilated ring.

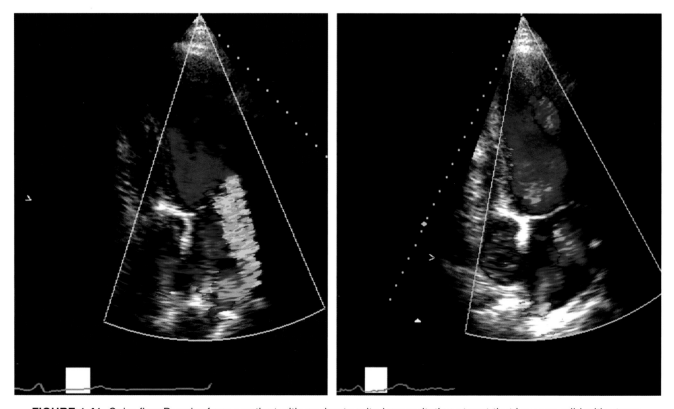

FIGURE 1.41. Color flow Doppler from a patient with moderate mitral regurgitation at rest that became mild with stress.

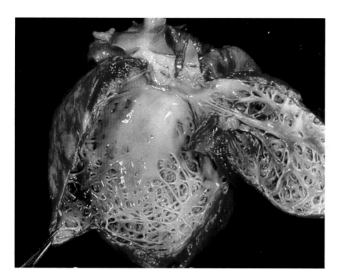

FIGURE 1.42. Pathology: dense, pale fibrous tissue lining the endocardium of the left ventricle and extending up to the mitral leaflets from a patient with endomyocardial fibrosis.

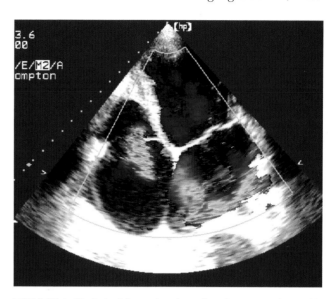

FIGURE 1.43. Apical four-chamber view from a patient with endomyocardial fibrosis. Note the significant fibrosis that is involving the right ventricular apex (brightness) and the mitral regurgitation secondary to left-sided involvement.

Management of Mitral Regurgitation

Mild and moderate mitral regurgitation are well tolerated and do not require intervention apart from prophylactic antibiotics for potential infection. Severe mitral regurgitation that causes significant symptoms in spite of medical therapy warrants mitral valve surgery. Mitral valve repair is particularly satisfactory for posterior leaflet prolapse and occasionally for anterior leaflet prolapse. Timing of surgery is critical. While it should be at the earliest opportunity for papillary muscle rupture, it could be delayed for 1 to 2 weeks in case of chordal

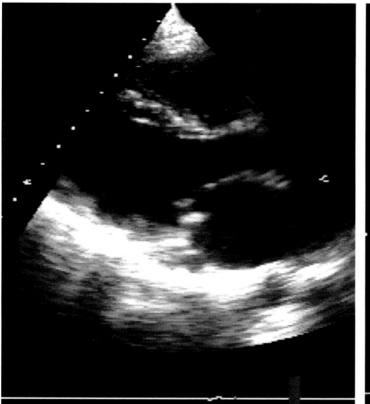

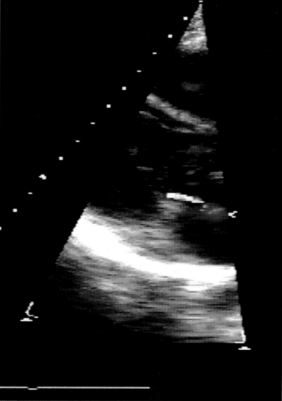

FIGURE 1.44. Parasternal long-axis views from a patient with severe mitral regurgitation after repair demonstrating significant fall in left ventricle cavity size.

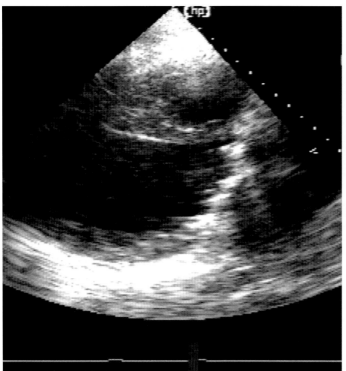
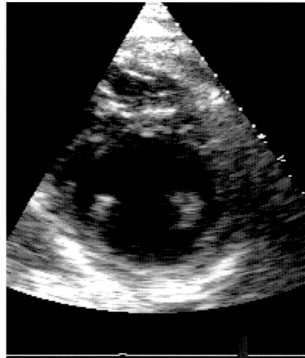

A

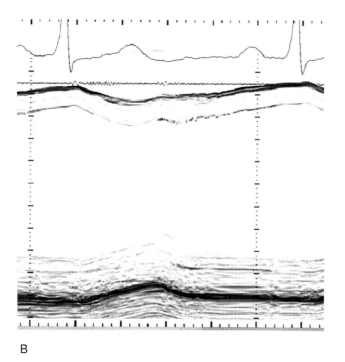

B

FIGURE 1.45. Parasternal long- and short-axis views of the left heart after mitral valve replacement for significant functional mitral regurgitation. Note the significant increase in left ventricle end-systolic dimension and poor overall systolic function.

rupture until hemodynamics settle. This does not justify delaying intervention until patients develop irreversible left ventricular disease, indicated by an increase in end-systolic volume.

The treatment of papillary muscle dysfunction is that of left ventricular disease with particular aim at reducing left ventricular diastolic pressures. Mitral valve replace-

ment in severe left ventricular disease should be avoided, as it adds to the disruption of ventricular geometry and hence functional performance. Instead an undersized mitral ring may be inserted to reduce the inflow diameter and hence the regurgitation, particularly in patients with dilated cardiomyopathy, whose ventricle is resistant to medical therapy. Stress echo may have a role in patient selection for surgical intervention. Mitral regurgitation that increases in severity with stress seems to deserve further attention compared to that which reduces with stress and with enhanced thickening of ventricular basal segment and shortening of the minor axis.

THE ROLE OF ECHOCARDIOGRAPHY IN PRE- AND PERIOPERATIVE PATIENT ASSESSMENT

Before Surgery

Transesophageal echocardiography is a major diagnostic tool, providing qualitative and quantitative information on the morphology and function of different components of the mitral valve. It provides on-line details on the exact cause of the mitral regurgitation, functional or organic. Severe valvar or subvalvar calcification in addition to anterior leaflet involvement reduces the likelihood for successful repair.[48,49] Pre-operative transthoracic echocardiography is equally important in assessing left ventricular size and function. The combination of the two should provide accurate information enough for decision making on the type of surgery–simple repair, repair and ring insertion, chordal reimplantation, or mitral valve replacement. To assess surgical outcome, left ventricular end-systolic volume of less than 60 mL/m^2, equivalent to end-systolic dimension of 5 cm, has been found to have a better postoperative value than dimensions of more than 5 cm. Left ventricular dysfunction caused by mitral regurgitation may require surgical correction even in the absence of significant symptoms. Such disturbances might worsen in some patients after mitral valve surgery, the reasons for which are not fully understood.[50]

Intraoperative Assessment

Intraoperative assessment provides early identification of postrepair valve dysfunction so that a second pump run can be established and the dysfunction corrected. A direct assessment of the mode of mitral valve repair can be provided, which includes direct leaflet repair, chordal replacement with Gore-Tex suture, or annuloplasty through insertion of a mitral ring. Intraoperative transesophageal technique helps in assessing left ventricular function before weaning off the bypass circulation. Moreover, it identifies any entrapped air in the cardiac chambers. Of course, all these findings should be interpreted in the light of specific circumstances–afterload effect, under-loaded or overloaded ventricles, and so on. In patients with combined left ventricular dysfunction in the setting of coronary artery disease and mitral regurgitation, intraoperative studies should identify the exact cause of early post-operative slow recovery, whether it is ventricular dysfunction, valve

regurgitation, or possibly graft occlusion that needs direct visualization and correction. The same indications for transesophageal echo postoperatively are applied in addition to early collection of extra cardiac fluid that may have significant hemodynamic effects, irrespective of its volume[51,52].

MITRAL VALVE SURGERY

Surgery requires open heart surgery and the use of cardiopulmonary bypass circulation. Less invasive approaches are now possible as outlined above and are available for repair and replacement.

Mitral Valve Repair

Mitral valve repair for mitral prolapse has now matured so that predictable results are widely available. Posterior leaflet repair is by far the commonest operation (80%) and is the most predictable. Good results have been reported with and without the use of a "ring." Anterior leaflet repair is more difficult, is less predictable, and usually requires the use of a "ring."

In primum inter-atrial communications and other forms of atrioventricular septal defect associated with left atrioventricular valve regurgitation, valve repair usually involves the suturing together of part of the superior and inferior bridging leaflets within the left ventricle. Repair of the so-called isolated cleft of the anterior leaflet of the mitral valve can usually be performed by inserting a patch on the anterior leaflet to bridge the cleft. The results of this technique are generally excellent and avoid the need for mitral valve replacement in virtually every case.

Mitral Valve Replacement

There is no ideal valve substitute. The choice lies between a mechanical bileaflet prosthesis and a porcine or bovine pericardial bioprosthesis. Mechanical valves have the advantage of durability but the disadvantage of life-long anticoagulation, although many of these patients are already committed to warfarin due to atrial fibrillation. Bioprosthetic valves degenerate. In the mitral position because of the high closing pressure, their life span can be as short as 5 years. Stentless mitral valves are under clinical investigation and include the mitral homograft and a glutaraldehyde-preserved pericardial valve, but medium-term results are not yet available.

Valve Replacement Complications

Structural Valve Failure

A paraprosthetic leak or structural valve failure can result from calcification, tear of leaflet from valve, leaflet per-

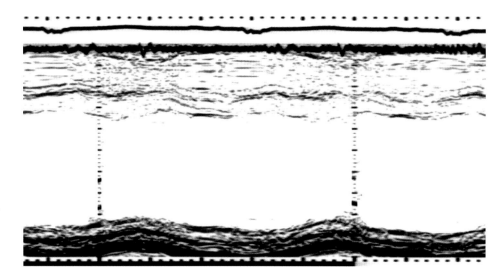

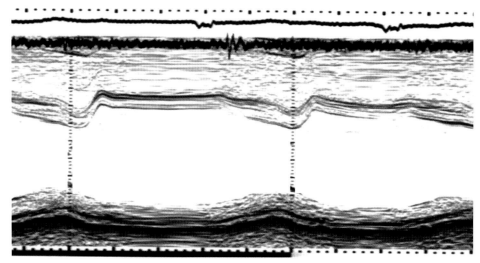

FIGURE 1.46. Left ventricle minor-axis M-mode from a patient with St Jude's mitral valve replacement. Note the normalized septal motion 12 months after surgery, suggesting significant para prosthetic leak.

foration, obstructed prosthesis due to thrombosis or calcification, thromboembolism, endocarditis, and conduction defects.

Para-prosthetic Regurgitation

Paraprosthetic regurgitation may vary from mild to severe. In the presence of mechanical valves, color Doppler in the transthoracic echo cannot display a uniform regurgitant jet due to the mechanical reflection and therefore may underestimate its importance. A normalized left ventricular septal motion suggests significant leak. Transesophageal echo, however, is much more sensitive, since the valve material does not distract the ultrasound beam. Although it tends to overestimate the regurgitation, it can locate the exact site of the leak. Combining left ventricular activity on the M-mode and transesophageal color flow provides a fairly accurate means of assessment.

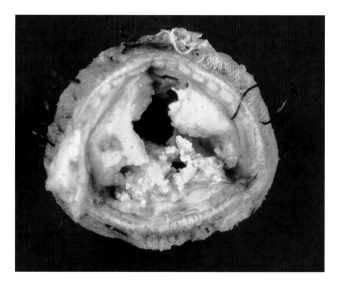

FIGURE 1.47. Pathologic specimen from a disintegrated Mitral valve showing calciprecation and tear xenograft.

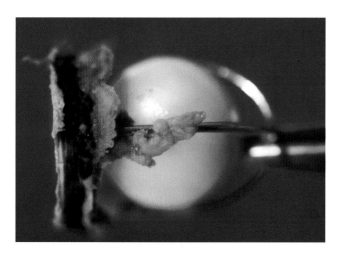

FIGURE 1.48. Starr-Edwards ball cage metallic valve excised from the mitral position. Note the ball in the cage with attached vegetation and clot.

Disintegrating Mitral Bioprosthesis

The expected durability of these valves in the mitral position is approximately 8 years. They should thus be followed up annually. Once they show signs of deterioration with rupture or tear of leaflets, they should be replaced as soon as possible, regardless of the severity of regurgitation.

Obstructed Mitral Prosthesis

Obstructed mitral prosthesis is due to thrombosis on the valve that prevents its movement. Rapid development of pulmonary edema in a patient with a mitral valve prosthesis suggests significant valve dysfunction with associated secondary pulmonary hypertension until proved otherwise. When confirmed, emergency valve replacement is the only management.

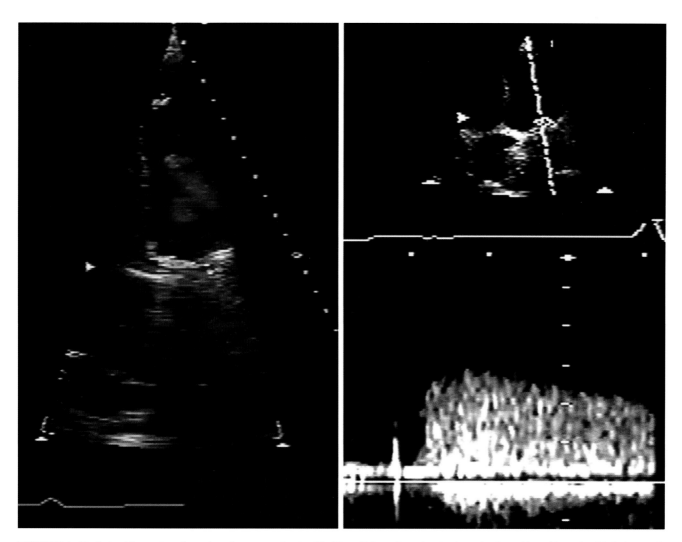

FIGURE 1.49. Apical four-chamber view from a patient with Starr-Edwards valve in the mitral position. Note the high forward-flow velocities, giving rise to a mean pressure drop of 20 mmHg on CW Doppler consistent with severe valve stenosis.

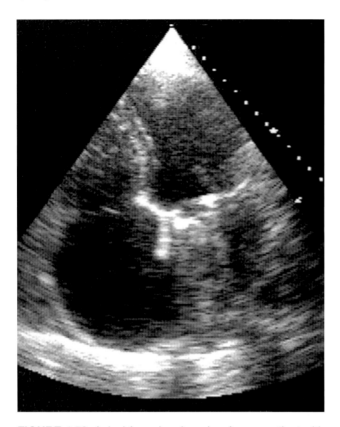

FIGURE 1.50. Apical four-chamber view from a patient with mitral valve and large vegetation on the valve.

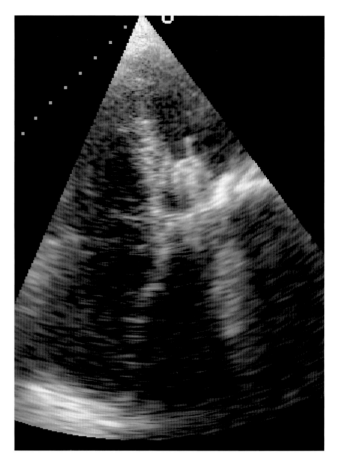

FIGURE 1.51. Apical four-chamber view from a patient with Starr-Edwards mitral prosthesis with small fibrin strands attached to it.

Endocarditis

Endocarditis is not uncommon. It is usually difficult to treat medically. Transthoracic echo may or may not show evidence of vegetation. Transesophageal echo provides clearer images of the valves. However, it should not be allowed to overestimate findings. Resistant infection may be eradicated only by valve replacement and debris clearing.

Fibrin Strands

Fibrin strands/thrombi can occur on mechanical valves and constitute no real clinical harm. They should be differentiated from vegetations.

REFERENCES

1. Daniels SJ, Mintz GS, Kotler MN. Rheumatic tricuspid valve disease: two-dimensional echocardiographic, hemodynamic, and angiographic correlations. *Am J Cardiol* 1983;51: 492–496.
2. Kilner Pj, Henein My, Gibson DG. Our tortuous heart in dynamic mode–an echocardiographic study of mitral flow and movement in exercising subjects. *Heart Vessels* 1997;12: 103–110.
3. Henein M, Lindqvist P, Francis D, et al. Tissue Doppler analysis of age-dependency in diastolic ventricular behaviour and filling: a cross-sectional study of healthy hearts (The Umea General Population Heart Study). *Eur Heart J* 2002;23: 162–171.
4. Come PC, Riley MF. M mode and cross-sectional echocardiographic recognition of fibrosis and calcification of the mitral valve chordae and left ventricular papillary muscles. *Am J Cardiol* 1982;49:461–466.
5. Naito M, Morganroth J, Mardelli TJ, et al. Rheumatic mitral stenosis: cross-sectional echocardiographic analysis. *Am Heart J* 1980;100:34–40.
6. Pellikka PA, Tajik AJ, Khandheria BK, et al. Carcinoid heart disease: clinical and echocardiographic spectrum in 74 patients. *Circulation* 1993;87:1188–1196.
7. Gibson DG. Valve disease. In: Weatherall DJ, Ledingham JG, Warrell DA, eds. *Oxford textbook of medicine.* New York: Oxford University Press, 1996:2451.
8. Smith MD, Handshoe R, Handshoe S, et al. Comparative accuracy of two-dimensional echocardiography and Doppler pressure half-time methods in assessing severity of mitral stenosis in patients with and without prior commissurotomy. *Circulation* 1986;73:100–107.
9. Kawahara T, Yamagishi M, Seo H, et al. Application of Doppler color flow imaging to determine valve area in mitral stenosis. *J Am Coll Cardiol* 1991;18:85–92.
10. Deng YB, Matsumoto M, Wang XF, et al. Estimation of mitral valve area in patients with mitral stenosis by the flow conver-

gence region method: selection of aliasing velocity. *J Am Coll Cardiol* 1994;24:683–689.

11. Nishimura RA, Rihal CS, Tajik AJ, et al. Accurate measurement of the transmitral gradient in patients with mitral stenosis: a simultaneous catheterization and Doppler echocardiographic study. *J Am Coll Cardiol* 1994;24:152–158.

12. Hatle L, Angelsen B, Tromsdal A. Noninvasive assessment of atrioventricular pressure half-time by Doppler ultrasound. *Circulation* 1979;60:1096–1104.

13. Hatle L, Angelsen BA. *Doppler ultrasound in cardiology*. 2nd ed. Philadelphia: Lea & Febiger, 1985.

14. Nakatani S, Masuyama T, Kodama K, et al. Value and limitations of Doppler echocardiography in the quantification of stenotic mitral valve area: comparison of the pressure half-time and the continuity equation methods. *Circulation* 1988; 77:78–85.

15. Shrestha NK, Moreno FL, Narciso FV, et al. Two-dimensional echocardiographic diagnosis of left-atrial thrombus in rheumatic heart disease. A clinicopathologic study. *Circulation* 1983;67:341–347.

16. Iliceto S, Antonelli G, Sorino M, et al. Dynamic intracavitary left atrial echoes in mitral stenosis. *Am J Cardiol* 1985;55: 603–606.

17. Gibson DG, Brown D. Measurement of instantaneous left ventricular dimension and filling rate in man, using echocardiography. *Br Heart J* 1973;35:1141–1149.

18. John Sutton MG, Traill TA, Ghafour AS, et al. Echocardiographic assessment of left ventricular filling after mitral valve surgery. *Br Heart J* 1977;39:1283–1291.

19. Desideri A, Vanderperren O, Serra A, et al. Long-term (9 to 33 months) echocardiographic follow-up after successful percutaneous mitral commissurotomy. *Am J Cardiol* 1992;69: 1602–1606.

20. Weyman AE, Heger JJ, Kronik TG, et al. Mechanism of paradoxical early diastolic septal motion in patients with mitral stenosis: a cross-sectional echocardiographic study. *Am J Cardiol* 1977;40:691–699.

21. Veyrat C, Kalmanson D, Farjon M, et al. Non-invasive diagnosis and assessment of tricuspid regurgitation and stenosis using one and two dimensional echo-pulsed Doppler. *Br Heart J* 1982;47:596–605.

22. Waller BF. Morphological aspects of valvular heart disease: part II. *Curr Probl Cardiol* 1984;9:1–74.

23. Abascal VM, Wilkins GT, O'shea JP, et al. Prediction of successful outcome in 130 patients undergoing percutaneous balloon mitral valvotomy. *Circulation* 1990;82:448–456.

24. Palacios IF, Block PC, Wilkins GT, et al. Follow-up of patients undergoing percutaneous mitral balloon valvotomy: analysis of factors determining restenosis. *Circulation* 1989;79:573–579.

25. Wilkins GT, Weyman AE, Abascal VM, et al. Percutaneous balloon dilatation of the mitral valve: an analysis of echocardiographic variables related to outcome and the mechanism of dilatation. *Br Heart J* 1988;60:299–308.

26. Pomerance A. Pathological and clinical study of calcification of the mitral valve ring. *J Clin Pathol* 1970;23:354–361.

27. Roberts WC. Morphologic features of the normal and abnormal mitral valve. *Am J Cardiol* 1983;51:1005–1028.

28. Savage DD, Garrison RJ, Castelli WP, et al. Prevalence of submitral (anular) calcium and its correlates in a general population-based sample (the Framingham Study). *Am J Cardiol* 1983;51:1375–1378.

29. Segal BL, Likoff W, Kingsley B. Echocardiography: clinical application in mitral regurgitation. *Am J Cardiol* 1967;19: 50–58.

30. Waller BF, Morrow AG, Maron BJ, et al. Etiology of clinically isolated, severe, chronic, pure mitral regurgitation: analysis of 97 patients over 30 years of age having mitral valve replacement. *Am Heart J* 1982;104(2 Pt 1):276–288.

31. Castello R, Lenzen P, Aguirre F, et al. Quantitation of mitral regurgitation by transesophageal echocardiography with Doppler color flow mapping: correlation with cardiac catheterization. *J Am Coll Cardiol* 1992;19:1516–1521.

32. Upton MT, Gibson DG. The study of left ventricular function from digitized echocardiograms. *Prog Cardiovasc Dis* 1978; 20:359–384.

33. Abbasi AS, Allen MW, Decristofaro D, et al. Detection and estimation of the degree of mitral regurgitation by range-gated pulsed Doppler echocardiography. *Circulation* 1980;61: 143–147.

34. Helmcke F, Nanda NC, Hsiung MC, et al. Color Doppler assessment of mitral regurgitation with orthogonal planes. *Circulation* 1987;75:175–183.

35. Miyatake K, Izumi S, Okamoto M, et al. Semiquantitative grading of severity of mitral regurgitation by real-time two-dimensional Doppler flow imaging technique. *J Am Coll Cardiol* 1986;7:82–88.

36. Spain MG, Smith MD, Grayburn PA, et al. Quantitative assessment of mitral regurgitation by Doppler color flow imaging: angiographic and hemodynamic correlations. *J Am Coll Cardiol* 1989;13:585–590.

37. Bargiggia GS, Tronconi L, Sahn DJ, et al. A new method for quantitation of mitral regurgitation based on color flow Doppler imaging of flow convergence proximal to regurgitant orifice. *Circulation* 1991;84:1481–1489.

38. Moises VA, Maciel BC, Hornberger LK, et al. A New method for noninvasive estimation of ventricular septal defect shunt flow by Doppler color flow mapping: imaging of the laminar flow convergence region on the left septal surface. *J Am Coll Cardiol* 1991;18:824–832.

39. Recusani F, Bargiggia GS, Yoganathan AP, et al. A new method for quantification of regurgitant flow rate using color Doppler flow imaging of the flow convergence region proximal to a discrete orifice. An in vitro study. *Circulation* 1991;83:594–604.

40. Eren M, Eksik A, Gorgulu S, et al. Determination of vena contracta and its value in evaluating severity of aortic regurgitation. *J Heart Valve Dis* 2002;11:567–575.

41. Klein AL, Obarski TP, Stewart WJ, et al. Transesophageal Doppler echocardiography of pulmonary venous flow: a new marker of mitral regurgitation severity. *J Am Coll Cardiol* 1991;18:518–526.

42. Nishimura RA, Tajik AJ. Determination of left-sided pressure gradients by utilizing Doppler aortic and mitral regurgitant signals: validation by simultaneous dual catheter and Doppler studies. *J Am Coll Cardiol* 1988;11:317–321.

43. Ren JF, Kotler MN, Depace NL, et al. Two-dimensional echocardiographic determination of left atrial emptying volume: a noninvasive index in quantifying the degree of nonrheumatic mitral regurgitation. *J Am Coll Cardiol* 1983;2:729–736.

44. Humphries WC, Jr., Hammer WJ, Mcdonough MT, et al. Echocardiographic equivalents of a flail mitral leaflet. *Am J Cardiol* 1977;40:802–807.

45. Mintz GS, Kotler MN, Segal BL, et al. Two-dimensional echocardiographic recognition of ruptured chordae tendineae. *Circulation* 1978;57:244–250.

46. Mintz GS, Kotler MN, Segal BL, et al. Two dimensional echocardiographic evaluation of patients with mitral insufficiency. *Am J Cardiol* 1979;44:670–678.

47. Panidis IP, Mcallister M, Ross J, et al. Prevalence and severity of mitral regurgitation in the mitral valve prolapse syndrome: a Doppler echocardiographic study of 80 patients. *J Am Coll Cardiol* 1986;7:975–981.

48. Castello R, Lenzen P, Aguirre F, et al. Quantitation of mitral regurgitation by transesophageal echocardiography with Doppler color flow mapping: correlation with cardiac catheterization. *J Am Coll Cardiol* 1992;19:1516–1521.

49. Klein AL, Bailey AS, Cohen GI, et al. Importance of sampling both pulmonary veins in grading mitral regurgitation by transesophageal echocardiography. *J Am Soc Echocardiogr* 1993;6:115–123.

50. Zile MR, Gaasch WH, Carroll JD, et al. Chronic mitral regurgitation: predictive value of preoperative echocardiographic indexes of left ventricular function and wall stress. *J Am Coll Cardiol* 1984;3(2 Pt 1):235–242.

51. Czer LS, Maurer G, Bolger AF, et al. Intraoperative evaluation of mitral regurgitation by Doppler color flow mapping. *Circulation* 1987;76(3 Pt 2):Iii108–Iii116.

52. Reichert SL, Visser CA, Moulijn AC, et al. Intraoperative transesophageal color-coded Doppler echocardiography for evaluation of residual regurgitation after mitral valve repair. *J Thorac Cardiovasc Surg* 1990;100:756–761.

2

Aortic Valve

ANATOMY

The aortic valve is a passive valve made up of three leaflets that assume the shape of half moons (semilunar). Opposite to the mitral valve there is no true aortic fibrous annulus but a complex root made up of the aortic wall sinuses, left ventricular myocardium, and interleaflet fibrous triangles. The ostia of the coronary arteries are located within the aortic sinuses.

AORTIC STENOSIS

Aortic stenosis can be localized at three levels: valvar, supravalvar, or subvalvar.

Causes

CONGENITAL AORTIC VALVE DISEASE

• **Congenital cusp malformation**: A single commissure is seen in infants and young children, whereas bicuspid or quadricuspid valves are usually discovered incidentally in young adults. The last two do not usually give rise to any significant hemodynamic abnormality before adulthood, as long as the pressure drop across the valve is not significant. The resulting turbulence at leaflet level adds to the predisposition of these valves to further deformation, fibrosis, calcification, and infective endocarditis.[1,2] In a bicuspid aortic valve the commissure is commonly transverse in position and rarely vertical. Mild aortic regurgitation and dilatation of the ascending aorta frequently co-exists with a bicuspid valve.[3] When the diagnosis is confirmed, suprasternal imaging is important to exclude aortic coarctation, which is also a common association. In congenital aortic stenosis, leaflet movement is limited at the tips rather than at the base, and therefore M-mode echocardiography may be misleading.

Bicuspid aortic valves are not intrinsically stenotic unless there is also dysplasia of the leaflets or other superimposed pathologic change. The valves may become stenotic due to sclerosis, or one of the leaflets may prolapse into the ventricle with subsequent insufficiency. Such valves are highly susceptible to infective endocarditis. The morphology of the leaflets also varies. The two leaflets can be of equal size, but more commonly, they are unequal. The larger leaflet almost always has a shallow raphe in its middle part.[1] Most larger leaflets are anterior, and both coronary arteries arise from the sinus above it.

• **Congenital aortic tubular stenosis:** this is a rare congenital disease that presents with uniformly narrowed aortic root and proximal ascending aorta. Management of this condition is complete resection and replacement of the aortic root and proximal (affected segment) ascending aorta. Aortic valve replacement alone in this condition does not absolve symptoms.

• **Subaortic stenosis:** this may be in the form of a fibrous membrane (ridge) below the aortic cusps or hypertrophied upper septum that bulges into the outflow tract. The former is a disease of the young that is usually in the shape of discrete, crescent-shaped fibrous shelf or membrane encircling the left ventricular outflow tract. It results in signs of ventricular hypertrophy and significant outflow tract gradient in the first three decades of life.[2] Subaortic fixed narrowing is commonly associated with some degree of aortic regurgitation, probably caused by the disturbed vortices in the outflow tract and proximal ascending aorta.[4,5] Other congenital cardiac conditions should always be excluded (e.g., atrial septal defect and coarctation of the aorta). When confirmed as the cause of symptoms, surgical excision is the best line of treatment,

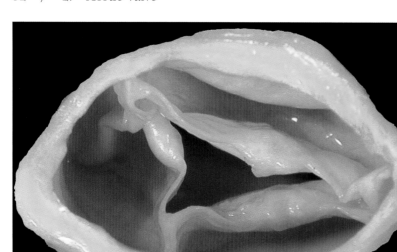

A

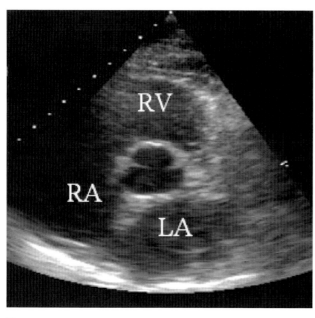

B

FIGURE 2.1. (A) Section in the ascending aorta showing a normal tricuspid aortic valve viewed from above. (B) Parasternal short-axis view of the aortic valve showing the three leaflets and their relation to the surrounding structures.

although it tends to recur unpredictably. Dynamic sub-aortic stenosis occurring early in life represents a component of hypertrophic cardiomyopathy. Muscular subaortic stenosis is more frequently seen in the elderly with a small left ventricular cavity irrespective of the cause of left ventricular hypertrophy.[6] When there is significant outflow tract narrowing it results in mid-systolic closure of the aortic valve. If the resting pressure drop (gradient) across the outflow tract is not significant in patients limited by exertional symptoms, pharmacologic stress seems an ideal diagnostic tool for establishing the relationship between potential outflow tract obstruction and symptoms. This condition is discussed in greater detail in Chapter 10.

Supra-aortic stenosis: This rare congenital anomaly involves fibrous narrowing of the proximal segment of the ascending aorta distal to the coronary sinuses. It should be diagnosed early in life from routine two-dimensional images, with the color Doppler showing localized aliasing at the site of narrowing confirming the diagnosis. Continuous-wave high Doppler velocity assesses the degree of stenosis. Supra-aortic stenosis occurs in association with Williams syndrome.[7–9]

ACQUIRED AORTIC STENOSIS

1. *Rheumatic aortic stenosis:* Like mitral valve disease, rheumatic aortic leaflet involvement is associated

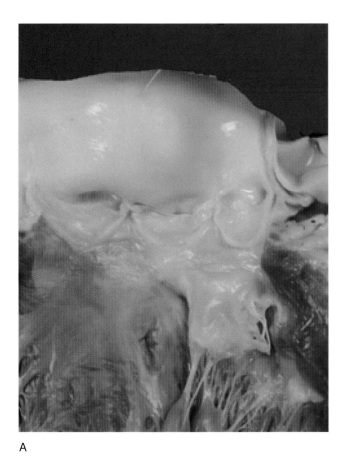

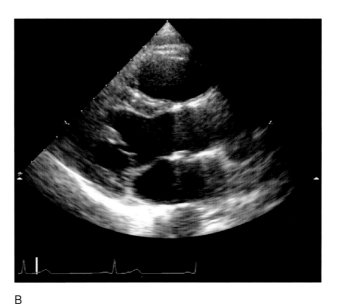

A

B

FIGURE 2.2. (A) Longitudinal section in the left ventricle and ascending aorta showing an opened aortic valve in direct continuity with the anterior leaflet of the mitral valve. (B) Parasternal long-axis view of the left ventricle and ascending aorta showing opened aortic valve in systole.

with commissural fusion, best seen in the short-axis view. As the disease progresses, the leaflets become fibrotic and calcify, resulting in valve stenosis. Rheumatic aortic valve disease is almost invariably associated with rheumatic mitral valve disease. The degree of aortic stenosis is usually clinically underestimated when associated with significant mitral stenosis. Isolated rheumatic aortic stenosis is very rare.

2. Senile or degenerative aortic stenosis: This results from calcium deposition on the aortic surface of the valve.[10] As with the mitral valve, calcification in the elderly affects the base and slowly involves the body of the leaflets, whereas with rheumatic disease the opposite occurs and the commissures fuse with calcification.[11] The calcium is deposited as large lumps within the body of each leaflet. Calcific aortic stenosis is an increasingly important disabling problem in an aging population, affecting 2% of people more than 65 years of age.[10]

Pathophysiology

Significant aortic stenosis with a pressure drop in excess of 70 mmHg represents a fixed resistance to left ventric-

ular ejection. It results in increased stroke work and hence hypertrophy that may be greater than in the coronary vascular bed, leading to subendocardial ischemia and later fibrosis. The latter is a progressive condition that leads to increased ventricular predisposition to dysfunction and arrhythmias. Aortic calcification may extend to the anterior (aortic) leaflet of the mitral valve. The calcification process may spread to the upper septum to cause conduction disturbances and possibly complete heart block. Later, with severe development of ventricular disease the cavity may dilate and its systolic function may deteriorate. This results in a rise in filling pressures, functional mitral regurgitation, and development of signs of heart failure and pulmonary congestion.

Assessment of Aortic Stenosis Severity

● **Extent of leaflet separation:** An average value of aortic leaflet separation with respect to the aortic root diameter on an M-mode recording gives an idea about the severity of stenosis. The normal value is on the order of 70%; mild stenosis, 50%; and moderate to severe stenosis, less than 30% of the aortic root diameter. This

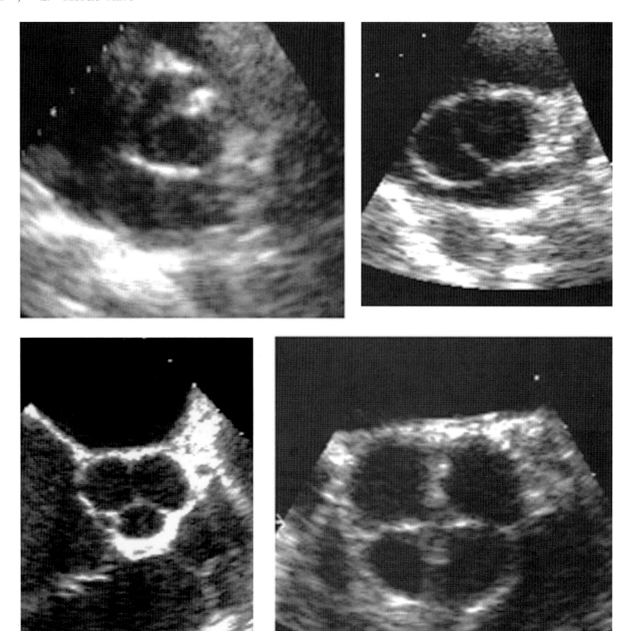

FIGURE 2.3. Parasternal short-axis view of the aortic valve showing different presentations of cusp formation.

method has its obvious limitations, with valve stenosis being overestimated in patients with severe leaflet calcification and those with significant left ventricular disease and low cardiac output.[12–14]

• *Continuous-wave Doppler:* Measuring peak pressure drop across the aortic valve provides instantaneous assessment. The modified Bernoulli equation (pressure drop across the aortic valve equals 4 times the recorded squared velocity: $\Delta P = 4V^2$) provides a direct estimation of aortic pressure drop (gradient).[15] This way of assessing aortic pressure has limitations, particularly when compared with catheter-obtained pressures. Continuous wave

pressure drop values are often higher than the peak-to-peak (left ventricular-aortic) pressure obtained by the pull-back technique, possibly because the aortic site of the latter is often the velocity recovery area in the ascending aorta, which results in underestimating the difference.[16,17] When comparing the mean aortic pressure, values of the two techniques are usually close. Continuous wave Doppler velocities may underestimate aortic pressure drop if the ultrasound beam is not parallel to the high-velocity jet (velocity varies inversely with cosine θ between the two).[18,19] In patients with severe left ventricular disease irrespective of its etiology, the modified

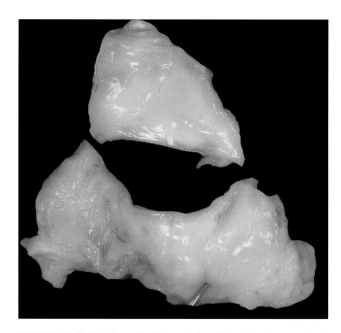

FIGURE 2.4. Section of a bicuspid aortic valve demonstrating leaflet morphology with one leaflet being larger than the other.

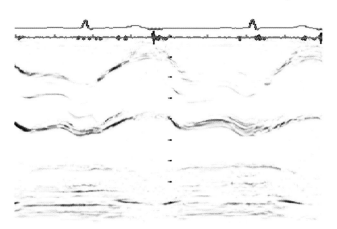

FIGURE 2.6. M-mode echogram from a patient with bicuspid aortic valve showing eccentric closure point, frequently seen in this condition.

Bernoulli equation may underestimate the degree of aortic stenosis. Thus the continuity equation is the best method for quantifying the severity of stenosis in such patients.[20]

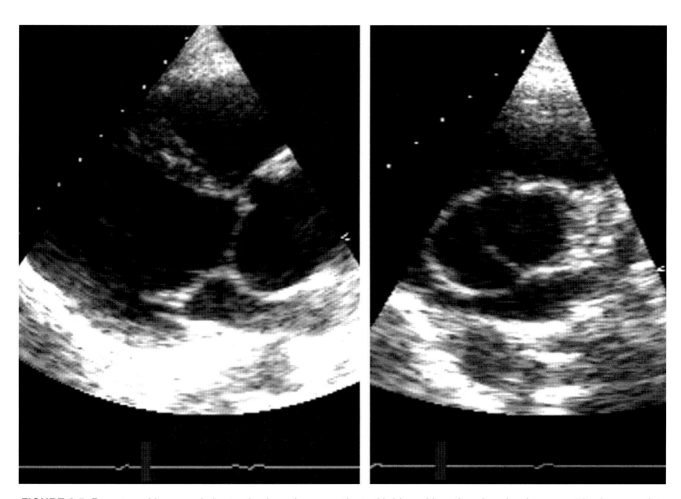

FIGURE 2.5. Parasternal long- and short-axis views from a patient with bicuspid aortic valve showing eccentric closure point.

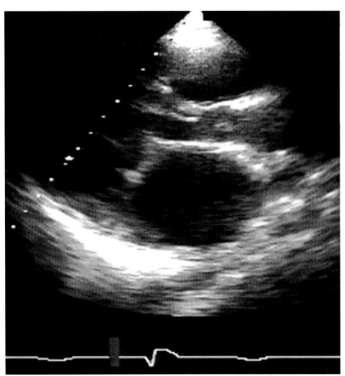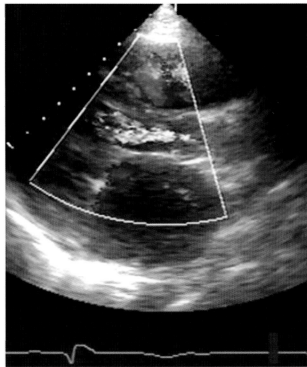

FIGURE 2.7. Parasternal long-axis view from a patient with tubular narrowing of the aortic root and proximal ascending aorta. Note the normal diameter of the ascending aorta distal to the site of narrowing.

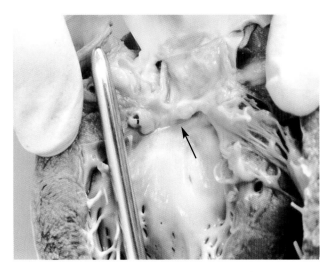

FIGURE 2.8. A section in the long axis of the left ventricle and outflow tract from a patient with subaortic stenosis. Note the fibrous ridge beneath the aortic cusps (arrow).

- **The continuity equation:** This is the best method for assessing valve area. The blood volume passing through the subvalvular region, and therefore the ratio of blood flow velocities between aortic and subaortic areas, is inversely proportional to the ratio of the cross-sectional area. The subaortic area is calculated as $(Diameter/2)^2 \times 3.14$. Aortic flow is measured from the velocity integral calculated from the continuous-wave Doppler and subaortic velocity integral from that of the pulsed-wave Doppler. Aortic flow = Aortic velocity integral × area = subvalvar velocity integral × area. Since ejection period is the same in the two areas, peak velocity may be used rather than integral. A velocity ratio of less than 0.25 (subaortic) is 94% sensitive in detecting severe aortic stenosis.[21–24] This method is ideal for assessing effective valve area in patients with poor ventricular systolic function and low-flow low-gradient state.

Color flow Doppler demonstrates the narrow jet width of aortic stenosis just beyond the aortic valve but does not help in quantifying the degree of stenosis.

Symptoms and Physiologic Disturbances

- **Breathlessness:** In patients with aortic valve disease, symptoms are mainly caused by the resulting ventricular disease. Breathlessness in aortic stenosis is due to raised left ventricular end-diastolic pressure and consequently raised left atrial pressure that initially appears on exertion, then later at rest, indicating severe additional left ventricular disease.[25]

- **Chest pain:** This is similar to that due to coronary artery disease but the underlying disturbed physiology is mismatch between the bulk of the myocardial mass and the coronary vascular bed as well as the direct effect of abnormal ventricular segmental relaxation on coronary flow in diastole. This has been shown to be associated

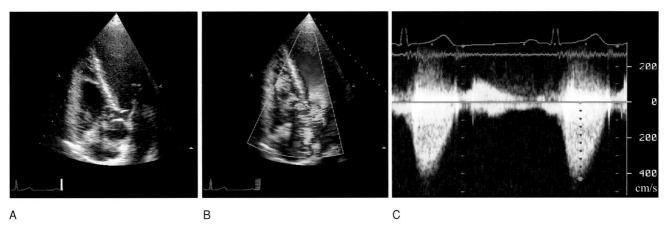

A   B   C

FIGURE 2.9. (A) Apical five-chamber view from a young patient with subaortic stenosis. Note the location of the membrane in relation to the valve cusps. (B) Color flow Doppler showing aliasing at the site of narrowing. (C) Continuous-wave Doppler from the same patient showing raised outflow tract pressure drop in the order of 70 mmHg.

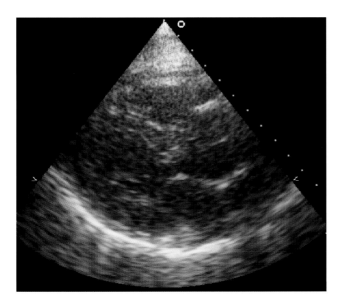

FIGURE 2.10. Parasternal long-axis view from an elderly lady with hypertrophied upper septum, bulging into the left ventricular outflow. Note the normal aortic valve cusps.

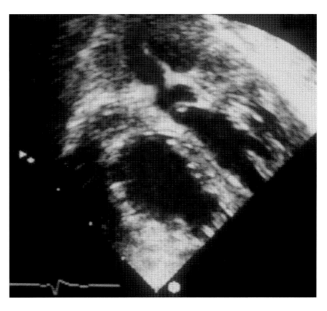

FIGURE 2.11. Parasternal long-axis view from a patient with supra-aortic stenosis.

with significant broadening of QRS duration that normalizes after valve replacement as does segmental ventricular function.[26]

● *Syncope:* Syncope is due to exertion-related hypotension as a result of the peripheral vasodilatation and the fixed resistance at the aortic valve level by stenosis, A-V conduction block by calcification, carotid sinus hypersensitivity, or periods of ventricular arrhythmia or even fibrillation. Similar mechanisms underlie the commonly known sudden death in patients with aortic stenosis.

● *Clinical signs:* A small Bernheim "a" wave might appear in the venous pulse associated with left atrial hypertrophy due to left ventricular hypertrophy. Two-

dimensional echocardiography has disproved the old belief that the Bernheim "a" wave represents right ventricular inlet obstruction and has confirmed it as a sign of atrial cross talk. The venous pressure remains normal (not raised) until late in the disease.[27]

Management of Aortic Stenosis

Mild aortic stenosis associated with normal carotid pulse and short systolic murmur with both components of the second heart sound audible is managed medically and followed up regularly with an echocardiogram for assessment of aortic pressure drop and left ventricular function. Prophylactic antibiotics are always recommended before

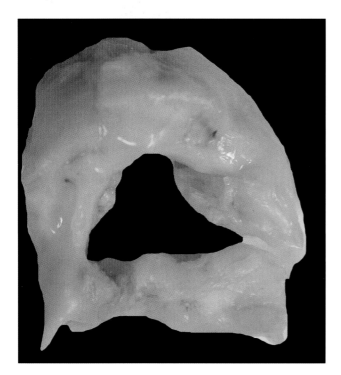

FIGURE 2.12. A picture of stenotic rheumatic aortic valve with fusion of the commissures, thickening, and calcification of the leaflets.

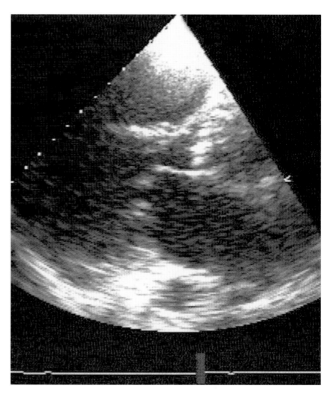

FIGURE 2.13. Parasternal long-axis view from a patient with combined rheumatic mitral and aortic valve disease.

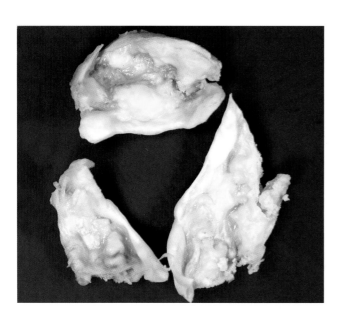

FIGURE 2.14. Pathology picture from an 80-year-old patient with senile degenerative calcification of the aortic valve. Note the nodular calcification in each leaflet.

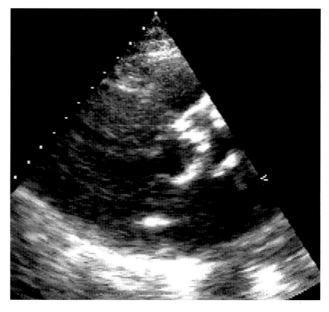

FIGURE 2.15. Parasternal long axis view from a patient with calcific aortic valve disease. Note the extent of calcification on the leaflets and the root.

dental and surgical procedures. Significant aortic stenosis confirmed by anatomic valve abnormality and a pressure drop across the valve of more than 60 mmHg (valve area of 0.9 cm^2 or less) in a symptomatic patient is recommended for intervention when cardiac output is normal.

A diagnostic coronary angiogram is always required in patients with aortic stenosis who are more than 40 years of age. Asymptomatic patients with accidental findings of aortic stenosis and a gradient of more than 60 mmHg may need to be objectively assessed with a provocation test.

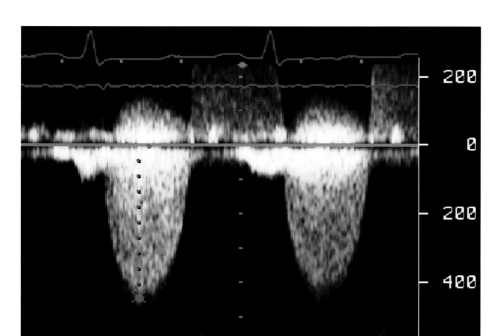

FIGURE 2.16. Continuous-wave Doppler recording from a patient with severe aortic stenosis and a pressure drop of 90 mmHg.

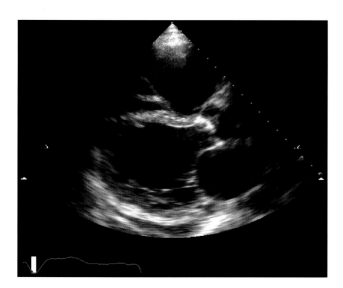

FIGURE 2.17. Parasternal long-axis view from a patient with calcified aortic valve and dilated ventricle with poor systolic function.

Symptom development with exercise has recently been suggested as indicating a need for surgery.[28] In patients with calcified valve leaflets but with low flow and low ressure drop, stress echocardiography helps identify those patients who need valve replacement. A valve area of less than 0.7 cm² that remains unchanged with stress is consistent with severe stenosis irrespective of the peak transvalvar pressure drop.[29]

Aortic Valvuloplasty

Aortic valvuloplasty is only advisable in infants and young children in whom the valve leaflets are thin and pliable, but in the majority a valve replacement is required at a later stage.[30] In the elderly, aortic valvuloplasty is not recommended in the management of stenotic valves. Open aortic valvotomy carries similar risks and benefits to valvuloplasty. The problem for the two procedures is the dysplastic valve leaflets, for which two-dimensional echo imaging provides more detailed analysis on the extent of disturbed anatomy and leaflet behavior. If ever needed, aortic valvuloplasty may serve as a bridge to complete valve replacement in patients with ignored aortic stenosis who are in late-stage heart failure.[31]

Aortic Valve Surgery

Aortic valve replacement is the only recommended procedure in adults, particularly with calcified cusps. The outcome is complete relief of breathlessness, angina, and syncope. Even in the presence of additional severe left ventricular disease aortic valve replacement is the only choice, the results of which are very successful, although the risk cannot be ignored. The lower the preoperative ejection fraction, the higher the perioperative mortality in these patients; thus optimal surgical timing is highly recommended.[32–35]

● *Mechanical or bioprosthetic valves:* These are the most common devices used. Their advantages and disadvantages have already been outlined. For those more than 60 years of age there is an increasing trend to use a bioprosthetic valve. The mean durability of the bioprosthetic valve is approximately 15 years, and the bleeding complications of long-term anticoagulation start to rise with age, reaching as high as six per 100 patients by 70 years

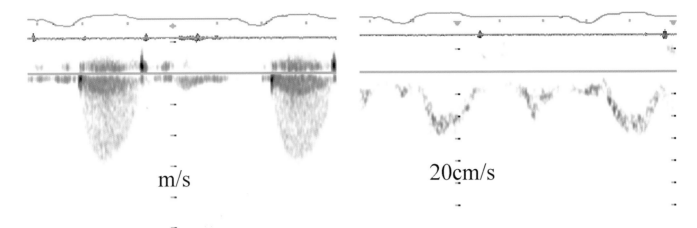

m/s

20cm/s

FIGURE 2.18. Continuous-wave Doppler (left) from the same patient and pulsed-wave Doppler velocities (right) of the subaortic area. Note the more than five times increase in velocities between the two areas, consistent with severe aortic stenosis.

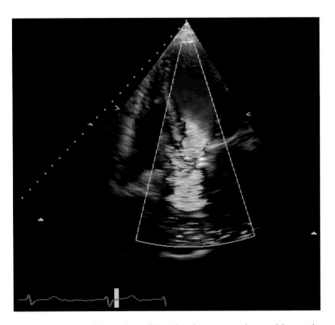

FIGURE 2.19. Color flow Doppler from a patient with aortic stenosis. Note the disturbed flow morphology due to the disrupted outflow tract by the calcified leaflets.

of age.[36–38] There is increasing interest in the use of stentless valves in the aortic position, particularly in patients with additional severe left ventricular disease. The recovery of ventricular function in these patients has been found to be much faster and more complete when they receive stentless valves than when they receive stented ones.[39–41] Stentless porcine valves have been developed in order to increase availability. These valves are treated, in the same way as the stented valves, with glutaraldehyde. The durability of these valves at 8 years is 90%, which is at least 10% better than current stented porcine valves. These data are derived from case series, some of which are case matched. Stentless valves have been shown to

have superior hemodynamics to stented valves early after operation and postoperatively to the second postoperative year. This has been shown in terms of improved diastolic function and reduction of left ventricular mass to the normal range.[42] It remains to be seen whether stentless valves are associated with increased long-term survival. They have also been shown to result in early recovery of function in patients with preoperative poor left ventricular function.

• **Homografts:** Long-term results of aortic homografts have proved encouraging, with freedom from valve degeneration at 15 years in 75%. Both homografts and autografts have advantages in the presence of endocarditis, as they contain no artificial material.[43,44] Both valves, once inserted, have significantly lower incidence of endocarditis than any other valve. However, they do degenerate eventually with calcification.

• **Pulmonary autograft or Ross operation:** This has unique features. As a living valve it is able to grow with the patient and therefore is particularly appropriate for patients before the end of puberty. It is also able to withstand high stress as seen during athletic exercise with heart rates above 170, where mechanical valves become increasingly inefficient.[45,46] Aortic autograft surgery is more complicated and is usually reserved for specialist centers and for patients with a life expectancy in excess of 20 years. Pulmonary valve homograft velocities tend to increase over the early postoperative months until it settles at a value of 2 to 3 m/s.

The Role of Echocardiography During Aortic Valve Surgery

Pre-operative echocardiographic examination aims at[47–49]

Assessing and quantifying the severity of aortic valve stenosis.

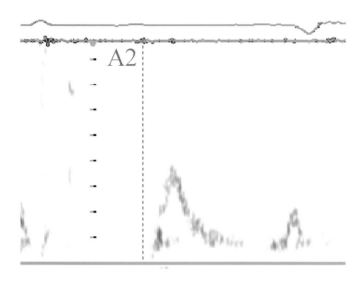

A2

FIGURE 2.20. Transmitral Doppler flow velocities from a patient with aortic stenosis limited by exertional breathlessness demonstrating restrictive filling pattern consistent with raised left atrial pressure.

Assessing the extent of left ventricular disease.

Measuring aortic root diameter to guide the size of the valve substitute.

Measuring the pulmonary valve annulus when pulmonary autograft procedure is anticipated.

Assessing aortic root and ascending aorta diameter that may be included in the surgical procedure.

Possibly suggesting the presence of additional coronary artery disease, based on the presence of myocardial scaring and/or segmental dyskinesia (however, it cannot confirm it).

Identifying additional valve lesions whether part of the same pathology or not.

• *Intraoperative echocardiographic study:* A transesophageal echocardiogram at the beginning of surgery usually confirms transthoracic findings, although pressure drop estimation is difficult due to the technical limi-

tation of aligning the continuous-wave Doppler beam with the left ventricular outflow tract axis. Its additional value is mainly for excluding other lesions before operation (i.e., the presence of a small ventricular septal defect or other aortic shunts in patients with congenital valve disease or those with prior history of endocarditis). At the end of the operation, echocardiographic examination helps in confirming perfect placement of the valve substitute and in excluding any paraprosthetic valve regurgitation that can be dealt with before closing the chest. It also assesses the amount of entrapped air inside the ventricle during the de-airing stage. In patients with difficulty being weaned from the bypass machine, echocardiography assesses the extent of ventricular

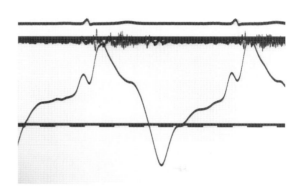

FIGURE 2.22. Jugular venous pulse from a patient with aortic stenosis and left ventricular hypertrophy showing Bernheim ''a'' wave followed by an X descent.

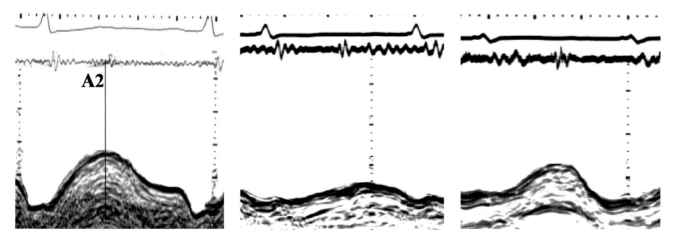

FIGURE 2.21. Septal left ventricular long-axis recording from a normal patient (left) and a patient with significant aortic stenosis before (middle) and after valve replacement (right). Note the normalization of long-axis amplitude of motion and lengthening velocities after surgery.

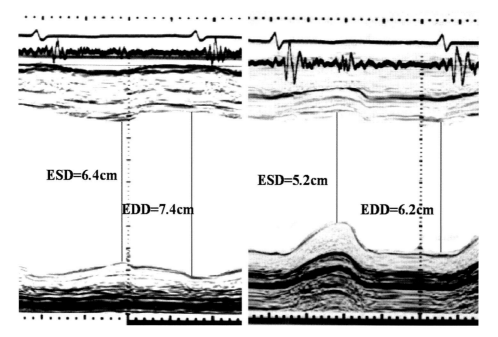

FIGURE 2.23. Left ventricular minor axis M-mode from a patient with severe aortic stenosis and poor left ventricular systolic function (left) and 5 days after valve replacement with a stentless valve substitute (right). Note the significant fall in end-systolic dimension and recovery of posterior wall systolic function.

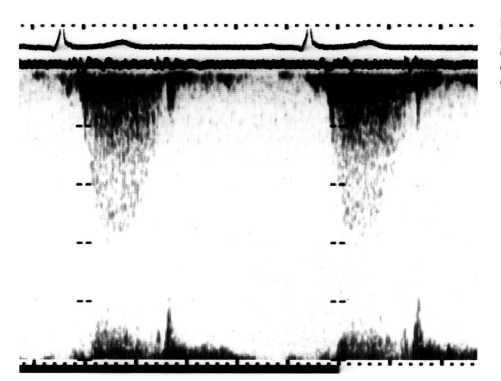

FIGURE 2.24. Pulmonary homograft peak velocity by continuous-wave Doppler demonstrating a peak velocity of 2.5 m/s.

loading. Finally, in patients with left or right ventricular disease due to compromised coronary filling, two-dimensional imaging together with Doppler provide excellent means for assessing the extent of ventricular impairment and coronary velocities.

• ***Post-operative echo examination:*** Echocardiography is the investigation of choice for assessing ventricular function in the early postoperative period. In patients with slow recovery, transthoracic or trans-

esophageal echo provide detailed evaluation of the valve as well as evaluation of ventricular function. Patients with high filling pressures may settle with vasodilators, whereas those with underfilled ventricles require fluid loading. Finally, a high-pressure pericardial collection irrespective of its volume may significantly contribute to the clinical deterioration of the early postoperative course. This should be drained to secure rapid recovery. Patients who develop high venous pressures who do not respond to diuretic therapy may have signs of postoperative tight pericardium, in the absence of pericardial effusion. A consistent increase in intrapericardial pressure leads to periodic (inspiratory) right heart filling and ejection followed by the left heart (being expiratory). This condition is benign and usually settles within days of the operation without a need for surgical intervention.

• *Long-term follow-up:* Echocardiography is the investigation of choice for the follow-up of patients after aortic valve surgery. Annual transthoracic echocardiographic examination with Doppler provides detailed assessment of valve function as well as left ventricular performance. It should help in discriminating between valve dysfunction and deterioration of ventricular function as two possible causes for symptoms in such patients.

AORTIC REGURGITATION

Etiology

Aortic regurgitation may result from different pathologies affecting either the valve leaflets or the aortic root:

• *Rheumatic involvement of the aortic valve:* This results in thickening of the cusps and fusion of the commissures with retraction of the leaflets and hence regurgitation.[25]

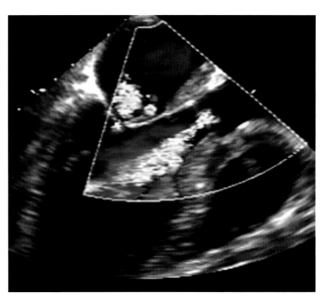

FIGURE 2.26. Transesophageal echo from a young patient with combined rheumatic mitral and aortic valve disease demonstrating aortic regurgitation.

• *Aortic leaflet prolapse:* Aortic prolapse is a rare presentation that results from myxomatous degeneration of the aortic leaflets and their diastolic prolapse into the outflow tract of the left ventricle. This is better viewed from the parasternal long-axis images as the leaflet tips meet below the aortic attachment level. Aortic prolapse may be associated with other conditions (e.g., mitral valve prolapse, bicuspid aortic valve disease, or Marfans disease). Aortic prolapse may also represent a consequence of aortic valvuloplasty for valve stenosis in infants and children.[50]

• *Aortic valve infection (endocarditis):* With infection, there is formation of vegetation on the surface of the leaflets, which can break off and embolize. The leaflets may also perforate. Valve infection complicated by vegetation may result in leaflet prolapse in diastole into the left ventricular outflow tract, causing aortic regurgitation. Aortic root abscess formation is associated with distortion of the valve leaflet and sinus morphology, and is much more commonly associated with conduction disturbances.[51]

• *Dilatation of aortic root:* This results from aneurysm of the ascending aorta, commonly seen with Marfan's syndrome, or isolated medial necrosis. Aneurysmal formation may rarely involve the coronary sinuses, resulting in blood stagnation and aortic regurgitation.[52,53] Aortic root dilatation may also be associated with more general connective-tissue disease (e.g., ankylosing spondylitis, rheumatoid arthritis, Reiters syndrome, or relapsing polychondritis).

• *Dissecting aneurysm:* This may involve the aortic root or proximal ascending aorta. The cause of aortic regurgitation in the two conditions may differ. Whereas in

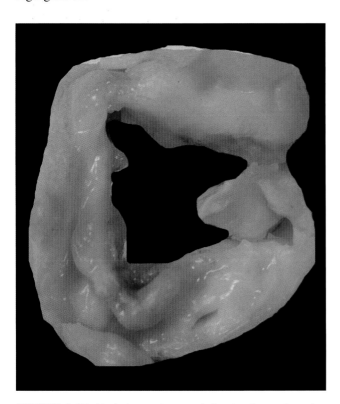

FIGURE 2.25. Pathology picture of rheumatic aortic valve from a patient with severe aortic regurgitation showing leaflet thickening and retraction due to the extensive fibrosis.

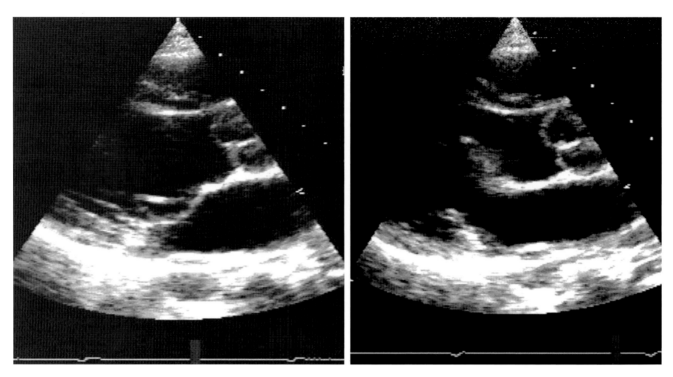

FIGURE 2.27. Parasternal long-axis view from a patient with aortic regurgitation secondary to leaflet prolapse. Note the level of leaflet closure with respect to their attachment level to the aorta.

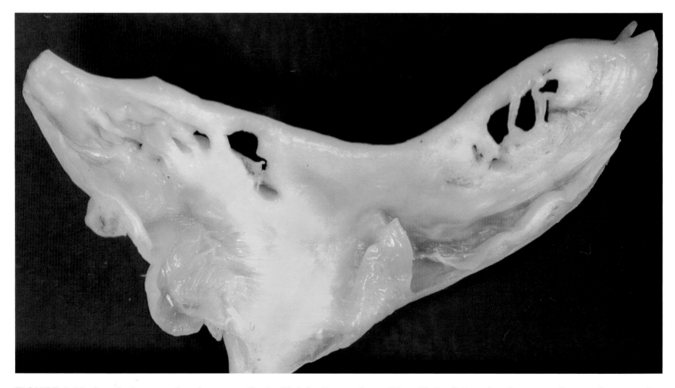

FIGURE 2.28. A pathology section from a patient with infective endocarditis with leaflet perforations causing aortic regurgitation.

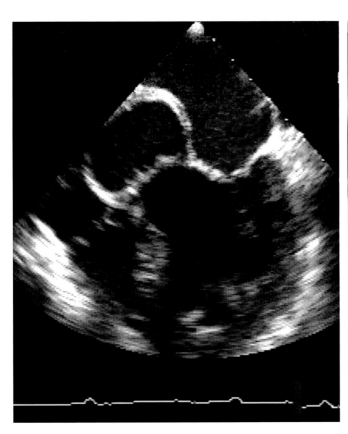 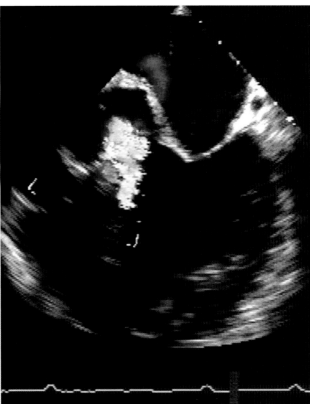

FIGURE 2.29. Transesophageal echocardiogram from a patient with severe aortic regurgitation secondary to bacterial endocarditis. Note the abscess cavity in the aortic root that changes its size and shape during the cardiac cycle; systole (left) and diastole (right).

the former the flap tends to hold the cusps opened in diastole, the dissection and false lumen in the latter tend to disturb the normal aortic vortices that close the valve cusps in early diastole.

• *Associated ventricular septal defect:* A small subaortic ventricular septal defect resulting in subaortic

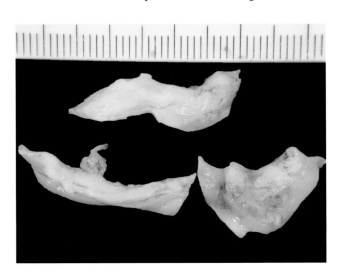

FIGURE 2.30. Pathologic specimen from a patient with aortic regurgitation secondary to infective endocarditis showing vegetation attached to the valve leaflet (arrow).

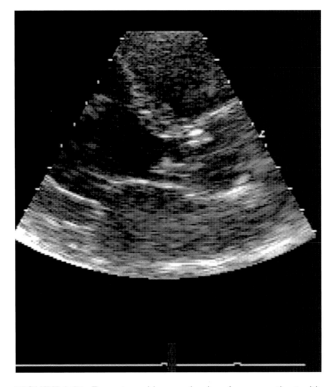

FIGURE 2.31. Parasternal long-axis view from a patient with infected aortic valve showing a 2-cm-long vegetation attached to the aortic cusp that moves freely in the aorta.

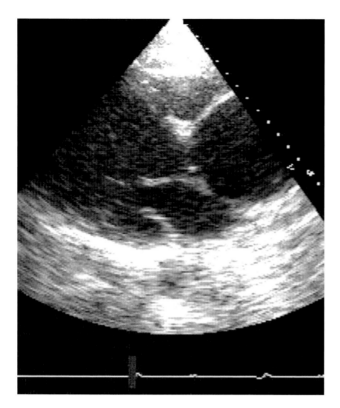

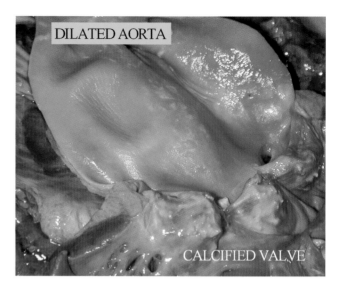

FIGURE 2.33. Pathologic section of the aortic root from a patient with a aneurysm showing generalized dilatation of the wall with calcification of the aortic valve leaflets.

FIGURE 2.32. Parasternal long-axis view of the left ventricular outflow tract and ascending aorta showing a fusiform aneurysm.

blood turbulence may be spontaneously closed by a prolapsing aortic leaflet. This results in significant failure of competent leaflet coaption and hence aortic regurgitation.

• *Syphilitic aortitis:* This causes an aortic aneurysm and dilatation of the valve area that may involve the coronary ostia.

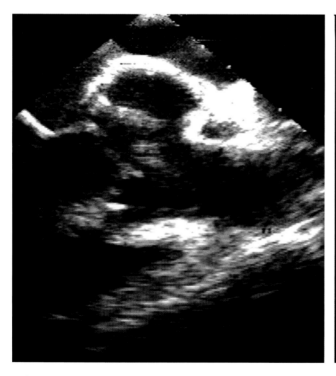

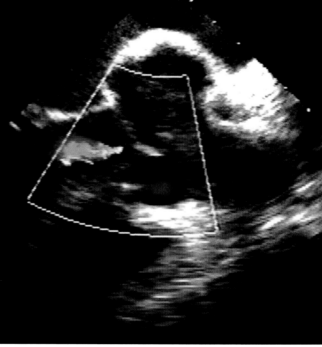

FIGURE 2.34. (A) Parasternal long-axis view from a patient with aneurysmal aortic sinuses with a small clot in the right coronary sinus (cauliflower appearance). (B) Mild aortic regurgitation.

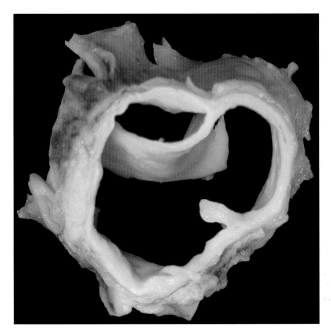

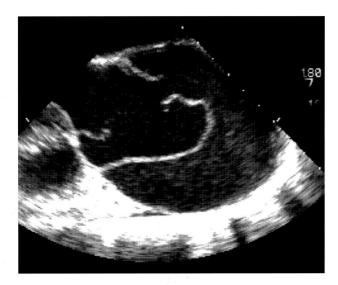

FIGURE 2.37. Transesophageal view from a patient with dissection of the ascending aorta 3 cm distal to the cusp level. Note the clotted false lumen.

FIGURE 2.35. Pathologic section from a patient with a dissection in the proximal ascending aorta forming a double-barreled aorta.

Pathophysiology

Aortic regurgitation is associated with a large left ventricular stroke volume that leads to cavity dilatation. At the same time, the duration of systole is increased, so that the time for coronary filling is correspondingly reduced. In severe regurgitation, the aortic-to-left-ventricular pressure difference in late diastole may be low enough to compromise coronary filling (coronary autoregulation no longer

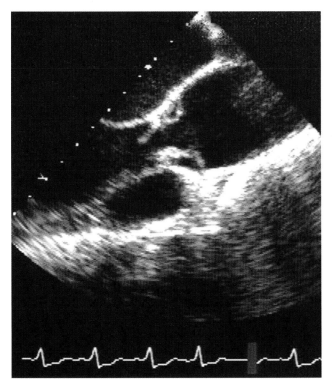

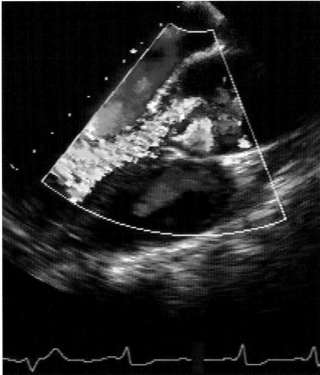

FIGURE 2.36. Parasternal long-axis view showing a proximal dissection of the aortic root with the flap bouncing back into the left ventricle in diastole (left), holding the cusps open and resulting in aortic regurgitation (right).

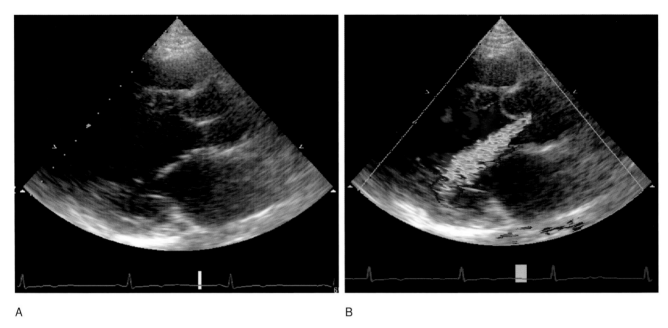

A   B

FIGURE 2.38. Parasternal long-axis view from a patient with aortic regurgitation. Note the prolapsing right coronary cusp closing off a small subaortic ventricular septal defect (left) and resulting in incompetent aortic valve (right).

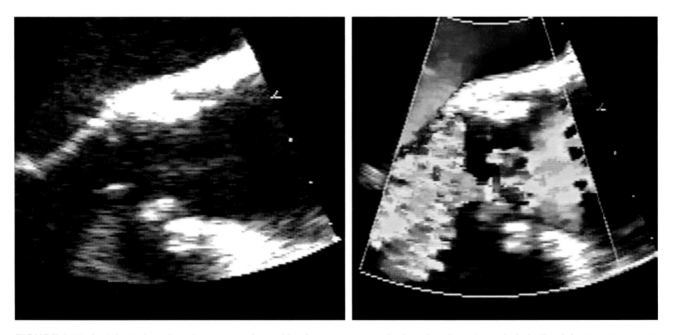

FIGURE 2.39. An infected aortic valve xenograft resulting in severe regurgitation showing a large hole in the right coronary cusp.

operates at aortic pressures of less than 40 mmHg), which results in ischemic myocardial manifestations.

Acute aortic regurgitation results mainly from cusp perforation caused by infection or from an aging homograft or xenograft. Although the left ventricular cavity becomes overloaded and active, overall ventricular function is maintained, since it does not dilate acutely. Acute severe regurgitation results in early mitral valve closure

(well before the onset of the QRS) and time-restricted left ventricular filling.[54] Of course, this should be differentiated from early mitral valve closure associated with first-degree heart block. As mentioned earlier, mid-diastolic equalization of aortic and left ventricular pressures has its effect on coronary circulation, perpetuating rapid deterioration of ventricular function. Although the left ventricle may not be able to dilate acutely, the large regurgitant

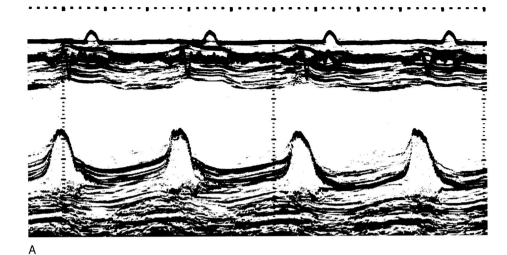

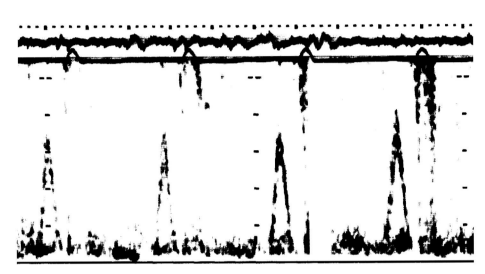

A

B

FIGURE 2.40. Mitral valve echogram from a patient with acute aortic regurgitation showing early diastolic mitral valve closure (top) and time-restricted filling (bottom).

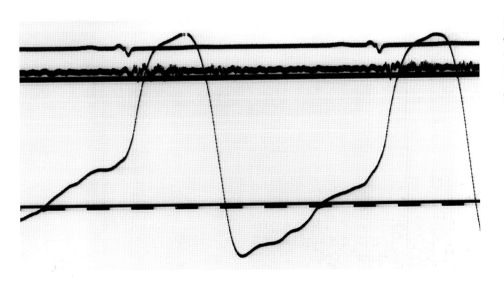

FIGURE 2.41. An apex-cardiogram from a patient with significant acute aortic regurgitation. Note the increase in end-diastolic pressure over the course of 12 months.

volume will result in raised diastolic pressures with its subsequent additional effect on subendocardial blood flow and function.

Clinical Picture and Physiologic Disturbances

Symptoms

Patients with chronic aortic regurgitation may be asymptomatic for many years. Symptoms develop only as the result of left ventricular disease. Exertional breathlessness is the main limiting symptom with aortic regurgitation that is caused by increased left ventricular diastolic pressure. In late stages, angina may be the result of coronary artery underperfusion. Aortic root dilatation may be associated with similar symptoms.[55]

Signs

All clinical signs are caused by large pulse volume; Water Hammer pulse, Corrigan's sign, DeMusset's sign, visible capillary pulsations in the nail beds (Quincke's), and Durozier's sign due to retrograde diastolic flow in the femoral artery.

The aortic systolic murmur heard in patients with significant aortic regurgitation is due to the large stroke volume rather than organic aortic leaflet stiffness and stenosis. P2 is loud when there is secondary pulmonary

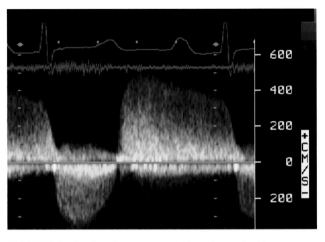

FIGURE 2.42. Continuous-wave Doppler velocities across the aortic valve from a patient with severe regurgitation and freely mobile leaflets. Note the raised forward velocities to 3 m/s resulting from the large stroke volume.

hypertension. A mid-diastolic murmur caused by a large aortic regurgitant jet hitting the anterior mitral leaflet may be heard at the apex (Austin-Flint) that mimics mitral stenosis. This is usually limiting leaflets movement in diastole and reversing its doming, resulting in functional narrowing of mitral valve opening and high velocities (diastolic murmur).[56]

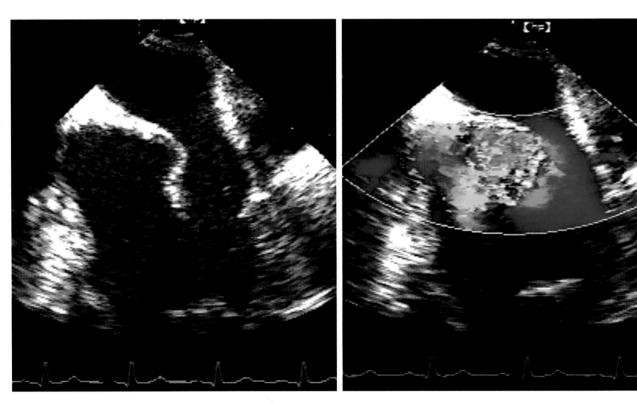

FIGURE 2.43. Transesophageal echocardiography from a patient with severe aortic regurgitation and mid-diastolic mitral stenotic murmur. Note the effect of the aortic regurgitation jet on anterior mitral leaflet morphology and narrowing of the left ventricular inflow tract in diastole (Austin-Flint murmur).

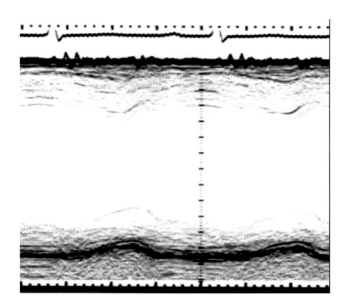

FIGURE 2.44. Left ventricular M-mode recording from a patient with long-standing severe aortic regurgitation who developed left ventricular disease. Note the significant increase in ventricular end-systolic diameter volume.

With development of left ventricular disease (increased end-systolic diameter of more than 5.0 cm) and reduced effective filling period due to the raised end-diastolic pressure, a third heart sound and mitral regurgitation murmur may be heard.

Signs of aortic regurgitation may be modified with other accompanying conditions:

• In infective endocarditis and cusp perforation the early diastolic murmur sounds musical in quality "seagull murmur." With homograft or xenograft degeneration, a loud systolic murmur may be heard, and a classical prolapsing and thickened leaflet is seen on two-dimensional echo images.

• In the presence of left ventricular disease, or rheumatic mitral stenosis or pulmonary hypertension, the collapsing pulse and other signs of severe aortic regurgitation may be lost, although the early diastolic murmur remains.

• With very severe aortic regurgitation when the valve is virtually absent, the regurgitant murmur may be inaudible, whereas the ventricular cavity is very active and the regurgitant jet diameter occupies almost the whole of the outflow tract.

Assessing Aortic Regurgitation Severity

• *Active left ventricular cavity:* An increase in left ventricular end-diastolic volume and fall in end-systolic volume is compatible with a significant overload. The main difference between aortic and mitral regurgitation is that in the former, ventricular loading occurs in early and mid diastole, whereas with mitral regurgitation it is pre-

dominantly early diastolic. An increase in left ventricular minor-axis dimension, end-systole of more than 5.0 cm, in the presence of any overload suggests independent ventricular disease even in the absence of significant symptoms. At this stage, recovery of ventricular function even after complete correction of the valve incompetence cannot be guaranteed.[57]

Coarse fluttering of anterior mitral leaflet: This is a common finding in aortic regurgitation. It is caused by the regurgitant jet interfering with the anterior leaflet opening in diastole. This sign, however, is not sensitive in estimating regurgitation severity.[58]

Color flow jet length: A rough assessment of aortic regurgitation is by measuring the distance of the regurgitant jet with respect to the valve level: subvalvar (mild), at mid ventricular cavity (moderate), and approaching the apex (severe). Although pulsed-wave Doppler technique is sensitive and specific, it has always been used to offer only a semiquantitative mean and therefore has become impractical for follow-up studies.[59,60]

Color flow jet diameter and area: This is an accurate way of assessing regurgitation severity, particularly with native valves. A broad jet of more than 12 mm or more than 65% of the aortic root diameter suggests severe regurgitation. Similarly, a color flow jet area that occupies more than half that of the left ventricular cavity on the apical view (>7.5 cm^2) suggests severe regurgitation, whereas an area of 1 cm^2 is compatible with trivial regurgitation. The major limitation of the latter is that the diameter and area, in particular, change over the course of diastole and may be affected by gain setting. Therefore for follow-up reasons fixed time measurements should be considered (early diastole).[61]

Continuous-wave Doppler: A rapid fall of aortic-to-left ventricular diastolic pressure by late diastole, particularly in the absence of raised left ventricular end-diastolic pressure, confirms severe regurgitation. A slow deceleration slope of less than 2 m/s^2 indicates mild regurgitation and a rapid slope of more than 4 m/s^2 indicates severe regurgitation. A pressure half time of less than 300 ms also suggests severe regurgitation. Left ventricular end-diastolic pressure can be calculated as the late diastolic aortic-ventricular pressure drop deducted from the systemic diastolic blood pressure. In patients in whom the aortic regurgitation jet is directed toward the right ventricle, apical continuous-wave recordings may be inappropriate, and the left parasternal window may be the optimal site.[62–65]

Diastolic flow reversal: In the descending aorta or femoral artery (Durozier's sign) this confirms significant aortic regurgitation.[66,67]

Continuity equation: Aortic regurgitation severity is the relative regurgitant volume to the left ventricular stroke volume. Therefore the ideal way for estimating the regurgitant fraction is by measuring mitral valve area and

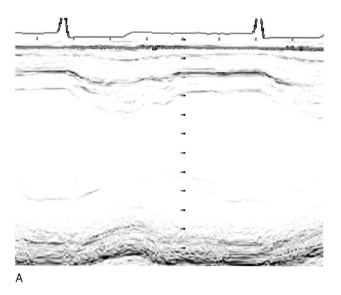

A

FIGURE 2.45. Left ventricular M-mode recordings from two patients with overloaded left ventricle caused by aortic regurgitation (A) and mitral regurgitation (B). Note the difference in loading pattern between the two; early and mid diastolic with aortic and mainly early diastolic with mitral regurgitation.

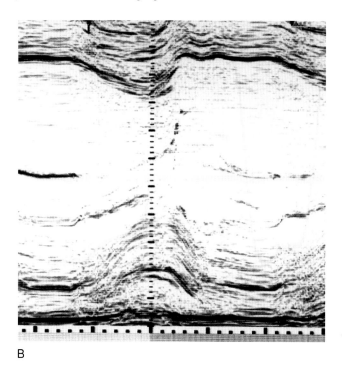

B

diastolic time flow integral and comparing it with that of the aortic valve. The difference would be taken as regurgitant fraction. The same method can be applied to measure the aortic regurgitant area. The velocity time integral at the valve level and valve area is compared with that 2 cm distal to the valve, and the valve regurgitant area is calculated. An area of 1.2 cm² suggests severe aortic regurgitation. Among the previous measures of aortic regurgitation, severity of regurgitant area is consid-

ered the only load-independent marker; however, it is less reliable than other measures, particularly with a dilated aorta.[68–71]

Management

Transthoracic echocardiography usually provides an excellent means of identifying the exact cause of aortic

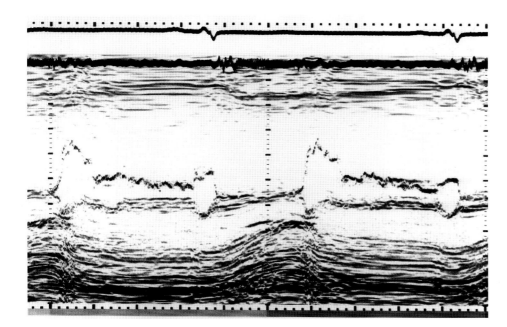

FIGURE 2.46. Mitral valve M-mode recording from a patient with aortic regurgitation. Note the course flutter of the anterior leaflet in diastole.

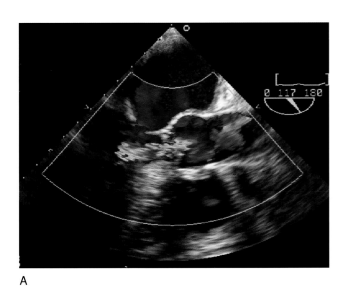

A

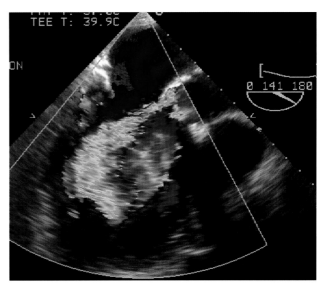

B

FIGURE 2.47. Color flow jet of aortic regurgitation showing mild severity (left) and severe regurgitation (right). Note the difference in jet distance with respect to the valve level.

regurgitation and any additional complications (e.g., left ventricular disease). It also assesses other valve anatomy and function, and hence excludes all other possible causes of the clinical findings and auscultation sounds. Even the proximal ascending aorta can be examined for aortic root abscess, aneurysm formation, or presence of a dissection. In patients with a limited transthoracic window, the transesophageal technique should provide detailed assessment of the aortic valve, root, and ascending aorta and identify the exact cause of valve regurgitation. Evidence for infection (vegetation or aortic root abscess) is rarely missed by this tech-

nique, but with thickened leaflets, additional evidence for infection is necessary in the absence of sizable vegetation.

Mild and moderate aortic regurgitation require prophylactic antibiotics. Severe aortic regurgitation in symptomatic patients needs aortic valve replacement. In asymptomatic patients, the condition could remain stable for years until signs of disease progression and left ventricular deterioration of function are demonstrated.[72,73] Calcium channel blockers (e.g., nifedipine) or angiotensin-converting enzyme inhibitors have been shown to delay the operation by a few years in asympto-

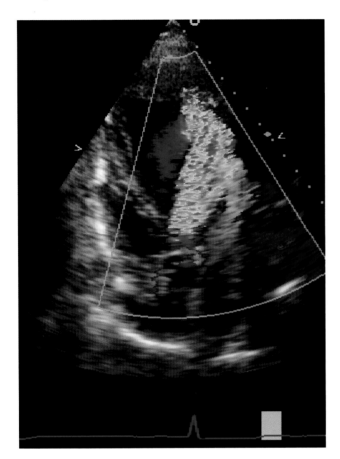

A

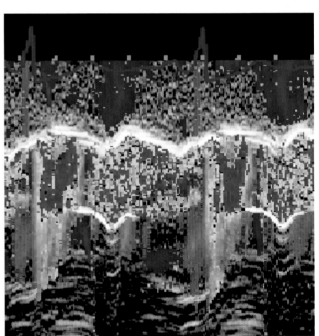

FIGURE 2.48. (A) Color flow jet of aortic regurgitation showing a broad jet of 12 mm of severe regurgitation. Note the corresponding difference in regurgitation area with respect to that of the left ventricle. (B, C) Color Doppler M-mode of the aortic root from two patients with mild (left) and severe (right) regurgitation. Note the difference in absolute and relative jet diameter with respect to the aortic root diameter.

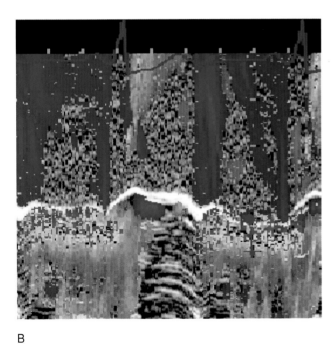

B

C

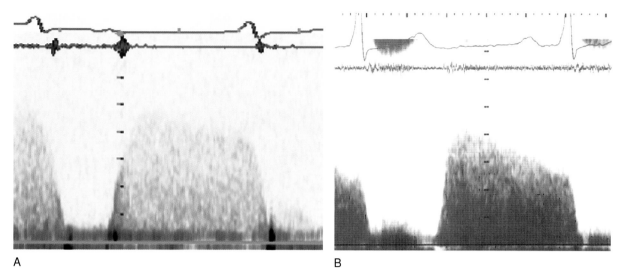

A   B

FIGURE 2.49. Continuous-wave Doppler recording of aortic regurgitation from two patients; mild (left) and severe (right). Note the fast deceleration, pressure half time, and the low aortic left ventricular pressure in late diastole with severe regurgitation.

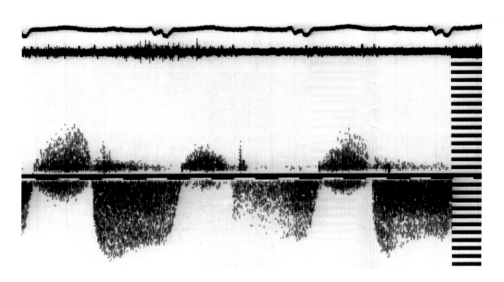

FIGURE 2.50. Continuous-wave Doppler from a patient with aortic regurgitation recorded from the left parasternal window demonstrating reversed signal.

matic patients. Cases of sudden death in patients with severe aortic regurgitation and left ventricular end-diastolic diameter of more than 7.0 cm have been reported. Progressive increase in left ventricular end-systolic diameter of more than 5.0 cm suggests the need for valve surgery even in the absence of symptoms. If ignored it may increase the operative mortality and result in a poor prognosis.[74–77] Acute aortic regurgitation, on the other hand, is a surgical emergency. Since it is always due to infective endocarditis, blood cultures should be taken, the organism isolated, and antibiotics started before urgent surgery. Vasodilators may help to stabilize the condition until surgery is available. Aortic regurgitation complicating acute dissection is another surgical emergency.

Other aortic pathologies (e.g., aneurysm or dissection) are always dealt with in the same session either by repair or by replacement. Recurrent aortic root and valve infection requires aortic root replacement, preferably by a homograft. As in aortic stenosis, in patients with aortic regurgitation and severe left ventricular disease, valve replacement with a low-resistance valve substitute (stentless) may result in faster recovery of ventricular function than is possible with a conventional stented one.[78]

Surgery for Aortic Regurgitation

In recent years there has been a growing interest in conserving the aortic valve. This has arisen partly because

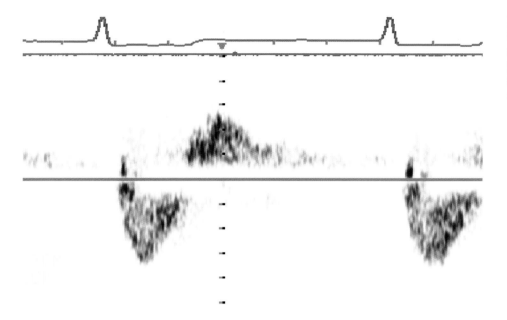

FIGURE 2.51. Pulsed-wave Doppler recording from the descending aorta from a patient with severe aortic regurgitation showing flow reversal in diastole.

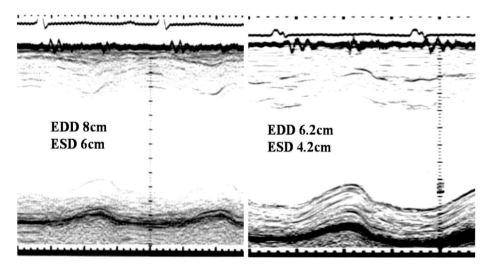

EDD 8cm
ESD 6cm

EDD 6.2cm
ESD 4.2cm

FIGURE 2.52. Left ventricular M-mode recording from a patient with severe aortic regurgitation and left ventricular disease before (left) and after (right) valve replacement surgery. Note the significant fall in cavity dimensions and improvement of systolic function as assessed by fractional shortening.

of the experience of aortic valve repair in acute and chronic Stanford type A dissection of the ascending aorta, and partly because in the Western world, disease of the aortic root has become the commonest cause of aortic regurgitation.[79]

Much recent interest has centered on the surgical management of Marfans syndrome. Before the era of open heart surgery, most patients with Marfans syndrome died of rupture of the aorta, often before the age of 30. In 1968, Bentall and DeBono described a composite graft-valve procedure in which a prosthetic valve was sewn into the proximal end of an artificial tubular graft, which in turn was anastomosed to the aortic annulus, with the coronary arteries anastomosed to the side of the graft.[80] This procedure completely removes the defective aortic segment most prone to dissection and rupture. After 30 years of experience with this operation, a recent multicenter retrospective report demonstrated the very con-

siderable success that has been achieved.[81] The 30-day mortality was 1.5% for 455 patients who underwent elective repair, 2.6% for the 117 patients who had an urgent repair, and 11.7% for the 103 patients who required emergency repair. Because nearly half the patients with aortic dissection had an aortic root diameter of 6.5 cm or less at the time of operation, it seems sensible to advocate prophylactic repair of aortic aneurysms in Marfan patients when the diameter of the aorta is well below that size.

Despite this, there are some disadvantages to the Bentall operation. These include all the known complications of mechanical prosthetic valves and the possibility of removing a potentially functional aortic valve. Another option is a technique of radical excision of the aortic root and implantation of the coronary ostia (Fagan 1983). Like the Bentall operation, this achieves the objective of removing the defective aortic wall, but in contrast, the patient's own valve leaflets are preserved, resulting in more normal valve function and the avoidance of the complications of an artificial valve. The long-term results of this procedure are excellent for elective operations.[82] Currently, in experienced units, prophylactic operation is recommended when the aortic root diameter reaches 5.0 cm. Until that time, patients are generally kept under close scrutiny with a combination of echocardiography and magnetic resonance angiography or spiral CT scans performed at 6-month intervals. In patients with a family history of a ruptured ascending aorta, elective surgery is recommended even if the diameter is less than 5 cm.[83] In all series so far reported, emergency repair of the ascending aorta invariably emerges as a strong predictor of early mortality.[84]

(For intraoperative echo assistance please refer to the sections dealing with aortic stenosis.)

REFERENCES

1. Beppu S, Suzuki S, Matsuda H, et al. Rapidity of progression of aortic stenosis in patients with congenital bicuspid aortic valves. *Am J Cardiol* 1993;71:322–327.
2. Pachulski RT, Chan KL. Progression of aortic valve dysfunction in 51 adult patients with congenital bicuspid aortic valve: assessment and follow up by Doppler echocardiography. *Br Heart J* 1993;69:237–240.
3. Hahn RT, Roman MJ, Mogtader AH, et al. Association of aortic dilation with regurgitant, stenotic and functionally normal bicuspid aortic valves. *J Am Coll Cardiol* 1992;19: 283–288.
4. Gewillig M, Daenen W, Dumoulin M, et al. Rheologic genesis of discrete subvalvular aortic stenosis: a Doppler echocardiographic study. *J Am Coll Cardiol* 1992;19:818–824.
5. Borow KM, Glagov S. Discrete subvalvular aortic stenosis: is the presence of upstream complex blood flow disturbances an important pathogenic factor? *J Am Coll Cardiol* 1992;19: 825–827.
6. Henein MY, O'Sullivan C, Sutton GC, et al. Stress-induced left ventricular outflow tract obstruction: a potential cause of dyspnea in the elderly. *J Am Coll Cardiol* 1997;30:1301–1307.
7. Nasrallah AT, Nihill M. Supravalvular aortic stenosis. Echocardiographic features. *Br Heart J* 1975;37:662–667.
8. Usher BW, Goulden D, Murgo JP. Echocardiographic detection of supravalvular aortic stenosis. *Circulation* 1974;49: 1257–1259.
9. Weyman AE, Caldwell RL, Hurwitz RA, et al. Cross-sectional echocardiographic characterization of aortic obstruction. 1. Supravalvular aortic stenosis and aortic hypoplasia. *Circulation* 1978;57:491–497.
10. Lindroos M, Kupari M, Heikkila J, et al. Prevalence of aortic valve abnormalities in the elderly: an echocardiographic study of a random population sample. *J Am Coll Cardiol* 1993;21: 1220–1225.
11. Brandenburg RO Jr, Tajik AJ, Edwards WD, et al. Accuracy of 2-dimensional echocardiographic diagnosis of congenitally bicuspid aortic valve: echocardiographic-anatomic correlation in 115 patients. *Am J Cardiol* 1983;51:1469–1473.
12. Chang S, Clements S, Chang J. Aortic stenosis: echocardiographic cusp separation and surgical description of aortic valve in 22 patients. *Am J Cardiol* 1977;39:499–504.
13. Lesbre JP, Scheuble C, Kalisa A, et al. [Echocardiography in the diagnosis of severe aortic valve stenosis in adults]. *Arch Mal Coeur Vaiss* 1983;76:1–12.
14. Williams DE, Sahn DJ, Friedman WF. Cross-sectional echocardiographic localization of sites of left ventricular outflow tract obstruction. *Am J Cardiol* 1976;37:250–255.
15. Hatle L, Angelsen BA, Tromsdal A. Non-invasive assessment of aortic stenosis by Doppler ultrasound. *Br Heart J* 1980;43: 284–292.
16. Berger M, Berdoff RL, Gallerstein PE, et al. Evaluation of aortic stenosis by continuous wave Doppler ultrasound. *J Am Coll Cardiol* 1984;3:150–156.
17. Currie PJ, Seward JB, Chan KL, et al. Continuous wave Doppler determination of right ventricular pressure: a simultaneous Doppler-catheterization study in 127 patients. *J Am Coll Cardiol* 1985;6:750–756.
18. Hatle L, Angelsen BA. *Doppler ultrasound in cardiology,* 2nd ed. Philadelphia: Lea & Febiger, 1985.
19. Lima CO, Sahn DJ, Valdes-Cruz LM, et al. Prediction of the severity of left ventricular outflow tract obstruction by quantitative two-dimensional echocardiographic Doppler studies. *Circulation* 1983;68:348–354.
20. Pellikka PA, Nishimura RA, Bailey KR, et al. The natural history of adults with asymptomatic, hemodynamically significant aortic stenosis. *J Am Coll Cardiol* 1990;15: 1012–1017.
21. Kosturakis D, Allen HD, Goldberg SJ, et al. Noninvasive quantification of stenotic semilunar valve areas by Doppler echocardiography. *J Am Coll Cardiol* 1984;3:1256–1262.
22. Richards KL, Cannon SR, Miller JF, et al. Calculation of aortic valve area by Doppler echocardiography: a direct application of the continuity equation. *Circulation* 1986; 73:964–969.
23. Zoghbi WA, Farmer KL, Soto JG, et al. Accurate noninvasive quantification of stenotic aortic valve area by Doppler echocardiography. *Circulation* 1986;73:452–459.
24. Oh JK, Taliercio CP, Holmes DR Jr, et al. Prediction of the severity of aortic stenosis by Doppler aortic valve area determination: prospective Doppler-catheterization correlation in 100 patients. *J Am Coll Cardiol* 1988;11:1227–1234.
25. Panidis IP, Segal BL. Aortic valve disease in the elderly. In: Frankl WS, Brest, AN, eds. *Valvular heart disease: comprehensive evaluation and management.* Philadelphia: FA Davis, 1985:289–311.
26. Collinson J, Flather M, Pepper JR, et al. Reversal of ventricular dysfunction and subendocardial ischaemia following aortic valve replacement in patients with severe aortic stenosis. *Circulation* 2000;102: 11–661.
27. Henein MY, Xiao HB, Brecker SJ, et al. Berheim "A" wave: obstructed right ventricular inflow or atrial cross talk? *Br Heart J* 1993;69:409–413.
28. Das P, Chambers J. Predictors Of outcome in asymptomatic aortic stenosis. *N Engl J Med* 2001;344:227–229.
29. Schwammenthal E, Vered Z, Moshkowitz Y, et al. Dobutamine echocardiography in patients with aortic stenosis and left ventricular dysfunction: predicting outcome as a function of management strategy. *Chest* 2001;119:1766–1777.
30. Cowley CG, Dietrich M, Mosca RS, et al. Balloon valvuloplasty versus transventricular dilation for neonatal critical aortic stenosis. *Am J Cardiol* 2001;87:1125–1127.
31. Buchwald AB, Meyer T, Scholz K, et al. Efficacy of balloon valvuloplasty in patients with critical aortic stenosis and car-

diogenic shock–the role of shock duration. *Clin Cardiol* 2001; 24:214–218.

32. Blitz LR, Gorman M, Herrmann HC. Results of aortic valve replacement for aortic stenosis with relatively low transvalvular pressure gradients. *Am J Cardiol* 1998;81:358–362.

33. Connolly HM, Oh JK, Orszulak TA, et al. Aortic valve replacement for aortic stenosis with severe left ventricular dysfunction. Prognostic indicators. *Circulation* 1997;95: 2395–2400.

34. Connolly HM, Oh JK, Schaff HV, et al. Severe aortic stenosis with low transvalvular gradient and severe left ventricular dysfunction: result of aortic valve replacement in 52 patients. *Circulation* 2000;101:1940–1946.

35. Pereira JJ, Lauer MS, Bashir M, et al. Survival after aortic valve replacement for severe aortic stenosis with low transvalvular gradients and severe left ventricular dysfunction. *J Am Coll Cardiol* 2002;39:1356–1363.

36. Hamamoto M, Bando K, Kobayashi J, et al. Durability and outcome of aortic valve replacement with mitral valve repair versus double valve replacement. *Ann Thorac Surg* 2003;75: 28–33.

37. John S, Ravikumar E, John CN, et al. 25-year experience with 456 combined mitral and aortic valve replacement for rheumatic heart disease. *Ann Thorac Surg* 2000;69:1167–1172.

38. Milano A, Guglielmi C, De Carlo M, et al. Valve-related complications in elderly patients with biological and mechanical aortic valves. *Ann Thorac Surg* 1998;66(6 Suppl):S82–S87.

39. Collinson J, Henein M, Flather M, et al. Valve replacement for aortic stenosis in patients with poor left ventricular function: comparison of early changes with stented and stentless valves. *Circulation* 1999;100(19 Suppl):II1–II5.

40. Jin XY, Zhang ZM, Gibson DG, et al. Effects of valve substitute on changes in left ventricular function and hypertrophy after aortic valve replacement. *Ann Thorac Surg* 1996;62: 683–690.

41. Jin XY, Pepper JR, Gibson DG, et al. Early changes in the time course of myocardial contraction after correcting aortic regurgitation. *Ann Thorac Surg* 1999;67:139–145.

42. Rajappan K, Melina G, Bellenger NG, et al. Evaluation of left ventricular function and mass after Medtronic freestyle versus homograft aortic root replacement using cardiovascular magnetic resonance. *J Heart Valve Dis* 2002;11:60–65.

43. Carr-White GS, Glennan S, Edwards S, et al. Pulmonary autograft versus aortic homograft for rereplacement of the aortic valve: results from a subset of a prospective randomized trial. *Circulation* 1999;100(19 Suppl):II103–II106.

44. Grocott-Mason RM, Lund O, Elwidaa H, et al. Long-term results after aortic valve replacement in patients with congestive heart failure. Homografts vs prosthetic valves. *Eur Heart J* 2000;21:1698–1707.

45. Oury JH, Doty DB, Oswalt JD, et al. Cardiopulmonary response to maximal exercise in young athletes following the Ross procedure. *Ann Thorac Surg* 1998;66(6 Suppl): S153–S154.

46. Porter GF, Skillington PD, Bjorksten AR, et al. Exercise hemodynamic performance of the pulmonary autograft following the Ross procedure. *J Heart Valve Dis* 1999;8: 516–521.

47. Laske A, Jenni R, Maloigne M, et al. Pressure gradients across bileaflet aortic valves by direct measurement and echocardiography. *Ann Thorac Surg* 1996;61:48–57.

48. Morocutti G, Gelsomino S, Spedicato L, et al. Intraoperative transesophageal echo-Doppler evaluation of stentless aortic xenografts. Incidence and significance of moderate gradients. *Cardiovasc Surg* 2002;10:328–332.

49. Sousa RC, Garcia-Fernandez MA, Moreno M, et al. [The contribution and usefulness of routine intraoperative transesophageal echocardiography in cardiac surgery. An analysis of 130 consecutive cases]. *Rev Port Cardiol* 1995;14:15–27.

50. Allen WM, Matloff JM, Fishbein MC. Myxoid degeneration of the aortic valve and isolated severe aortic regurgitation. *Am J Cardiol* 1985;55:439–444.

51. Krivokapich J, Child JS, Skorton DJ. Flail aortic valve leaflets: M-mode and two-dimensional echocardiographic manifestations. *Am Heart J* 1980;99:425–437.

52. Depace NL, Nestico PF, Kotler MN, et al. Comparison of echocardiography and angiography in determining the cause of severe aortic regurgitation. *Br Heart J* 1984;51:36–45.

53. Imaizumi T, Orita Y, Koiwaya Y, et al. Utility of two-dimensional echocardiography in the differential diagnosis of the etiology of aortic regurgitation. *Am Heart J* 1982; 103:887–896.

54. Botvinick EH, Schiller NB, Wickramasekaran R, et al. Echocardiographic demonstration of early mitral valve closure in severe aortic insufficiency. Its clinical implications. *Circulation* 1975;51:836–847.

55. Morganroth J, Perloff JK, Zeldis SM, et al. Acute severe aortic regurgitation: pathophysiology, clinical recognition, and management. *Ann Intern Med* 1977;87:223–232.

56. Gibson DG. Valve disease. In: Weatherall DJ, ed. *Oxford textbook of medicine.* Oxford: Oxford Medical Publications, 1996: 2451.

57. Henry WL, Bonow RO, Rosing DR, et al. Observations on the optimum time for operative intervention for aortic regurgitation. II. Serial echocardiographic evaluation of asymptomatic patients. *Circulation* 1980;61:484–492.

58. Robertson WS, Stewart J, Armstrong WF, et al. Reverse doming of the anterior mitral leaflet with severe aortic regurgitation. *J Am Coll Cardiol* 1984;3(2 Pt 1):431–436.

59. Esper RJ. Detection of mild aortic regurgitation by range-gated pulsed Doppler echocardiograhy. *Am J Cardiol* 1982;50: 1037–1043.

60. Ciobanu M, Abbasi AS, Allen M, et al. Pulsed Doppler echocardiography in the diagnosis and estimation of severity of aortic insufficiency. *Am J Cardiol* 1982;49:339–343.

61. Tribouilloy C, Shen WF, Slama M, et al. Assessment of severity of aortic regurgitation by M-mode colour Doppler flow imaging. *Eur Heart J* 1991;12:352–356.

62. Beyer RW, Ramirez M, Josephson MA, et al. Correlation of continuous-wave Doppler assessment of chronic aortic regurgitation with hemodynamics and angiography. *Am J Cardiol* 1987;60:852–856.

63. Labovitz AJ, Ferrara RP, Kern MJ, et al. Quantitative evaluation of aortic insufficiency by continuous wave Doppler echocardiography. *J Am Coll Cardiol* 1986;8:1341–1347.

64. Masuyama T, Kodama K, Kitabatake A, et al. Noninvasive evaluation of aortic regurgitation by continuous-wave Doppler echocardiography. *Circulation* 1986;73:460–466.

65. Masuyama T, Kitabatake A, Kodama K, et al. Semiquantitative evaluation of aortic regurgitation by Doppler echocardiography: effects of associated mitral stenosis. *Am Heart J* 1989;117:133–139.

66. Hoffmann A, Pfisterer M, Stulz P, et al. Non-invasive grading of aortic regurgitation by Doppler ultrasonography. *Br Heart J* 1986;55:283–285.

67. Quinones MA, Young JB, Waggoner AD, et al. Assessment of pulsed Doppler echocardiography in detection and quantification of aortic and mitral regurgitation. *Br Heart J* 1980;44:612–620.

68. Enriquez-Sarano M, Seward JB, Bailey KR, et al. Effective regurgitant orifice area: a noninvasive Doppler development of an old hemodynamic concept. *J Am Coll Cardiol* 1994; 23:443–451.

69. Kitabatake A, Ito H, Inoue M, et al. A new approach to noninvasive evaluation of aortic regurgitant fraction by two-dimensional Doppler echocardiography. *Circulation* 1985;72: 523–529.

70. Reimold SC, Ganz P, Bittl JA, et al. Effective aortic regurgitant orifice area: description of a method based on the conservation of mass. *J Am Coll Cardiol* 1991;18:761–768.

71. Zhang Y, Nitter-Hauge S, Ihlen H, et al. Measurement of aortic regurgitation by Doppler echocardiography. *Br Heart J* 1986; 55:32–38.

72. Acar J, Michel PL, Luxereau P, et al. How to manage patients with severe left ventricular dysfunction and valvular regurgitation. *J Heart Valve Dis* 1996;5:421–429.

73. Borer JS. Aortic valve replacement for the asymptomatic patient with aortic regurgitation: a new piece of the strategic puzzle. *Circulation* 2002;106:2637–2639.

74. Bonow RO, Dodd JT, Maron BJ, et al. Long-term serial changes in left ventricular function and reversal of ventricular dilatation after valve replacement for chronic aortic regurgitation. *Circulation* 1988;78(5 Pt 1):1108–1120.

75. Bonow RO, Lakatos E, Maron BJ, et al. Serial long-term assessment of the natural history of asymptomatic patients with chronic aortic regurgitation and normal left ventricular systolic function. *Circulation* 1991;84:1625–1635.

76. Borow KM, Green LH, Mann T, et al. End-systolic volume as a predictor of postoperative left ventricular performance in volume overload from valvular regurgitation. *Am J Med* 1980; 68:655–663.

77. Carabello BA, Spann JF. The uses and limitations of end-systolic indexes of left ventricular function. *Circulation* 1984; 69:1058–1064.

78. Jin XY, Pillai R, Westaby S. Medium-term determinants of left ventricular mass index after stentless aortic valve replacement. *Ann Thorac Surg* 1999;67:411–416.

79. Gott VL, Greene PS, Alejo DE, et al. Replacement of the aortic root in patients with Marfan's syndrome. *N Engl J Med* 1999;340:1307–1313.

80. Bentall H, De Bono A. A Technique for complete replacement of the ascending aorta. *Thorax* 1968;23:338–339.

81. David TE, Feindel CM. An aortic valve-sparing operation for patients with aortic incompetence and aneurysm of the ascending aorta. *J Thorac Cardiovasc Surg* 1992;103:617–621.

82. Yacoub MH, Gehle P, Chandrasekaran V, et al. Late results of a valve-preserving operation in patients with aneurysms of the ascending aorta and root. *J Thorac Cardiovasc Surg* 1998;115: 1080–1090.

83. Coady MA, Rizzo JA, Hammond GL, et al. What is the appropriate size criterion for resection of thoracic aortic aneurysms? *J Thorac Cardiovasc Surg* 1997;113:476–491.

84. Lepore V, Jeppsson A, Radberg G, et al. Aortic Surgery in patients with Marfan syndrome: long-term survival, morbidity and function. *J Heart Valve Dis* 2001;10:25–30.

3

Tricuspid Valve

ANATOMY

The morphologically right atrioventricular valve has three leaflets (tricuspid): septal, inferior (mural), and anterosuperior, which are separated from each other by anteroseptal, superoinferior, and inferoseptal commissures, respectively. The inferior leaflet takes its origin exclusively from the diaphragmatic parietal wall of the ventricle and is often called the mural leaflet. Each commissure is usually supported by the corresponding papillary muscle. The most characteristic and distinguishing feature of the tricuspid valve is the direct attachment of the cords from the septal leaflet to the septum. These chordal attachments to the septal surface are never seen in the morphologic left ventricle except when the tricuspid valve straddles and inserts on the left ventricular septal aspect. The reason for this complex arrangement of chordae tendinae is that the atrioventricular valves must close during systole, and these prevent them from ballooning into the atria.

TRICUSPID STENOSIS

Etiology

Tricuspid valve stenosis is less prevalent than mitral stenosis. A number of diseases may contribute to the physiologic presentation of tricuspid stenosis.

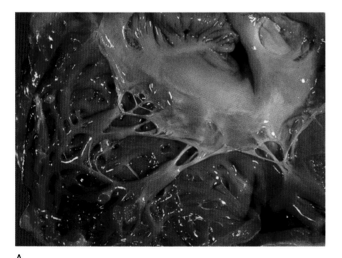

A

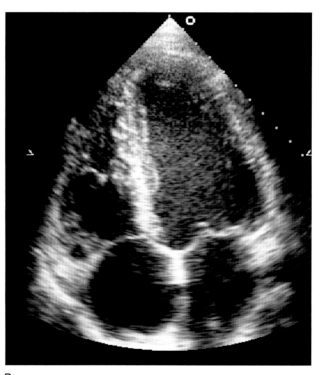

B

FIGURE 3.1. (A) Section of the right heart showing the anatomy of the tricuspid valve and its relation to the right atrium and ventricle. (B) Two-dimensional image of the right heart from the apical view demonstrating the tricuspid septal and anterosuperior leaflets and the trabecular right ventricular apex.

61

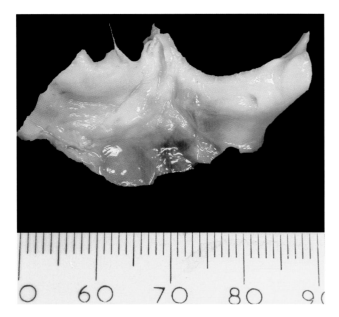

FIGURE 3.2. Pathology section from a patient with rheumatic tricuspid valve leaflet showing generalised thickening.

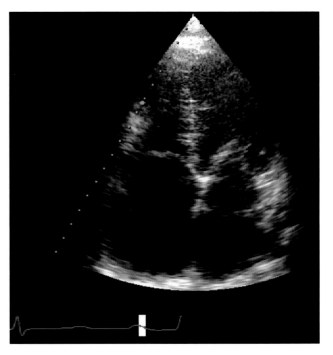

FIGURE 3.3. Apical four-chamber view from a patient with rheumatic mitral and tricuspid valve disease. Note the restricted cusp movement and the valve doming in diastole.

• *Rheumatic valve disease:* This is the most common cause of tricuspid stenosis. The cusps are thickened and the commissures fused so that the valve area becomes small and the valve leaflets dome toward the right ventricle in diastole. In contrast to mitral disease, the subvalvar apparatus is not usually involved.[1–3] As the disease progresses, the right atrium dilates and becomes congested. This is always associated with some degree of tricuspid regurgitation.

• *Carinoid disease:* This is a colonic tumor that secretes 5-hydroxytryptamine, which circulates with the blood and affects usually the right heart. The tricuspid valve leaflets become fibrosed and fused so that their movement and opening are restricted.[4,5]

• *Right ventricular pacing:* Tricuspid stenosis may infrequently complicate right ventricular pacing. A

pacing wire that perforates one of the three leaflets causes local inflammation, fibrosis, and leaflet stiffness. This can easily be missed by echocardiography if right-sided flow velocities are not carefully studied. Color flow Doppler of the tricuspid valve should give an indication of valve narrowing, and continuous-wave Doppler usually confirms significantly raised forward-flow velocities. A severe degree of stenosis caused by pacing wires may require valve replacement and insertion of an epicardial lead.[6]

• *Functional tricuspid stenosis:* When tricuspid valve leaflets are morphologically normal, raised right

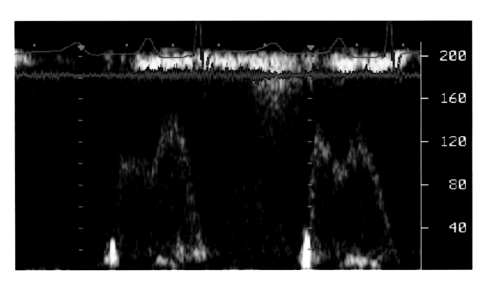

FIGURE 3.4. Continuous-wave Doppler across the tricuspid valve from the same patient showing high velocities and a mean pressure drop of 4 mmHg.

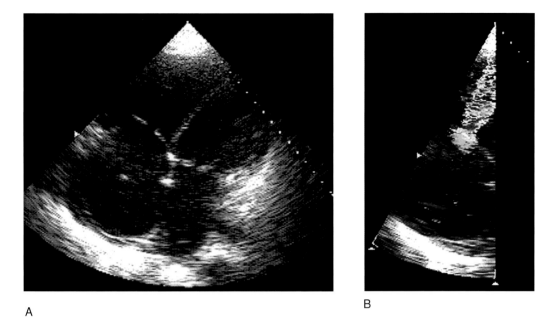

A   B

FIGURE 3.5. (A) Apical four-chamber view from a patient with carcinoid tricuspid valve disease showing restricted valve opening in diastole and raised flow velocities. (B) Color flow Doppler of tricuspid valve forward velocities from the same patient demonstrating aliasing (high velocities) at the leaflet level consistent with restricted valve opening.

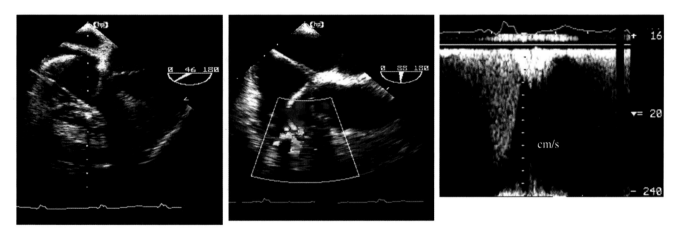

FIGURE 3.6. Transesophageal echo of the right heart showing extensive fibrosis at the site of crossing of the pacemaker lead through the tricuspid valve leaflets. Note the extent of valve fibrosis (left) resulting in physiologic stenosis shown by aliasing color Doppler (center) and raised flow velocities > of more than 2 m/s (right).

ventricular inflow velocities can be caused by a number of pathologies:

1. *A large atrial septal defect.* With significant left-to-right shunt that increases the right atrial stroke volume, right ventricular filling velocities increase. This does not usually result in conventional signs of tricuspid stenosis. After closure of the atrial septal defect transtricuspid velocities normalize.

2. *Localized pericardial effusion behind the right atrium.* With progressive increase in a localized effusion pressure the right atrial free wall may collapse and narrow the inflow tract of the right ventricle, thus resulting in significantly raised velocities. Irrespective of the volume of the pericardial collection, the localized raised pressure is the direct cause of functional tricuspid stenosis. Draining the pericardial effusion results in complete normalization of valve function and flow velocities.

3. *Right atrial myxoma.* Although rare with respect to its incidence in the left atrium when present, the tumor narrows the right ventricular inflow tract, causing raised filling velocities. This disturbed physiology normalizes completely after excision of the tumor.

4. *Right atrial secondaries.* Tumors of different histologic entities may spread hematologically directly to

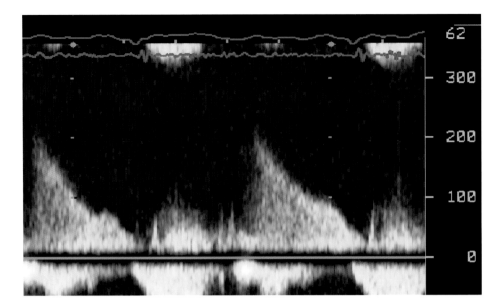

FIGURE 3.7. Transtricuspid flow velocities from a patient with atrial septal defect. Note the raised velocities up to 2 m/s before closure.

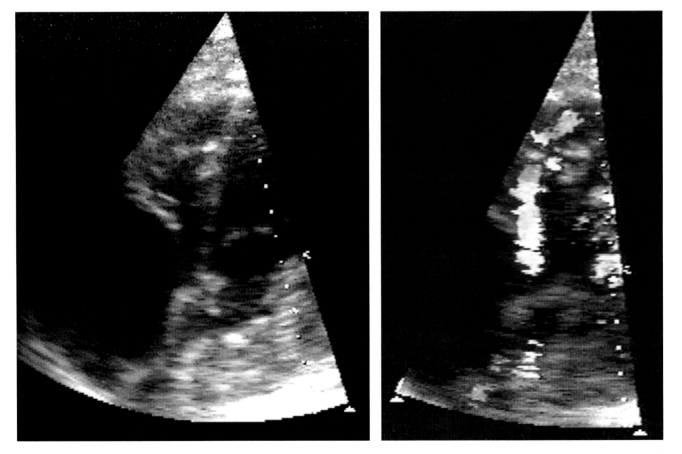

FIGURE 3.8. Apical four-chamber view from a patient with localized pericardial effusion behind the right atrium. Note the collapse of the right atrial free wall (left) narrowing the inflow tract of the right ventricle (left) and resulting in color aliasing just below the transtricuspid valve level.

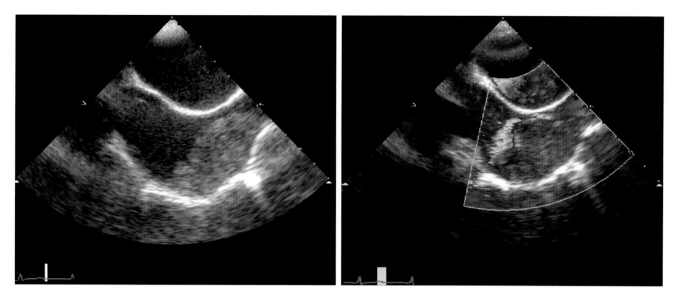

FIGURE 3.9. Secondaries invading the right atrium causing narrowed inflow and high velocities (colour Doppler).

the right atrium (e.g., ovarian sarcoma, renal carcinoma, lymphoma). Large right atrial secondaries may occupy a considerable part of the atrium and interfere with right ventricular inflow tract and filling.

Pathophysiology

Regardless of the etiology, the physiologic picture of tricuspid stenosis shares a raised transvalvar pressure drop and increased flow velocities. Although this pressure drop is much less than the corresponding one across the mitral valve, it results in raised right atrial pressures and systemic venous congestion of varying severity.[7–9] Jugular venous pressure is usually raised, demonstrating a slow early diastolic descent consistent with high-resistance inflow tract of the right ventricle. Long-standing tricuspid stenosis may result in worsening systemic venous congestion, liver dysfunction, and ascites.

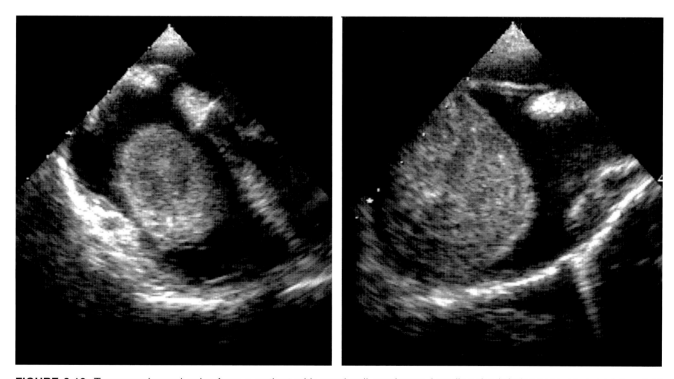

FIGURE 3.10. Transesophageal echo from a patient with renal cell carcinoma invading the inferior vena cava and the right atrium.

Management

Echocardiography is the ideal tool for determining the exact cause of tricuspid stenosis. Conventional two-dimensional imaging helps in assessing right ventricular inflow tract, tricuspid leaflet morphology, and function as well as right atrial size. In addition, extra-cardiac causes that may distort the right atrial cavity shape and function can be detected (pericardial effusion). Disturbed normal color flow Doppler pattern along the vertical axis of the right atrium helps in identifying the level of narrowing. This is usually confirmed by pulsed and continuous-wave Doppler, particularly when right ventricular filling velocities are raised. Transesophageal echo is ideal for delineating a clear image of the tricuspid valve leaflets and function. The atrial septum is clearly seen and the extent

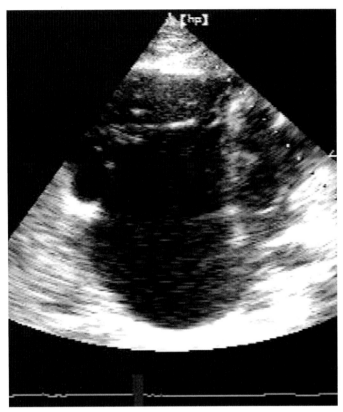

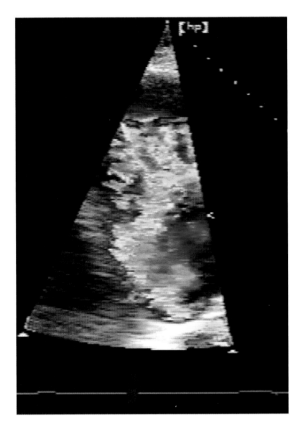

A

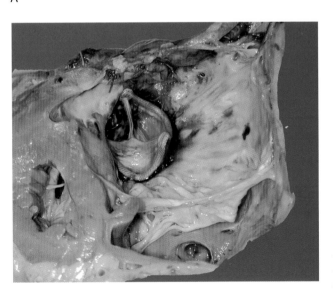

B

FIGURE 3.11. (A) Apical four-chamber view from an adult with Ebstein's anomaly and severe tricuspid regurgitation. (B) View from the right ventricle shows thickened ballooned and enlarged tricuspid valve leaflets that are displaced down into to the right ventricle. There is also replacement of the mitral valve by a Carpentier Edwards prosthesis.

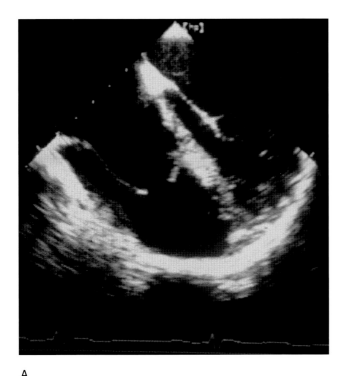
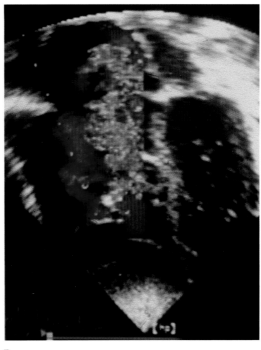

A

B

FIGURE 3.12. (A) Transesophageal and (B) transthoracic echo from a patient with Ebstein's anomaly showing dilated right heart, apical displacement of the septal tricuspid leaflet (left) and severe regurgitation (right) on color flow Doppler.

of tumor invasion of the atrial wall can be assessed. Blood-borne tumor spread can also be assessed by careful study of the inferior vena cava on the transesophageal echo images of the right atrium.

Treatment

● *Medical:* Systemic venous congestion is usually managed with diuretics. However, a balance should be preserved, since with the fixed narrowing of the inflow tract right ventricular filling relies on the raised right atrial pressure. Radical cure can not be achieved without correcting the organic lesion.

● *Surgical:* Tricuspid valvotomy should be considered at the time of surgery for other valves, particularly with a rheumatic etiology. When missed, it underestimates the surgical success for other lesions (e.g., mitral stenosis). In severe rheumatic tricuspid stenosis, valve replacement is the only option, although this procedure does result in some degree of stenosis from the inserted prosthetic valve. Successful drainage of localized pericardial effusion alleviates the associated functional disturbance. Whenever feasible and appropriate, removal of the right atrial space-occupying lesion (tumor) should result in complete recovery of right heart function as long as it had not invaded the cavity wall.

TRICUSPID REGURGITATION

Etiology

● *Congenital:* The most common cause of congenital tricuspid regurgitation is Ebstein's anomaly. The

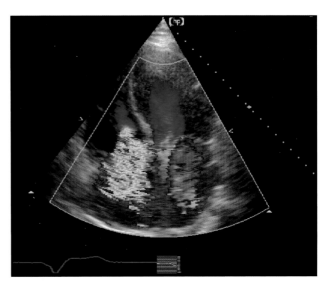

FIGURE 3.13. Apical four- chamber view from a patient with pulmonary hypertension showing dilated right heart and tricuspid regurgitation on color Doppler.

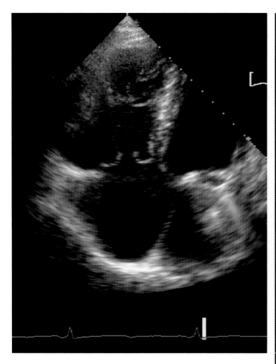
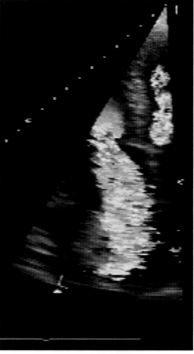
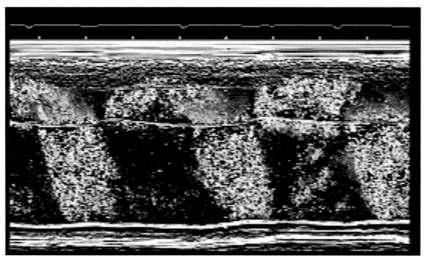

FIGURE 3.14. Apical views from a patient with rheumatic mitral valve disease showing involved tricuspid leaflets in the disease process. Note the thickened, short, and failing-to-coapt leaflets in systole (left), resulting in severe regurgitation on color flow Doppler (right) that approaches the back of the right atrium on color flow M-mode (bottom).

important echocardiographic features of Ebstein's malformation are displacement of the hinge point of the septal and mural (inferior) leaflets of the tricuspid valve from the atrioventriuclar junction into the inlet portion of the right ventricle. In most cases the valve leaflets are dysplastic, but in the more severe cases the septal or mural leaflets are virtually absent, and characteristically the anterosuperior leaflet is large with a so-called "sail-like motion." Mild to moderate valve regurgitation is commonly encountered, and an atrial septal defect within the oval fossa usually results in right-to-left interatrial shunting. Well-recognized associated anomalies include not only an atrial septal defect but also pulmonary stenosis and ventricular septal defect. Ebstein's malformation of the mitral valve is extremely rare, and involvement of the left atrioventricular valve is more likely to be found in congenitally corrected transposition of the great arteries.

- *Functional:* Tricuspid regurgitation frequently occurs with dilatation of the right ventricular cavity and tricuspid ring. It is also seen in patients with pulmonary hypertension irrespective of its etiology or in the terminal stage of congestive heart failure.

- *Rheumatic disease:* Severe tricuspid regurgitation has been increasingly recognized after mitral valve replacement for rheumatic disease, in the absence of significant left-sided disease or pulmonary hypertension. Recent evidence suggests an organic rheumatic cusp involvement and ring dilatation in this condition.[10]

- *Endocarditis:* Isolated tricuspid valve endocarditis is less common than other valves, but when present, it

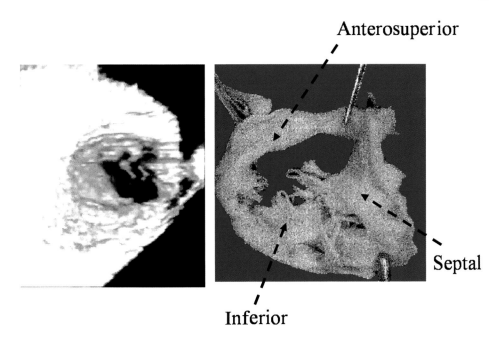

Anterosuperior

Septal

Inferior

FIGURE 3.15. Pathologic section from the same patient showing thickened and fibrosed tricuspid leaflets with fused commissures along with the corresponding three-dimensional images (en face view).

may complicate an infected central line or develop in intravenous drug users.[11,12]

● **Endomyocardial fibrosis:** Although rare, right-sided endomyocardial fibrosis distorts the inflow tract of the right ventricle and predisposes to severe tricuspid regurgitation. A similar picture is seen with carcinoid syndrome.[13]

● **Pacemaker insertion:** Significant tricuspid regurgitation may develop complicating pacemaker insertion, particularly when the lead perforates one of the leaflets. Leaflet fibrosis and retraction develop, resulting in failure of coaption and significant valve incompetence.

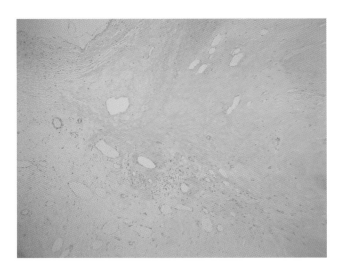

FIGURE 3.16. Histologic section from the septal leaflet demonstrating vascularization and patchy fibrosis consistent with long-standing inflammatory process.

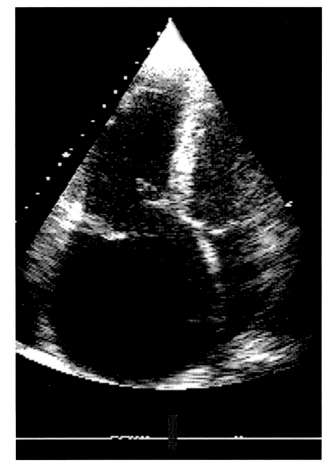

FIGURE 3.17. Apical two-dimensional views of the right heart from a drug user showing vegetation attached to the anterosuperior leaflet of the tricuspid valve and resulting in leaflet prolapse and failure of coaption.

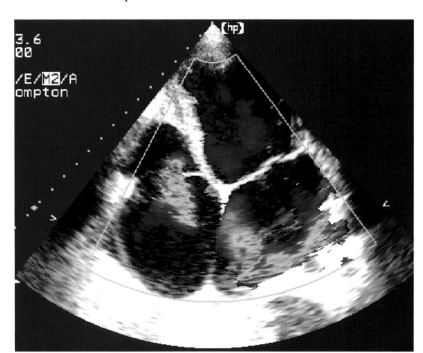

FIGURE 3.18. Apical two-dimensional images from a patient with endomyocardial fibrosis showing distorted right ventricular inlet, fibrosed subvalvar apparatus, and tricuspid regurgitation.

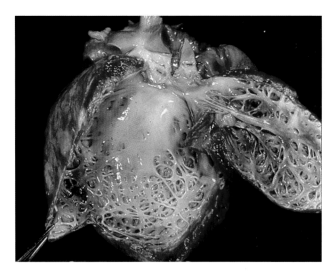

FIGURE 3.19. Pathologic section from a patient with endomyocardial fibrosis demonstrating extensive subendocardial fibrosis.

- **Leaflet prolapse:** Mid-systolic tricuspid valve prolapse may be associated with that of the mitral valve. An example of the association of the two-valve dysfunction is seen in Marfans syndrome, although tricuspid regurgitation is usually insignificant compared with mitral regurgitation.[14–16]

- **Cardiomyopathy:** Long-standing ischemic myocardial disease of the left ventricle may also involve the right ventricle, particularly in patients with prior right ventricular infarction. Progressive ischemic deterioration of the right ventricle may result in dilatation of the basal segment and tricuspid ring and consequently development of significant regurgitation. A similar picture may be seen in the late stage of idiopathic dilated cardiomyopathy involving the right heart.

- **Radiotherapy:** Tricuspid regurgitation is an uncommon complication that may appear many years after radiotherapy to the chest. The exact mechanism of valvular regurgitation is poorly understood.

Pathophysiology

Mild tricuspid regurgitation is common even in 30% of normal people with no cardiac disease. Severe tricuspid regurgitation, irrespective of its etiology, results in signs and symptoms of raised systemic venous pressure. Raised right atrial pressure is transmitted to the vena cava. A systolic V wave "from the right ventricle" is seen in the vena cava with the right atrium functioning as a conduit. The systolic wave is followed by a deep, wide-angled early diastolic 'Y' descent when the tricuspid valve opens and the right ventricle fills. Long-standing tricuspid regurgitation results in hepatic congestion and fluid retention, and eventually renal impairment. With severe tricuspid regurgitation, the systolic murmur may not be audible because of laminar regurgitation flow.

Assessment of Tricuspid Regurgitation

- **Color flow Doppler:** This detects the presence of tricuspid regurgitation, although its absence does not exclude it. A dilated right atrium and a broad regurgitation jet that approaches the vena cava suggests significant incompetence. A tricuspid regurgitation jet area of more than 40% that of the right atrium is consistent with significant regurgitation.[17]

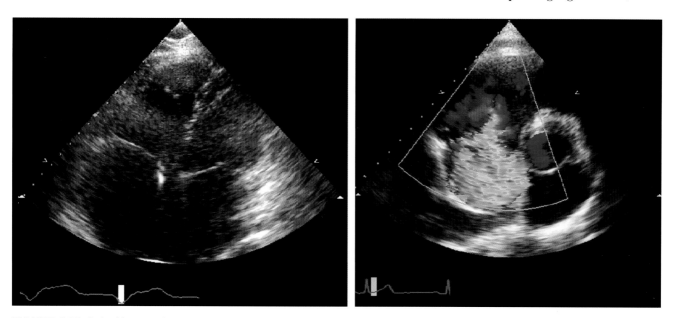

FIGURE 3.20. Apical images from a patient with fluid retention after pacemaker insertion. Note the thickened valve leaflets (left) and the severe regurgitation (right) resulting from localized fibrosis.

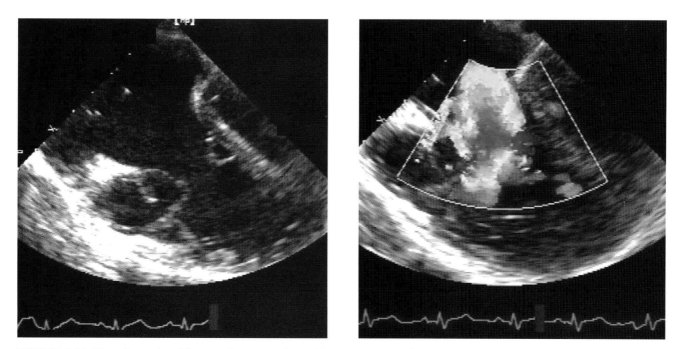

FIGURE 3.21. Two-dimensional images from a patient with congenitally deformed Tricuspid valve leaflets (left), resulting in severe regurgitation (right).

● *Proximal isovelocity convergence technique:* The same principle as mentioned in the assessment of mitral regurgitation can be applied to determine severity of tricuspid incompetence.

● *Continuous-wave Doppler:* This registers the pressure drop between the right ventricle and the atrium in systole using the modified Bernoulli equation. In the absence of pulmonary valve or infundibular stenosis, adding right atrial pressure (approximately 10 mmHg) to the transtricuspid pressure drop can be used to estimate pulmonary artery systolic pressure. Normally with mild functional regurgitation, the higher the pressure drop across the tricuspid valve, the longer it takes to decelerate in early diastole (i.e., after end-ejection). With severe regurgitation and absence of retrograde tricuspid leaflet resistance, the continuous-wave trace becomes more triangular, peaking in early systole and stopping close to end-ejection (P2). This shape represents a reversed V

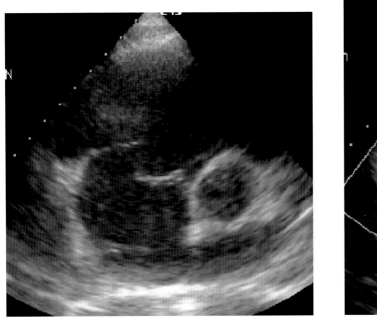
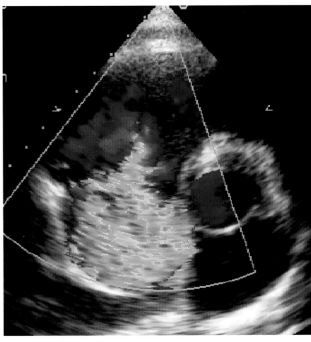

A   B

FIGURE 3.22. Modified parasternal view from a patient with tricuspid valve prolapse causing severe regurgitation. Notice the failure of leaflet coaption.

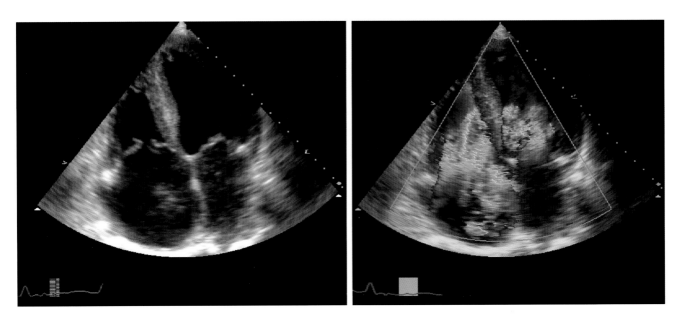

FIGURE 3.23. Apical four-chamber view from a patient with ischemic cardiomyopathy showing dilated four chambers (left) and severe tricuspid regurgitation on the color Doppler picture (right).

wave in the jugular venous pulse due to pressure equalization between the right atrium and right ventricle. In addition, the pressure drop across the valve may fall to as low as 5- to 10 mmHg due to the increased right atrial pressure. Equalization of forward and backward flow areas suggests free regurgitation. The combination of this picture along with systolic flow reversal in the superior vena cava and inferior vena cava or hepatic veins and early diastolic forward flow corresponding to the deep "Y" descent of the venous pulse confirms the diagnosis of severe regurgitation.[18–20]

• **Reversed septal movement:** With severe right ventricular volume overload from the tricuspid regurgitation the interventricular septal movement becomes reversed

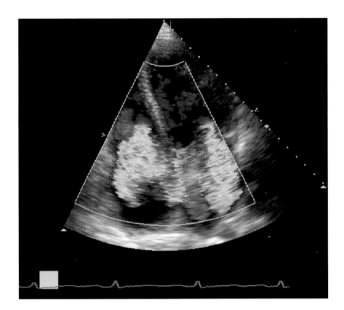

FIGURE 3.24. Two-dimensional image of the tricuspid valve from a patient, 10 years after radiotherapy. Note the dilated ring, and severe tricuspid regurgitation.

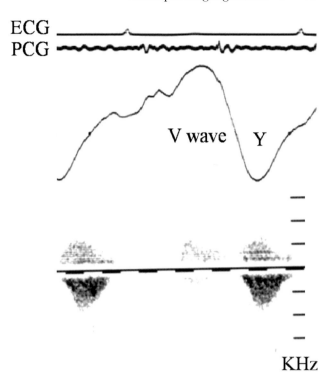

FIGURE 3.25. Jugular venous pulse from a patient with severe tricuspid regurgitation. Note the prominent systolic V wave on the pulse (top) associated with systolic flow reversal in the superior vena cava (bottom). This is followed by a deep broad early diastolic Y descent.

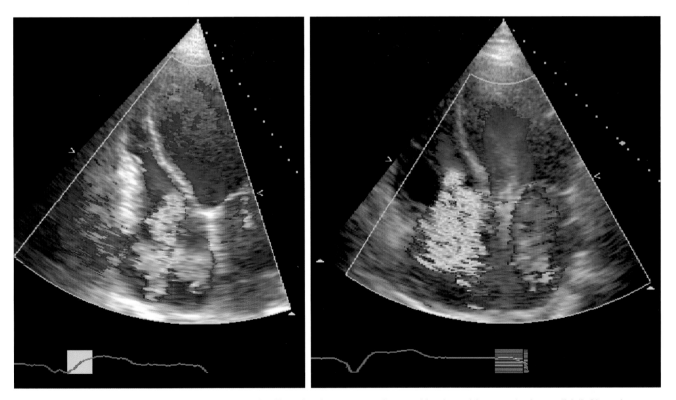

FIGURE 3.26. Two-dimensional images and color Doppler from two patients with tricuspid regurgitation, mild (left) and severe (right). Note the difference in right atrial size and jet area and diameter.

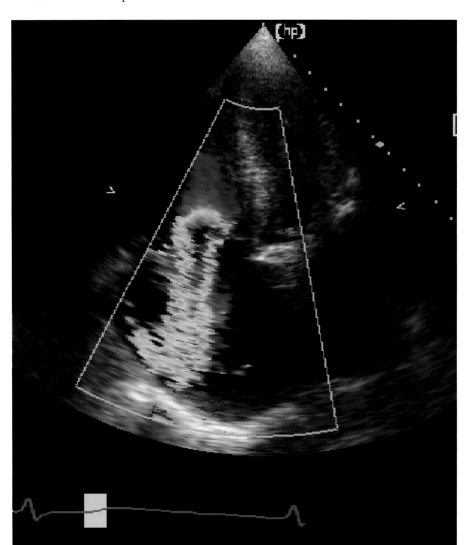

FIGURE 3.27. Color flow Doppler of severe tricuspid regurgitation from a patient demonstrating Proximal isovelocity technique at the site of leaflet tips.

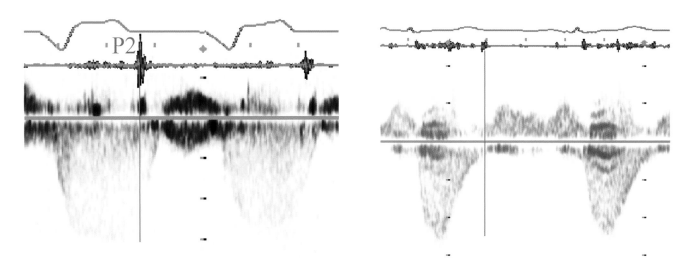

FIGURE 3.28. Continuous-wave Doppler recordings from two patients with tricuspid regurgitation, mild (left) and severe (right). Note the low-pressure drop and the equalization of right ventricular and atrial pressures in early diastole with severe regurgitation.

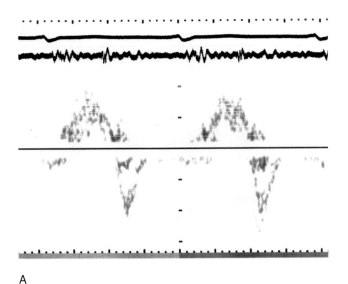

A

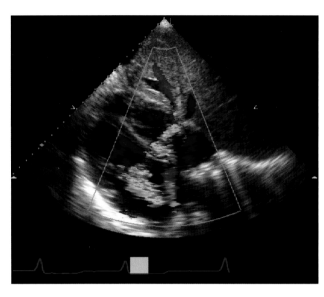

B

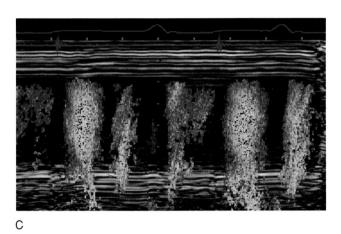

C

FIGURE 3.29. (A) Pulsed-wave Doppler velocities from a patient with severe tricuspid regurgitation demonstrating flow reversal in the inferior vena cava. (B) Respective color Doppler flow reversal in inferior vena cava. (C) Colour M-mode Doppler showing flow reversal in hepatic veins (red).

and the septum functions as part of the right ventricle in systole. This can easily be demonstrated on M-mode images of the left ventricular minor axis.

Treatment

Medical treatment by diuretics aims at controlling the fluid retention. It may result in significant fall in right ventricular size and hence the extent of tricuspid regurgitation. Moderately severe regurgitation is reasonably well tolerated compared with mitral regurgitation. Tricuspid regurgitation secondary to rheumatic mitral valve disease may subside after successful mitral valve surgery, although direct inspection of the tricuspid valve is always recommended for possible plication and repair in an attempt to avoid future incompetence. If the regurgitation is very severe and the fluid retention requires very large doses of diuretics, large enough to cause significant metabolic consequences, valve repair or replacement may be considered.

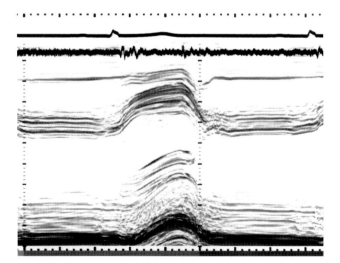

FIGURE 3.30. M-mode recording of left ventricular minor axis from a patient with severe tricuspid regurgitation demonstrating reversed septal movement.

Surgical Procedures

Tricuspid valve replacement is usually indicated when a prior repair has failed. The repair procedures are less predictable than mitral repair, but like the mitral valve it can be performed with or without a supporting ring. Many young patients with Ebsteins anomaly are symptom-free, but excellent results of surgical repair have been reported in symptomatic patients. A frequent complication of tricuspid valve replacement is heart block due to the close proximity of the atrioventricular node to the tricuspid annulus. It is therefore wise to place permanent epicardial electrodes at the time of surgery. These can be easily connected to a pacing box, thus avoiding the problems of running an endocardial lead through a prosthetic valve. Large right atria are usually complicated by arrhythmia (commonly atrial flutter). Trials to control such arrhythmia by right atrial reduction surgery (Maze operation) have been attempted with good results, particularly in Ebsteins anomaly.

REFERENCES

1. Daniels SJ, Mintz GS, Kotler MN. Rheumatic tricuspid valve disease: two-dimensional echocardiographic, hemodynamic, and angiographic correlations. *Am J Cardiol* 1983;51:492–496.
2. Guyer DE, Gillam LD, Foale RA, et al. Comparison of the echocardiographic and hemodynamic diagnosis of rheumatic tricuspid stenosis. *J Am Coll Cardiol* 1984;3:1135–1144.
3. Shimada R, Takeshita A, Nakamura M, et al. Diagnosis of tricuspid stenosis by M-mode and two-dimensional echocardiography. *Am J Cardiol* 1984;53:164–168.
4. Pellikka PA, Tajik AJ, Khandheria BK, et al. Carcinoid heart disease. clinical and echocardiographic spectrum in 74 patients. *Circulation* 1993;87:1188–1196.
5. Ross EM, Roberts WC. The carcinoid syndrome: comparison of 21 necropsy subjects with carcinoid heart disease to 15 necropsy subjects without carcinoid heart disease. *Am J Med* 1985;79:339–354.
6. Heaven DJ, Henein MY, Sutton R. Pacemaker lead related tricuspid stenosis: a report of two cases. *Heart* 2000;83:351–352.
7. Denning GK, Henneke KH, Rudolph W. Assessment of tricuspid stenosis by Doppler echocardiography. *J Am Coll Cardiol* 1987 [9]. Abstract.
8. Parris TM, Panidis JP, Ross J, et al. Doppler echocardiographic findings in rheumatic tricuspid stenosis. *Am J Cardiol* 1987;60:1414–1416.
9. Veyrat C, Kalmanson D, Farjon M, et al. Non-invasive diagnosis and assessment of tricuspid regurgitation and stenosis using one and two dimensional echo-pulsed Doppler. *Br Heart J* 1982;47:596–605.
10. Henein MY, Sheppard M, Ho Y, et al. Evidence for rheumatic valve disease in patients with severe tricuspid regurgitation long after mitral valve surgery-role of 3D reconstruction. *J Heart Valve Dis* 2003;12:566–572.
11. Ginzton LE, Siegel RJ, Criley JM. Natural history of tricuspid valve endocarditis: a two dimensional echocardiographic study. *Am J Cardiol* 1982;49:1853–1859.
12. Bates ER, Sorkin RP. Echocardiographic diagnosis of flail anterior leaflet in tricuspid endocarditis. *Am Heart J* 1983;106(1 Pt 1):161–163.
13. Howard RJ, Drobac M, Rider WD, et al. Carcinoid heart disease: diagnosis by two-dimensional echocardiography. *Circulation* 1982;66:1059–1065.
14. Chandraratna PN, Lopez JM, Fernandez JJ, et al. Echocardiographic detection of tricuspid valve prolapse. *Circulation* 1975;51:823–826.
15. Rippe JM, Angoff G, Sloss LJ, et al. Multiple floppy valves: an echocardiographic syndrome. *Am J Med* 1979;66:817–824.
16. Schlamowitz RA, Gross S, Keating E, et al. Tricuspid valve prolapse: a common occurrence in the click-murmur syndrome. *J Clin Ultrasound* 1982;10:435–439.
17. Suzuki Y, Kambara H, Kadota K, et al. Detection and evaluation of tricuspid regurgitation using a real-time, two-dimensional, color-coded, Doppler flow imaging system: comparison with contrast two-dimensional echocardiography and right ventriculography. *Am J Cardiol* 1986;57:811–815.
18. Currie PJ, Seward JB, Chan KL, et al. Continuous wave Doppler determination of right ventricular pressure: a simultaneous Doppler-catheterization study in 127 patients. *J Am Coll Cardiol* 1985;6:750–756.
19. Sakai K, Nakamura K, Satomi G, et al. [Hepatic vein blood flow pattern measured by Doppler echocardiography as an evaluation of tricuspid valve insufficiency]. *J Cardiogr* 1983;13:33–43.
20. Chan KL, Currie PJ, Seward JB, et al. Comparison of three Doppler ultrasound methods in the prediction of pulmonary artery pressure. *J Am Coll Cardiol* 1987;9:549–554.

Pulmonary Valve

ANATOMY

The pulmonary valve lies anterior and to the left of the aortic valve. The three pulmonary leaflets assume the shape of half moons (semilunar) and are similar but usually not equal in size. The right and left coronary sinuses of the aorta always face the pulmonary valve. The leaflets are thinner and more delicate than the aortic leaflets. Unlike the aortic valve, the pulmonary valve sits on a complete muscular ring of the infundibulum and is not in direct continuity with the tricuspid valve. It is thickest along the closing edge. The delicate, pocketlike leaflets are formed primarily of collagen and therefore open and close passively, with little elastic recoil. In the middle of the free edge of each leaflet is a fibrous mound, the nodule of Arrantius. Coaptation of the three nodules ensures complete central closure of the valve orifice during ventricular diastole.

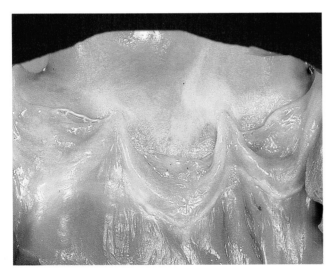

FIGURE 4.1. Section in the right ventricular outflow tract showing the pulmonary valve with three semi lunar leaflets.

In adults, the pulmonary valve is better viewed from the parasternal short-axis window with anterior angulation. It can occasionally be seen from the suprasternal and subcostal views. Normal transpulmonary valve blood velocity is on the order of 75 cm/s in mid ejection.[1]

PULMONARY STENOSIS

Pulmonary stenosis can be at three levels: valvular, subvalvar, and supravalvar.

Valvular Stenosis

Pulmonary valve stenosis is almost always congenital in origin. It is very rarely rheumatic. Congenital pulmonary stenosis is associated with doming leaflets with total fusion and a single orifice in the middle. In tetralogy of Fallot, pulmonary valve leaflets are often dysplastic, small and thickened, and the valve may have only two leaflets.[2] In systole, the leaflets appear doming in the center of the pulmonary artery and are unable to move parallel to the arterial wall as they normally do.[3] In diastole, leaflets may look completely normal, since they are not really thickened. Pulmonary stenosis is commonly associated with post-stenotic dilatation of the pulmonary artery, which itself may suggest the presence of pulmonary stenosis. Contrary to what occurs with the aortic valve, it is uncommon for the pulmonary valve leaflets to calcify with time.[4] Balloon valvuloplasty is the ideal procedure for managing congenital pulmonary stenosis in children and early adulthood, but the procedure may be complicated by some degree of pulmonary regurgitation, particularly in the long term.[5]

Rheumatic pulmonary stenosis is extremely rare. Other rare causes of pulmonary valve stenosis are carcinoid disease,[6] where kinins released by the carcinoid

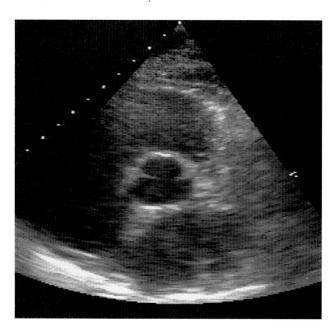 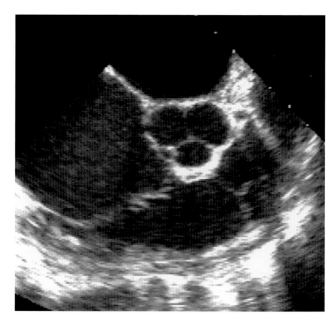

FIGURE 4.2. Short-axis view of the aortic valve demonstrating normal-looking pulmonary valve leaflets and pulmonary artery diameter. Transthoracic (left) and transesophageal (right) views.

tumor in the gastrointestinal tract cause superficial fibrosis of both the tricuspid and the pulmonary valve.

Subvalvar Pulmonary Stenosis

Subvalvar pulmonary stenosis is commonly caused by infundibular stenosis or a two-chambered right ventricle either in isolation or together with valvar stenosis or tetralogy of Fallot.[9] Subvalvar pulmonary stenosis can easily be seen on two-dimensional images and confirmed by color Doppler. When it occurs alone, it is often associated with post-stenotic dilatation. It may also be part of other disease conditions such as hypertrophic cardiomyopathy that involves the right heart. Rare causes of subvalvar stenosis include tumors, both primary (angiosarcoma or fibroma) and secondary (melanoma).

Supravalvar Pulmonary Stenosis

Supravalvar pulmonary stenosis occurs in the proximal segment of the pulmonary artery, in the form of either single or multiple narrowings,[10,11] as in Williams syndrome. A typical example occurs following banding of the pulmonary artery as part of the management of significant intracardiac shunting such as multiple ventricular septal defects.[12] However, supravalvar stenosis may also involve only the pulmonary artery branches and spare the main trunk.[13] Once again, color flow Doppler indicates the site of narrowing and continuous-wave Doppler can be used to assess the severity of stenosis.

Pulmonary Stenosis Severity

Color flow Doppler shows the level at which maximum aliasing occurs: valvar, subvalvar, or supravalvar. Continuous-wave Doppler is the ideal technique for registering peak pulmonary valve velocities that can be translated into a pressure drop by applying the modified Bernoulli equation. A pressure drop of more than 75 mmHg is considered severe stenosis.[7,8] Severe pulmonary stenosis is usually associated with some degree of right ventricular hypertrophy and dysfunction. Significant impairment of right ventricular systolic function and consequently reduction in stroke volume may underestimate the severity of pulmonary stenosis when relying solely on the pulmonary velocities.

PULMONARY REGURGITATION

Isolated congenital pulmonary regurgitation is rare. In adult congenital heart practice, pulmonary regurgitation is often seen long after pulmonary valvotomy or pulmonary valvuloplasty. It is particularly common after repair of tetralogy of Fallot.[14] The degree of pulmonary regurgitation varies from mild to severe. Significant pulmonary regurgitation may occur secondary to pulmonary artery dilatation and may complicate endocarditis.[15] This is, however, a rare cause of pulmonary regurgitation.

Assessment of Pulmonary Regurgitation

A color flow jet diameter of more than 7.5 mm suggests significant pulmonary regurgitation when compared with MRI assessment.[16]

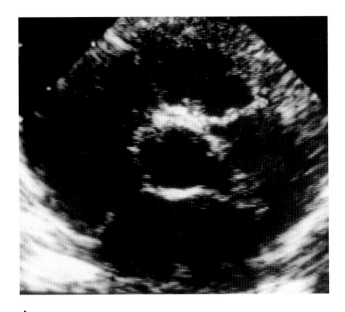

A

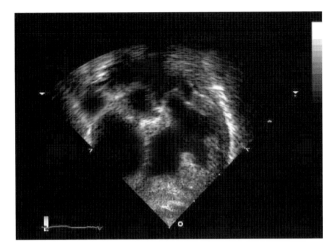

B

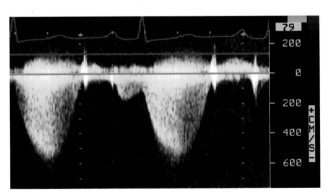

C

FIGURE 4.3. Subcostal views from a patient with deformed pulmonary valve showing stiff and (A) fibrosed leaflets and (B) systolic doming causing valve stenosis. (C) Pathologic section from a patient with bicuspid pulmonary valve.

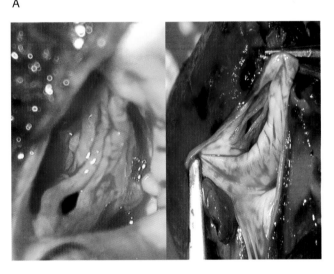

FIGURE 4.4. Continuous-wave Doppler velocities across a stenotic pulmonary valve registering a value of 4.5 m/s equivalent to a pressure drop of 81 mmHg.

Continuous-wave Doppler velocities are more accurate in discriminating between mild and significant regurgitation.[16,17] A pulmonary regurgitation signal that shows a sharp decline to meet the baseline (i.e., pressure equalization in mid diastole or before the Q wave of the succeeding cycle) is consistent with significant regurgitation. Mild regurgitation demonstrates a measurable retrograde pressure drop between the pulmonary artery and the right ventricle in late diastole. Severe pulmonary regurgitation is usually associated with right ventricular dilatation and increased activity (i.e., to accommodate the increased right ventricular stroke volume).

The degree of pulmonary regurgitation can be assessed using the pulmonary regurgitation index. The pulmonary regurgitation index represents the ratio between the pulmonary regurgitation duration from continuous-wave Doppler and total diastolic time expressed as a percent. A

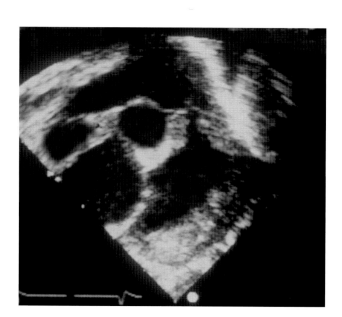
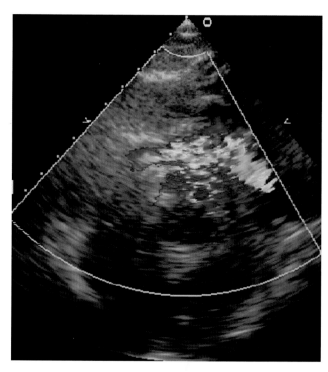

FIGURE 4.5. Subcostal views demonstrating subvalvar (infundibular) pulmonary stenosis. Note the level of narrowing below the valve leaflets.

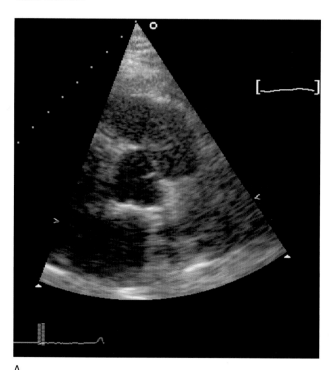

A

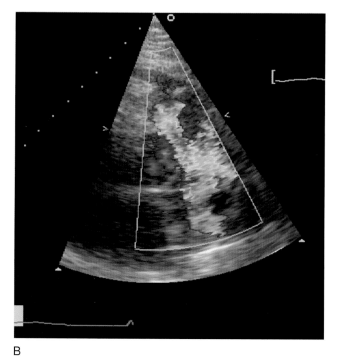

B

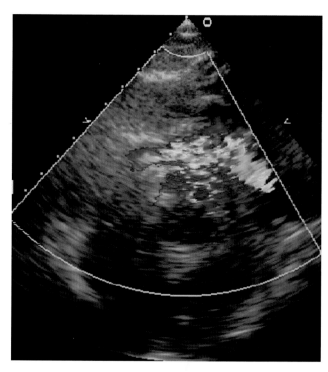

C

FIGURE 4.6. (A) Two-dimensional images of the pulmonary valve demonstrating subvalvar pulmonary stenosis caused by secondaries (melanoma). (B) Color flow Doppler demonstrating the stenosis level beneath the valve. (C) Continuous-wave Doppler showing peak right ventricular outflow tract velocities of 2.0 m/s.

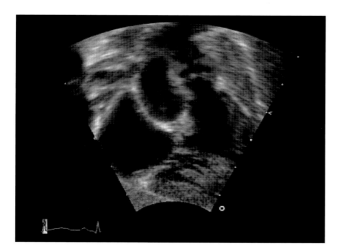

FIGURE 4.7. Subcostal views showing supravalvar pulmonary stenosis of the main pulmonary trunk.

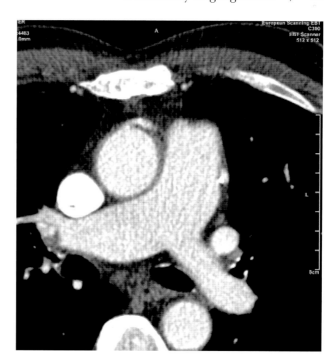

FIGURE 4.8. Electron beam angiography corresponding to parasternal short-axis view from a patient with narrowed left pulmonary artery with respect to a normal right branch.

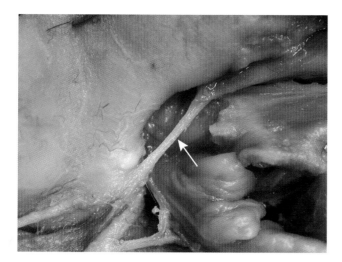

FIGURE 4.9. Section in the pulmonary trunk showing threadlike pulmonary artery. No valve was present at the distal end.

pulmonary regurgitation index of less than 74% is suggestive of significant regurgitation. In patients with a fast heart rate, this index may underestimate the pulmonary regurgitation, and in those with severe right ventricular disease and raised end-diastolic pressure it may overestimate pulmonary regurgitation severity as the pulmonary artery and right ventricular diastolic pressures will equalize in mid diastole. In patients with atrial fibrillation, an

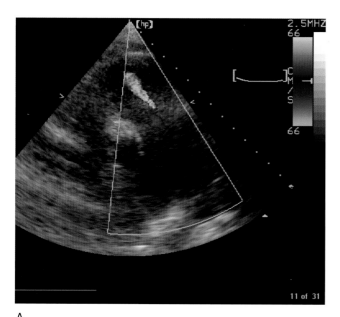

A

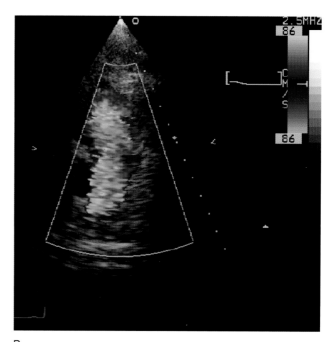

B

FIGURE 4.10. Parasternal short-axis view from two patients with pulmonary regurgitation, mild (left) and severe (right); post-pulmonary valvotomy as shown by color flow Doppler. Note the narrow pulmonary regurgitation jet in diastole with mild and broad jet (>8 mm) with severe pulmonary regurgitation.

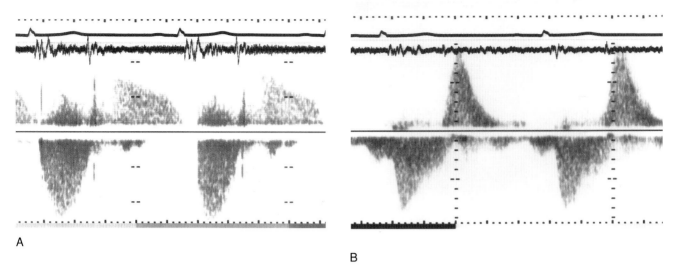

A

B

FIGURE 4.11. Continuous-wave Doppler velocities from two patients with pulmonary regurgitation, mild (left) and severe (right). Note the equalization of pulmonary artery and right ventricular pressures in mid diastole in the patient with severe regurgitation.

average of five cycles should be considered for estimating pulmonary regurgitation index.

Complications

Right Ventricular Dilatation

Long-standing pulmonary regurgitation is usually well tolerated by the right ventricle, probably due to the low pressure difference between the pulmonary artery and the right ventricular cavity. Even in patients with severe pulmonary regurgitation the right ventricular cavity may remain completely normal in size and function. However, follow-up of such patients may reveal varying degrees of

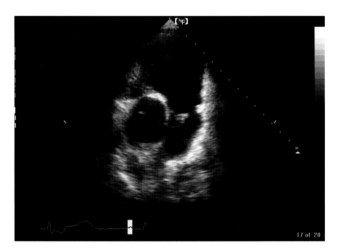

FIGURE 4.13. Short axis of the aortic valve and right ventricular outflow tract demonstrating dilated right ventricle.

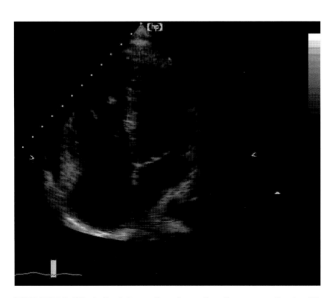

FIGURE 4.12. Apical four-chamber view from a patient with severe pulmonary regurgitation showing a slightly dilated right ventricular cavity but maintained function.

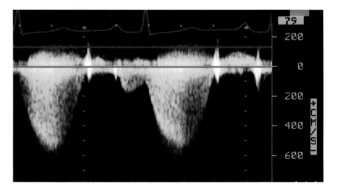

FIGURE 4.14. Transpulmonary continuous-wave Doppler from a patient with Noonan's syndrome and pulmonary stenosis showing A wave consistent with restrictive right ventricular physiology. The appearance of an A wave in the pulmonary flow.

right ventricular dilatation (remodeling) and eventually dysfunction. Serial measurements of the right ventricular outflow tract diameter (from the long and short axes) and inflow tract (from the apical four-chamber view) can be used for monitoring changes in ventricular size in patients with pulmonary regurgitation.

Right Ventricular Dysfunction

In some patients with long-standing regurgitation, particularly in the presence of right ventricular dilatation, the intrinsic characteristics of the myocardium may change and become stiff (incompliant). The same physiology is frequently observed in patients with small right ventricular size, particularly those with critical pulmonary stenosis and previous valvotomy. In this situation, the right ventricle may not proportionally dilate.[18] Right ventricular physiology becomes restrictive with (a) an A wave in the pulmonary flow velocity (recorded by pulsed-wave Doppler) consistent with direct propagation of atrial contraction velocity to the pulmonary artery with the right ventricle itself functioning as a conduit in late diastole, (b) a giant A wave on jugular venous pulse, (c) a dominant E wave on right ventricular filling pattern with short deceleration time.

Restrictive right ventricular physiology is commonly associated with varying degrees of tricuspid regurgitation and dilatation of the pulmonary artery. Atriogenic tricus-

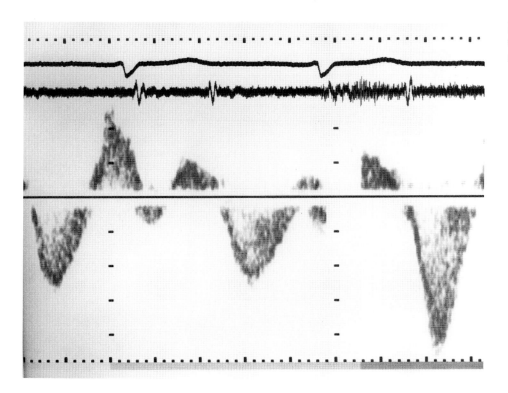

FIGURE 4.15. Superior vena caval flow in the same patient showing giant pressure A wave.

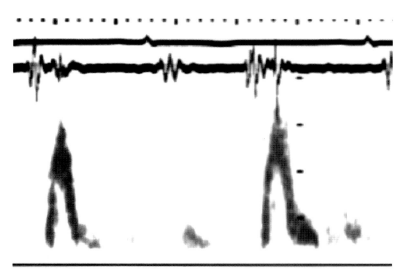

FIGURE 4.16. Right ventricular filling pattern from a patient with restrictive physiology showing dominant E wave with very short deceleration time. Peak E wave coincides with the onset of the third heart sound on the phonocardiogram.

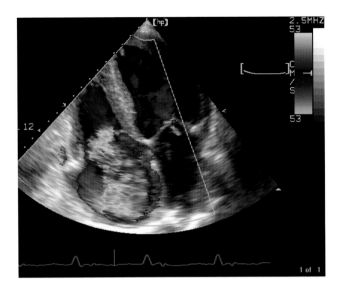

FIGURE 4.17. Apical four-chamber view from a patient with right ventricular disease complicated by tricuspid regurgitation seen by color Doppler.

pid regurgitation may develop late in the disease process, particularly in patients with a long pulmonary regurgitation interval that provokes long tricuspid regurgitation. The effect of this advanced ventricular dysfunction is compromised right ventricular filling time and limited stroke volume and exercise intolerance.[19] While similar disturbances on the left side can be corrected by Dual chamber pacing and shortening of the atrioventricular delay, no attempts have been proposed to correct long tricuspid regurgitation.

Arrhythmia

Untreated significant pulmonary regurgitation may result in atrial or even ventricular arrhythmias. Early correction of the organic valve disease may protect the patient from any further deterioration of atrial and ventricular function and subsequently development of arrhythmias.

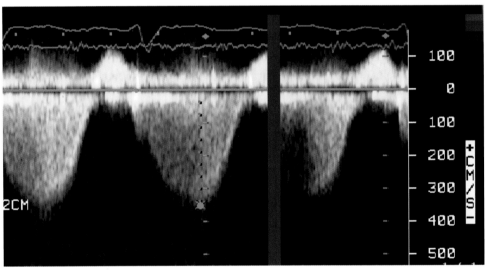

A

FIGURE 4.18. Continuous-wave Doppler from a patient with late-stage right ventricular disease demonstrating tricuspid regurgitation with atriogenic component (top) that limits total right ventricular filling time (bottom).

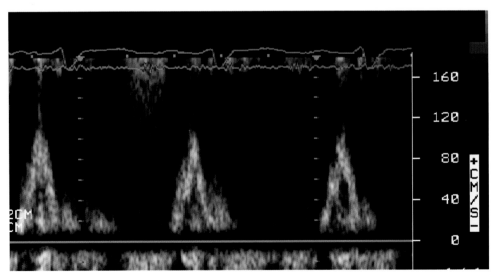

B

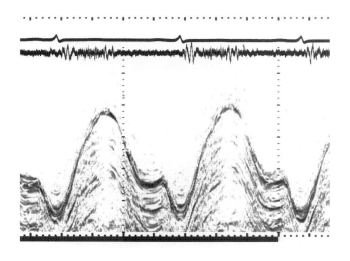

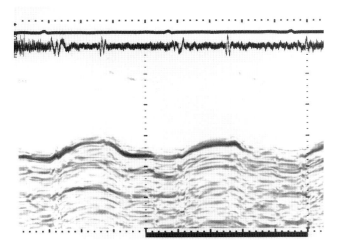

FIGURE 4.19. M-mode recording of Right ventricular free wall long axis from a normal subject (top) and a patient with severe right ventricular disease (bottom). Note the significant drop in amplitude and velocities, particularly in early diastole.

Assessment of Right Ventricular Function

Quantification of right ventricular function is not always easy because of its complex anatomy. Long-axis movement can easily be studied by recording tricuspid ring movement in systole and diastole using both M-mode and tissue Doppler techniques. Right ventricular free wall (long-axis) amplitude has been shown to correlate with overall systolic function assessed by ejection fraction.[20] Also, in early diastole various degrees of functional impairment can be demonstrated by the lengthening velocity and the presence of incoordination (post-ejection shortening). Finally, late diastolic amplitude of backward movement of the long axis (toward the atrium) can be used as a marker for assessing right atrial function. Normal right ventricular long-axis amplitude is approximately 2.5 ± 0.25 cm.[21] Myocardial tissue Doppler velocities can be used to assess right ventricular free wall

function, again in systole and diastole. Normal values range from 9 ± 2 cm/s for systolic velocity to 10 ± 2 cm/s for early diastolic lengthening velocity.

Complications of Restrictive Right Ventricular Disease

The following list some complications of restrictive right ventricular disease:

1. Cyanosis. Restrictive right ventricular physiology with increased diastolic pressure results in raised right atrial pressure and possible shunt reversal at atrial level across an atrial septal defect or even a small patent foramen ovale. Patients may experience transient ischemic attacks or cyanosis. Contrast echocardiography with a biological contrast (mixed blood and saline) is often useful in confirming the presence of an atrial shunt, particularly with Valsalva maneuver, when the air bubbles cross the septum and appear in the right atrium.

2. Right heart failure. Reduced right ventricular function and increased right atrial pressure will be reflected on the systemic circulation and result in salt and water retention and signs and symptoms of right ventricular decompensation.

3. Arrhythmia. The increased atrial size and pressure in patients with stiff right ventricle may trigger different forms of arrhythmia: fibrillation or flutter.

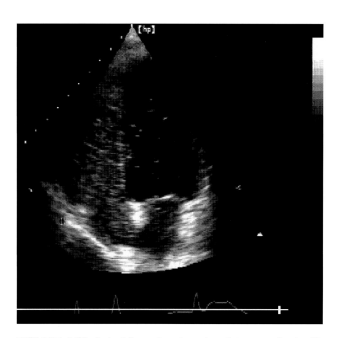

FIGURE 4.20. Apical four-chamber view from a patient with restrictive right ventricular disease and cyanosis demonstrating right-to-left shunt at the atrial level using echo contrast.

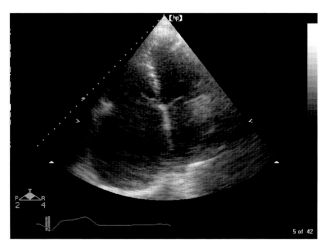

FIGURE 4.21. Apical four-chamber view from a patient with stiff right ventricle and arrhythmia demonstrating disproportionately large right atrium.

Management

Although pulmonary valve replacement may be a long-term solution for severe pulmonary regurgitation, there is no consensus regarding the exact time for surgical intervention. Decision making should be based on individual cases and considering other factors (e.g., the presence of early signs of right ventricular disease). Pulmonary valve replacement by a homograft has proved a very satisfactory operation with excellent clinical outcome. Transvalvar velocities may show some increase over the early postoperative period but remain stable afterward.

Recently, transcatheter pulmonary valve replacement has been investigated, and preliminary results are promising.[22]

As is the case in restrictive left ventricular physiology, treatment with an angiotensin-converting enzyme inhibitor may have a substantial role in balancing overall cardiac physiology in patients with restrictive right ventricular disease, but the current literature is lacking the evidence to support this proposal.

REFERENCES

1. Griffith JM, Henry WL. An ultrasound system for combined cardiac imaging and Doppler blood flow measurement in man. *Circulation* 1978;57:925–930.
2. Weyman AE, Hurwitz RA, Girod DA, et al. Cross-sectional echocardiographic visualization of the stenotic pulmonary valve. *Circulation* 1977;56:769–774.
3. Leblanc MH, Paquet M. Echocardiographic assessment of valvular pulmonary stenosis in children. *Br Heart J* 1981;46: 363–368.
4. Nishimura RA, Pieroni DR, Bierman FZ, et al. Second natural history study of congenital heart defects. pulmonary stenosis: echocardiography. *Circulation* 1993;87(2 Suppl):I73–I79.
5. Masura J, Burch M, Deanfield JE, et al. Five-year follow-up after balloon pulmonary valvuloplasty. *J Am Coll Cardiol* 1993;21:132–136.
6. Pellikka PA, Tajik AJ, Khandheria BK, et al. Carcinoid heart disease. clinical and echocardiographic spectrum in 74 patients. *Circulation* 1993;87:1188–1196.
7. Lima CO, Sahn DJ, Valdes-Cruz LM, et al. Noninvasive prediction of transvalvular pressure gradient in patients with pulmonary stenosis by quantitative two-dimensional echocardiographic Doppler studies. *Circulation* 1983;67:866–871.
8. Johnson GL, Kwan OL, Handshoe S, et al. Accuracy of combined two-dimensional echocardiography and continuous wave Doppler recordings in the estimation of pressure gradient in right ventricular outlet obstruction. *J Am Coll Cardiol* 1984;3:1013–1018.
9. Caldwell RL, Weyman AE, Hurwitz RA, et al. Right ventricular outflow tract assessment by cross-sectional echocardiography in tetralogy of Fallot. *Circulation* 1979;59:395–402.

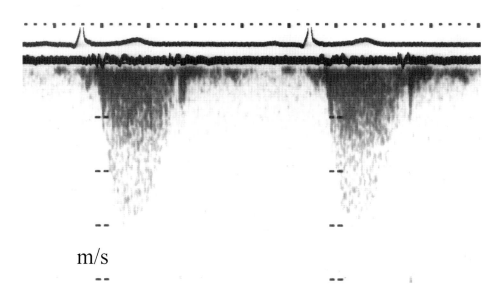

FIGURE 4.22. Continuous-wave Doppler recording from a patient with pulmonary homograft 12 months after surgery showing a peak velocity of 3 m/s.

m/s

10. French JW. Aortic and pulmonary artery stenosis: improvement without intervention? *J Am Coll Cardiol* 1990;15:1631–1632.

11. Wren C, Oslizlok P, Bull C. Natural history of supravalvular aortic stenosis and pulmonary artery stenosis. *J Am Coll Cardiol* 1990;15:1625–1630.

12. Foale RA, King ME, Gordon D, et al. Pseudoaneurysm of the pulmonary artery after the banding procedure: two-dimensional echocardiographic description. *J Am Coll Cardiol* 1984;3(2 Pt 1):371–374.

13. Rodriguez RJ, Riggs TW. Physiologic peripheral pulmonic stenosis in infancy. *Am J Cardiol* 1990;66(20):1478–1481.

14. Brand A, Dollberg S, Keren A. The prevalence of valvular regurgitation in children with structurally normal hearts: a color Doppler echocardiographic study. *Am Heart J* 1992;123:177–180.

15. Panidis IP, Kotler MN, Mintz GS, et al. Clinical and echo-cardiographic correlations in right heart endocarditis. *Int J Cardiol* 1984;6:17–34.

16. Li W, Davlouros P, Gibson DG, et al. Assessment of pulmonary regurgitation in adults with repaired tetralogy of Fallot–comparison between Doppler echocardiography and MRI. *Circulation* 2001;104[II]:431. Abstract.

17. Miyatake K, Okamoto M, Kinoshita N, et al. Pulmonary regurgitation studied with the ultrasonic pulsed Doppler technique. *Circulation* 1982;65:969–976.

18. Hayes CJ, Gersony WM, Driscoll DJ, et al. Second natural history study of congenital heart defects. Results of treatment of patients with pulmonary valvar stenosis. *Circulation* 1993;87(2 Suppl):I28–I37.

19. Rowe SA, Zahka KG, Manolio TA, et al. Lung function and pulmonary regurgitation limit exercise capacity in post-operative tetralogy of Fallot. *J Am Coll Cardiol* 1991;17:461–466.

20. Kaul S, Tei C, Hopkins JM, et al. Assessment of right ventricular function using two-dimensional echocardiography. *Am Heart J* 1984;107:526–531.

21. Florea VG, Florea ND, Sharma R, et al. Right ventricular dysfunction in adult severe cystic fibrosis. *Chest* 2000;118:1063–1068.

22. Bonhoeffer P, Boudjemline Y, Saliba Z, et al. Transcatheter implantation of a bovine valve in pulmonary position: a lamb study. *Circulation* 2000;102:813–816.

Valve Substitutes

Valve replacement with various substitutes in patients with severe valve dysfunction has been practiced for the last 40 years, particularly in those patients with unrepairable valve deformation.[1] Artificial valve substitutes are essentially of two types: mechanical and bioprostheses.

Mechanical valves are either of the ball-cage type (Starr-Edwards), single disk (Bjork-Shiley), or bileaflet prosthesis (St. Jude). Although mechanical valves are durable and correct the organic valve dysfunction, they have a number of potential complications, usually infection; endocarditis, particularly of the sewing ring; hemolysis; dehiscence that results in severe regurgitation; and thrombosis. They also require lifelong anticoagulation, and this itself has potential complications.[2–5]

Bioprosthetic valves or tissue valves [e.g., Hancock porcine valve or Toronto (Stentless) porcine valve] are recommended for all patients in whom long-term anticoagulation cannot be afforded and for patients living in countries where regular anticoagulation control is doubtful. They too have their disadvantages, being made of tissue. Bioprostheses are subject to infection, calcification, and significant dysfunction. The major disadvantage, however, is that they do not last as long as mechanical valves. Once degeneration is detected urgent life-saving valve replacement is usually necessary.[6–9]

Even if clinical details of the mechanical valve are not available to the sonographer, the chest x-ray may give an

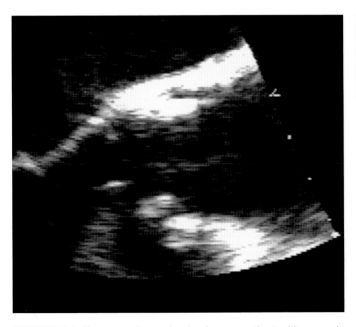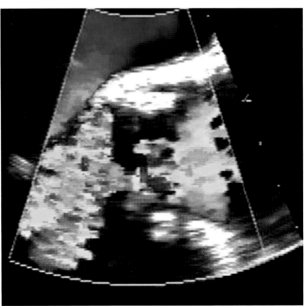

FIGURE 5.1. Transesophageal echo from a patient with a porcine aortic valve. Note the degeneration of the valve leaflets that results in severe mitral regurgitation (right).

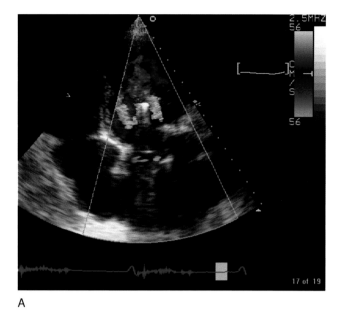

A

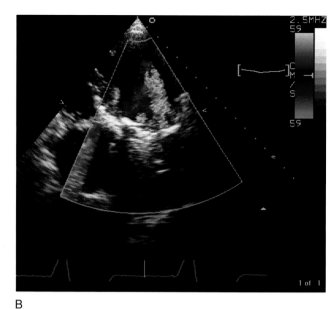

B

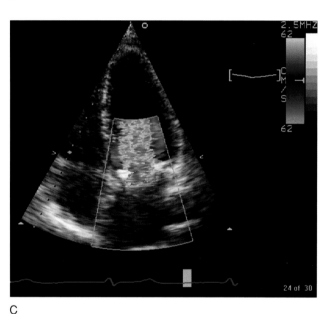

C

FIGURE 5.2. Color flow Doppler recording from three mitral prosthetic valves taken from the transthoracic apical four-chamber views. Note the two jets characterizing a ball–cage valve, eccentric jet with Bjork-Shiley, and central single jet with bileaflet valve.

idea about the valve shape and struts.[10] Echocardiographic two-dimensional imaging is an excellent tool for assessing valve movement and function.[11,12] Color Doppler significantly adds to the use of echocardiography in the follow-up of such patients, particularly for demonstrating characteristic flow patterns. Color Doppler typically displays two separate jets with a Starr-Edwards ball-cage prosthesis (particularly in the mitral position), an eccentric single jet with the tilted disk (Bjork-Shiley) valve, and a single central jet with the bileaflet valve.[13–15]

One disadvantage of color flow Doppler is that it fails to detect valve regurgitation jet from transthoracic images because of the mechanical ultrasound artefact that distracts the image. However, in severe paraprosthetic valve regurgitation, careful angling of the imaging probe should demonstrate the exact site of the dehiscence and the mitral regurgitation jet.

Transesophageal echo is more sensitive than transthoracic echo in detecting the presence and assessing the severity of paraprosthetic valve regurgitation. However, careful interpretation of images should be considered to avoid overestimation of the severity of the incompetence. The same limitations apply to prosthetic valves in the aortic position.[16–19]

M-mode echocardiography has become limited in its use in studying prosthetic valve function, simply because it does not provide an accurate quantitative assessment of the mechanical valve apart from the simple display of the M-mode reflection of the moving part of the valve.[20] However, M-mode provides a unique way for assessing the ventricular response to valve regurgitation. Normally,

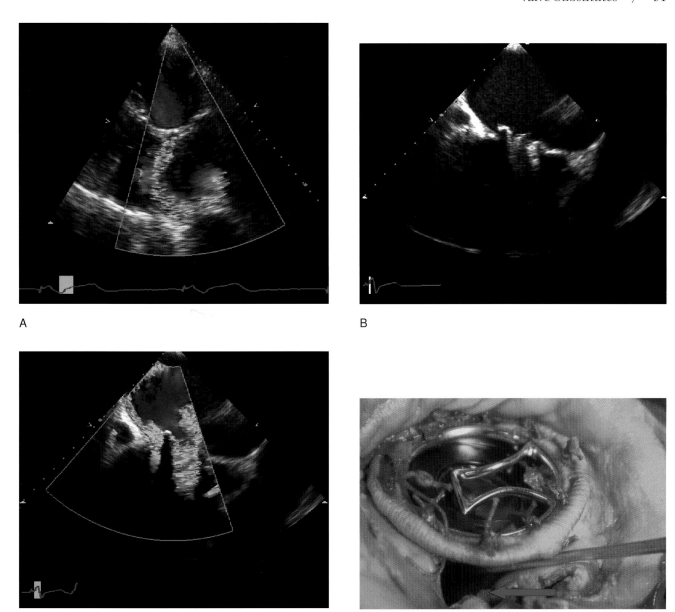

A

B

C

D

FIGURE 5.3. Transthoracic and transesophageal echo from a patient with dehisced mechanical mitral valve. Note the location of the dehiscent site at the lateral wall. Pathologic specimen from a patient with mechanical mitral valve and paravalvular leak caused by slippage of stitches.

the septal wall of the left ventricle becomes reversed after valve replacement surgery. In patients with severe para-prosthetic valve regurgitation, M-mode recording of left ventricular minor axis demonstrates a normalized septal movement and an active left ventricular cavity, consistent with significant left ventricular overload.

Furthermore, in patients with double valve replacement in whom color flow Doppler may not be conclusive in confirming the origin of the ventricular overload, an M-mode of left ventricular minor axis is usually of great help in differentiating between significant mitral and aortic regurgitation. Although left ventricular increase in

dimension is exclusively early diastolic with mitral regurgitation, it occurs all the way through early and mid diastole, with significant aortic regurgitation.

Continuous-wave Doppler has now become the ideal tool to provide accurate assessment of mechanical valve function. Continuous-wave Doppler measures peak forward-flow velocities across the mechanical valve that can be converted into pressure drop (gradient) using the modified Bernoulli equation $4V^2$, particularly with high velocities. All artificial valves are somewhat stenotic, since they operate on a fixed valve area, unlike native valves. However, a comparative increase in velocities and

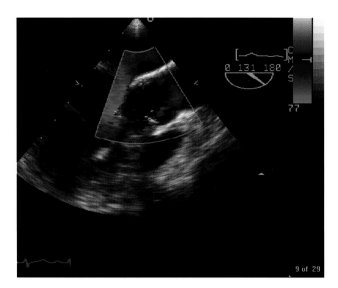

FIGURE 5.4. Transesophageal echo of left ventricular outflow tract and aortic valve demonstrating mild paraprosthetic aortic regurgitation on color flow Doppler.

pressure drop during follow-up with respect to postoperative values suggests the presence of valve stenosis.[21,22]

The pressure drop across valves is also affected by its location and the driving pressure of the column of blood passing through it. For instance, the same St. Jude mechanical valve operates at a peak pressure drop of 15 mmHg in the mitral position but operates at a pressure drop of 5 to 6 mmHg in the tricuspid position.[23]

Most mechanical valves have a small degree of functional regurgitation corresponding to the amount of blood displaced when the valve opens and closes. This may

appear only as a weak continuous wave Doppler signal. With severe para-prosthetic regurgitation, the continuous-wave Doppler signal is strong and the duration of mitral regurgitation is short, thus making the valve opening click very close to the second heart sound.[24,25]

HOMOGRAFTS

Homografts are only feasible for aortic valve replacement either directly in the aortic position or in the pulmonary position as part of Ross procedure (Aortic autograft). Assessment of aortic valve homograft function is exactly the same as that for the native valve in Chapter 2. In particular circumstances the mitral valve can be replaced by a reversed pulmonary valve, the so-called "top hat" operation, and the pulmonary valve is replaced by a homograft or a stentless valve substitute. This operation is ideal for patients in whom optimum anticoagulation cannot be achieved. Although not generally practiced, it has proved a great success in the small number of patients in whom it has been used.

The same technique can be used in tricuspid valve disease, in patients with severe tricuspid regurgitation, particularly those who have a contraindication to anticoagulants.

ENDOCARDITIS

All valve substitutes, particularly mechanical and bioprostheses, are subject to infection, since they are made of foreign material. Infection may occur in the form of vegetation deposition or may be localized to the sewing

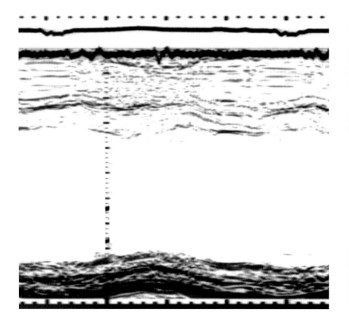
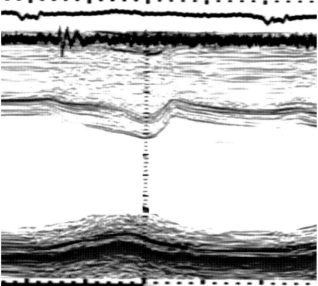

FIGURE 5.5. M-mode recording of left ventricular minor axis from a patient 1 year after valve replacement showing reversed septal movement (left). The same patient 4 years later after developing severe paraprosthetic mitral regurgitation (right). Note the dilatation of the ventricle and the extent of cavity activity.

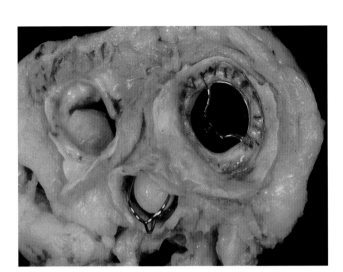

A

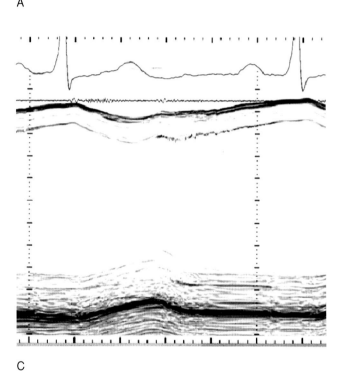

C

FIGURE 5.6. (A) Pathologic section from a patient with a Bjork-Shiley valve in the mitral position, Starr-Edwards in the aortic position, and annuloplasty ring around the tricuspid valve leaflets. (B, C) M-mode recording of left ventricular minor axis from two patients, one with severe mitral regurgitation and the other with severe aortic regurgitation. Note the difference in the pattern of left ventricular filling and increase in dimension. Although it is exclusively early diastolic in mitral regurgitation, it is early and mid diastolic in aortic regurgitation.

B

ring. Infection in the sewing ring is not usually apparent on two-dimensional images, even on transesophageal images. The decision about whether to replace a valve suspected of being infected is therefore usually made on clinical grounds. Persistent clinical evidence for endocarditis justifies valve replacement with a homograft, particularly in the aortic position, to clear up the site of infection.

MANAGEMENT

Aortic valve replacement by any substitute is the common practice for severe aortic valve disease. Although in highly specialized centers homograft banks are available, in others mechanical valves are the ones most commonly used. For severe mitral regurgitation various repair techniques have proved their success in preserving the native valve. Nevertheless, the frequency of replacing a mitral valve with a prosthesis for mitral regurgitation in the United States is much higher than in Europe, 80% versus 50%. With artificial valves regular follow-up is needed. Irrespective of technical expertise a suggested annual follow-up of the valve function and the ventricular function is generally recommended. In patients with valve substitutes who present with acute heart failure, valve dysfunction should be considered the first differential diagnosis until proved otherwise. When clinical diagnosis of endocarditis is made, the artificial valve is the first to be

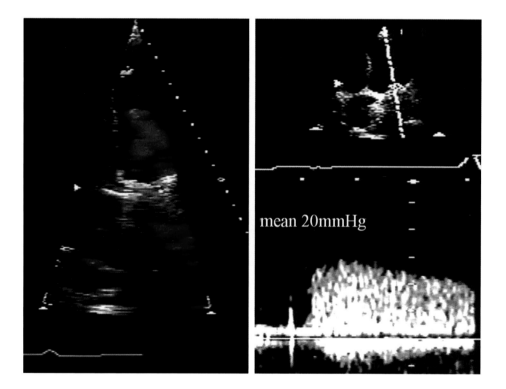

FIGURE 5.7. Continuous-wave Doppler of transmechanical aortic valve velocities 5 years after surgery, when the patient developed signs of heart failure and a pressure drop of 70 mmHg. Note the loud systolic murmur on the phonocardiogram.

m/s

mean 20mmHg

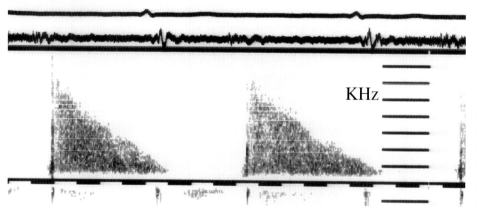

KHz

FIGURE 5.8. Continuous-wave Doppler of transmechanical mitral valve Starr-Edwards prosthesis from a patient showing severe stenosis (top) compared to another with normally functioning valve (bottom). Note the normal steep drop in transvalvular filling velocities.

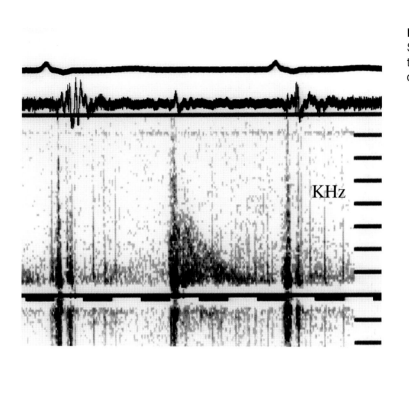

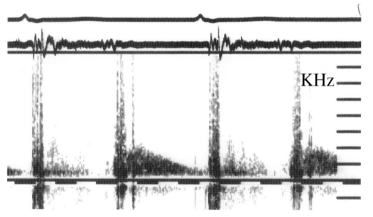

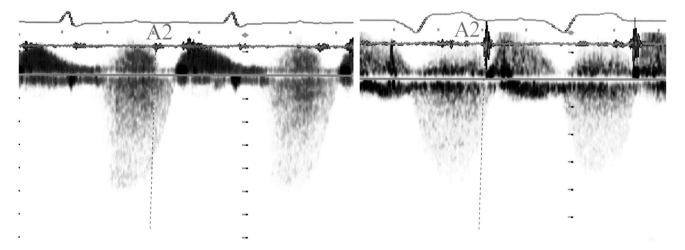

FIGURE 5.10. Continuous-wave Doppler demonstrating paraprosthetic mitral regurgitation from two patients, mild functional (left) and severe (right). Note the early ending of the regurgitation trace with respect to A2 in the patient with severe incompetence.

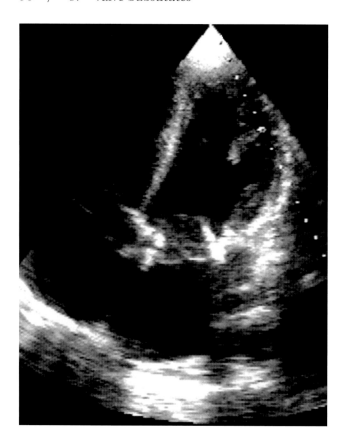

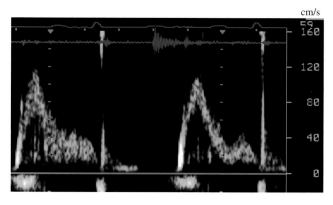

FIGURE 5.11. Apical four-chamber view from a patient with top hat procedure (pulmonary autograft in the mitral position). Note the normal transvalvar flow pattern and continuous-wave velocities.

FIGURE 5.12. Apical four-chamber view from a patient with porcine mitral valve, showing large vegetation attached to the valve.

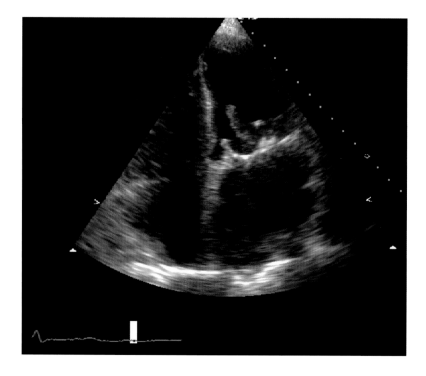

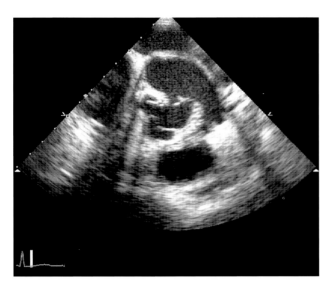
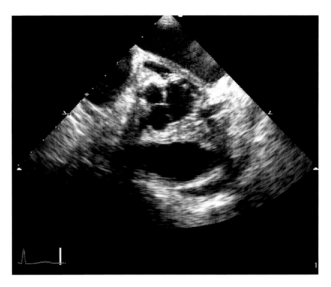

A   B

FIGURE 5.13. Transesophageal echo from a patient with clinical evidence for bacterial endocarditis showing an area of dehiscence between the mitral valve prosthesis and aortic root in systole (A) and diastole (B).

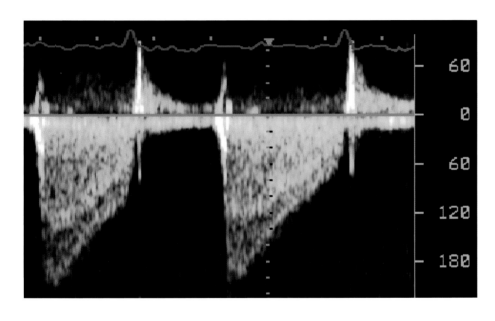

FIGURE 5.14. Transesophageal echo from a patient with Starr-Edwards mitral valve prosthesis showing double envelope continuous-wave velocity display consistent with partial valve narrowing.

blamed unless clear evidence for infection of another valve is provided.

REFERENCES

1. Harken DE, Soroff HS, Taylor WJ. Partial and complete prosthesis in aortic insufficiency. *J Thorac Cardiovasc Surg* 1960;40:744–762.
2. Beaudet RL, Poirier NL, Guerraty AJ, et al. Fifty-four months' experience with an improved tilting disk valve (Medtronic-Hall). *Thorac Cardiovasc Surg* 1983;31(Spec 2):89–93.
3. Bjork VO, Holmgren A, Olin C, et al. Clinical and haemodynamic results of aortic valve replacement with the Bjork-Shiley tilting disc valve prosthesis. *Scand J Thorac Cardiovasc Surg* 1971;5:177–191.
4. Nicoloff DM, Emery RW, Arom KV, et al. Clinical and hemodynamic results with the St. Jude Medical cardiac valve prosthesis. A three-year experience. *J Thorac Cardiovasc Surg* 1981;82:674–683.
5. Simon EB, Kotler MN, Segal BL, et al. Clinical significance of multiple systolic clicks from Starr-Edwards prosthetic aortic valves. *Br Heart J* 1977;39:645–650.
6. Cooper DM, Stewart WJ, Schiavone WA, et al. Evaluation of normal prosthetic valve function by Doppler echocardiography. *Am Heart J* 1987;114:576–582.
7. Fawzy ME, Halim M, Ziady G, et al. Hemodynamic evaluation of porcine bioprostheses in the mitral position by Doppler echocardiography. *Am J Cardiol* 1987;59:643–646.
8. Hoffmann A, Weiss P, Dubach P, et al. Progressive functional deterioration of bioprostheses assessed by Doppler ultrasonography. *Chest* 1990;98:1165–1168.

9. Ryan T, Armstrong WF, Dillon JC, et al. Doppler echocardiographic evaluation of patients with porcine mitral valves. *Am Heart J* 1986;111:237–244.

10. Mehlman DJ. A guide to the radiographic identification of prosthetic heart valves: an addendum. *Circulation* 1984;69: 102–105.

11. Kotler MN, Mintz GS, Panidis I, et al. Noninvasive evaluation of normal and abnormal prosthetic valve function. *J Am Coll Cardiol* 1983;2:151–173.

12. Nanda NC, Cooper JW, Mahan EF III, et al. Echocardiographic assessment of prosthetic valves. *Circulation* 1991;84(3 Suppl):I228–I239.

13. Kapur KK, Fan P, Nanda NC, et al. Doppler color flow mapping in the evaluation of prosthetic mitral and aortic valve function. *J Am Coll Cardiol* 1989;13:1561–1571.

14. Sprecher DL, Adamick R, Adams D, et al. In vitro color flow, pulsed and continuous wave Doppler ultrasound masking of flow by prosthetic valves. *J Am Coll Cardiol* 1987;9:1306–1310.

15. Zoni A, Botti G, Morozzi L. Color Doppler imaging in mitral prostheses: normal flow pattern of Bjork-Shiley valve. *Am J Noninvas Cardiol* 1989;3:261–264.

16. Hixson CS, Smith MD, Mattson MD, et al. Comparison of transesophageal color flow Doppler imaging of normal mitral regurgitant jets in St. Jude Medical and Medtronic Hall cardiac prostheses. *J Am Soc Echocardiogr* 1992;5:57–62.

17. Khandheria BK, Seward JB, Oh JK, et al. Value and limitations of transesophageal echocardiography in assessment of mitral valve prostheses. *Circulation* 1991;83:1956–1968.

18. Nellessen U, Schnittger I, Appleton CP, et al. Transesophageal two-dimensional echocardiography and color Doppler flow velocity mapping in the evaluation of cardiac valve prostheses. *Circulation* 1988;78:848–855.

19. Taams MA, Gussenhoven EJ, Cahalan MK, et al. Transesophageal Doppler color flow imaging in the detection of native and Bjork-Shiley mitral valve regurgitation. *J Am Coll Cardiol* 1989;13:95–99.

20. Feldman HJ, Gray RJ, Chaux A, et al. Noninvasive in vivo and in vitro study of the St. Jude mitral valve prosthesis. Evaluation using two dimensional and M mode echocardiography, phonocardiography and cinefluoroscopy. *Am J Cardiol* 1982;49:11101–11109.

21. Burstow DJ, Nishimura RA, Bailey KR, et al. Continuous wave Doppler echocardiographic measurement of prosthetic valve gradients. A simultaneous Doppler-catheter correlative study. *Circulation* 1989;80:504–514.

22. Reisner SA, Meltzer RS. Normal values of prosthetic valve Doppler echocardiographic parameters: a review. *J Am Soc Echocardiogr* 1988;1:201–210.

23. Marti V, Carreras F, Borras X, et al. Doppler echocardiographic findings in normal-functioning St. Jude Medical and Bjork-Shiley mechanical prostheses in the tricuspid valve position. *Am J Cardiol* 1991;67:307–309.

24. Chen YT, Kan MN, Chen JS, et al. Detection of prosthetic mitral valve leak: a comparative study using transesophageal echocardiography, transthoracic echocardiography, and auscultation. *J Clin Ultrasound* 1990;18:557–561.

25. Flachskampf FA, O'Shea JP, Griffin BP, et al. Patterns of normal transvalvular regurgitation in mechanical valve prostheses. *J Am Coll Cardiol* 1991;18:1493–1498.

6 Endocarditis

Endocarditis is an infectious process that particularly affects the heart valves. It is most commonly caused by bacterial infection or, more rarely, by fungi. Endocarditis of the left-sided valve is more common than that of the right, which is mainly seen in intravenous drug users.

The differential diagnosis of infective endocarditis is that of patients presenting with long-standing fever that is of unclear etiology and that may be resistant to antibiotics. Prolonged fever with a prior history of heart valve disease raises the possibility of endocarditis until otherwise proved. Clinical signs of endocarditis (e.g., splinter hemorrhages) strongly support the suspicion of left-sided valve infection and formation of "vegetations." Vegetations are the most commonly seen echocardiogarphic evidence of infective endocarditis.[1,2] Echocardiography is the ideal imaging investigation to confirm the diagnosis of vegetation on the valves. However, very small vegetations less than 3 mm in diameter may be missed on a routine transthoracic echocardiographic study.[3] This limits the sensitivity of the technique to 80% for detecting evidence for valve infections.[4,5] In the presence of strong clinical suspicion of endocarditis and inconclusive transthoracic echo images, transesophageal examination is always recommended, particularly in patients with prosthetic valves. In patients with suspected aortic root infection who present with a long PR interval or acute heart block, transesophageal echo has a sensitivity of 90% for confirming the diagnosis of infective endocarditis.[6,7]

In addition to its diagnostic value, echocardiography also assesses the degree of valve dysfunction that results from the infection. This is mainly in the form of incompetence[8,9] and may have important implications on the clinical outcome. A vegetation of more than 10 mm caused by *Staphylococcus aureus* infection carries significant morbidity and mortality with respect to other infections.[9,10] Patients with no vegetations and not more than mild mitral or aortic regurgitation have a low risk.[9]

MITRAL VALVE ENDOCARDITIS

The echocardiographic presentation of mitral valve infection varies. Irregularly thickened leaflets, particularly on the atrial side, may represent a mild degree of leaflet infection.[11] The presence of extensive mitral apparatus calcification significantly reduces the sensitivity of echocardiographic images in diagnosing valve infection. Large vegetations on the mitral valve may make the leaflets flail and may result in significant regurgitation.[12,13] Differentiation of mitral valve vegetations from myxomatous degeneration may be difficult. Mitral valve endocarditis may present in the form of leaflet perforation, resulting in variable degrees of mitral regurgitation.

Suspected prosthetic mitral valve infection should be carefully assessed by the transesophageal approach. Even the absence of clear vegetation does not exclude the diagnosis of infective endocarditis, particularly when there is a strong clinical evidence. In these cases the infection may be confined only to the prosthesis sewing ring. This carries the risk of acute dehiscence and severe mitral regurgitation that requires emergency surgery.

AORTIC VALVE ENDOCARDITIS

Like mitral endocarditis, thickened aortic valve leaflets in the presence of calcification may complicate the image and make confirmation of a diagnosis difficult.[14,15] However, a sizable vegetation that makes one of the aortic valve leaflets flail and fail to coapt with the other leaflets causing significant aortic regurgitation confirms the diagnosis. The sensitivity of aortic regurgitation can be assessed by color Doppler and the activity of the left ventricular shortening. Premature mitral valve closure suggests severe acute aortic regurgitation secondary to endocarditis. This condition usually requires emergency surgical intervention.[16]

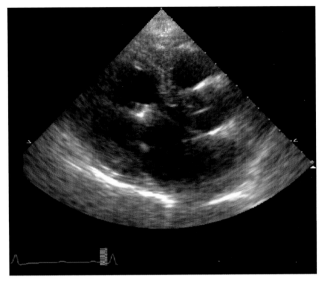

A

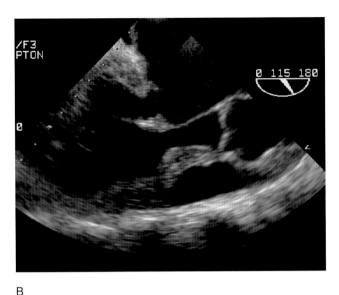

B

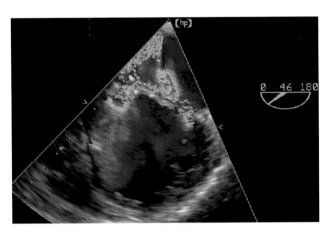

C

FIGURE 6.1. (A) Parasternal long-axis view of the mitral valve from a patient with infective endocarditis showing a large vegetation attached to the anterior mitral leaflet. (B) Transesophageal echo from a patient with vegetation attached to anterior leaflet. (C) Transesophageal echo showing anterior leaflet perforation complicating endocarditis.

Infection of the aortic valve may extend to involve the aortic root and to cause abscess formation. This is most commonly associated with staphylococcal infection. Aortic root infection may be localized to one segment or become generalized around the root in the form of multiple small compartments that are either separated or connected.[17] Diagnosis of such a condition is best made from the parasternal short-axis view of the aortic root on either transthoracic or transesophageal images. A cavity attached to the aortic root that changes size and shape during the different phases of the cardiac cycle suggests an abscess formation that is in direct continuity with the root. Continuous systolic and diastolic flow through the cavity raises the possibility of fistula formation. The commonest location of the fistula is between the left ventricular outflow tract and the left atrium.[18,19]

Aortic valve and root infection may spread to the nearby structures, in particular the mitral valve, resulting in infected anterior leaflet (jet lesion).[20] When found on careful echocardiographic examination, it suggests a pos-

sible need for surgical repair of the mitral valve at the time of aortic valve and root surgery. Although careful aortic root examination by transthoracic approach is informative, transesophageal images may provide more precise details that may have important surgical implications.

Patients with a recurrent infection of and around an aortic prosthetic valve should receive a complete clearance of the root and insertion of a homograft in order to eradicate the infection.

RIGHT HEART ENDOCARDITIS

Endocarditis involving the right heart is much rarer than that involving the left heart.[21] The commonest cause of right heart infection is the presence of pacemaker wires, right heart catheters, or intravenous drug injection.[22] Vegetations affecting the tricuspid valves may be larger than those affecting the left heart valves. This is possibly because of the difference in the valve size (area) and

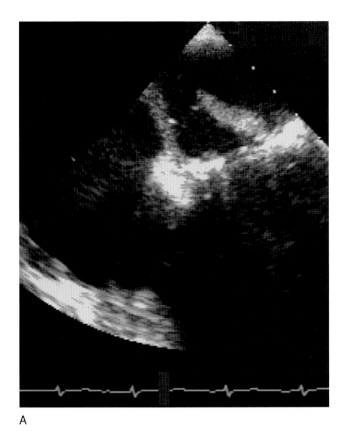

A

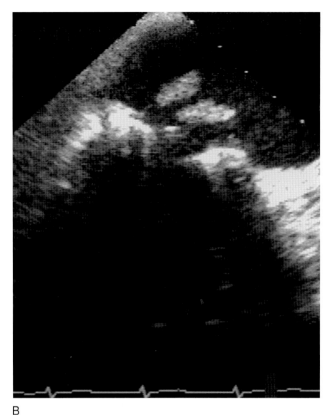

B

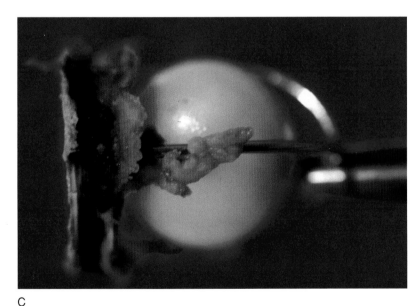

C

FIGURE 6.2. (A, B) Transesophageal echo from a patient with infected prosthetic mitral valve showing a large vegetation on the atrial side of the valve attached to the ring. (C) Starr-Edwards mitral valve with vegetation and clot attached to the strut.

chamber pressure.[23,24] While left-sided symptoms and signs are systemic, those associated with a right side infection are mainly respiratory (e.g., dry cough, pleurisy, pulmonary embolism).[25] Patients with right-sided infection tend to respond well to antibiotics. Therefore the need for valve replacement or surgical repair is usually much less than with the left-sided infection.[24] Transthoracic echocardiography is quite appropriate in confirming tricuspid valve vegetations, particularly with the use of

modified apical views. Transesophageal imaging may add to the accuracy of the echo diagnosis, in particular in patients with right-sided leads or catheters.

Pulmonary valve infection is very rare[26] and usually only occurs in the presence of congenital pulmonary valve disease as a substrate for infection. When present, the infection may be associated with some degree of pulmonary regurgitation that can be accurately assessed from parasternal transthoracic views as well as transesophageal ones.

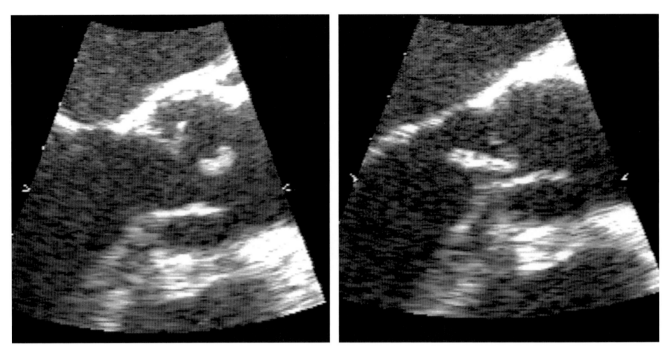

FIGURE 6.3. Transesophageal echo from a patient with infective endocarditis affecting the aortic valve. Note the large vegetation attached to the left coronary cusp, prolapsing into the left ventricular outflow tract in diastole.

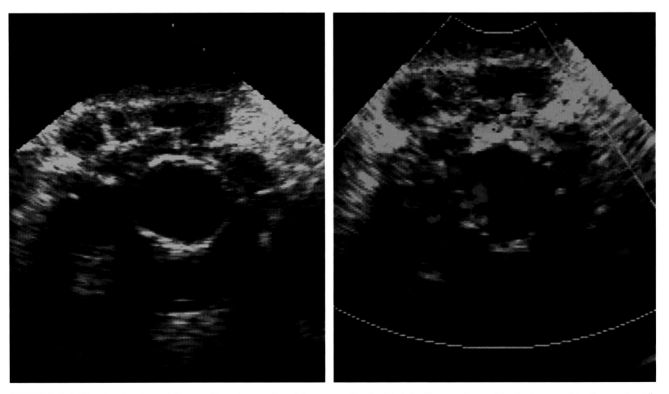

FIGURE 6.4. Short-axis view of the aortic valve and root from a patient with infective endocarditis that spread to the root wall. Note the 1-cm thickness of the aortic root wall and the multiple small cavities around the root with blood flow inside.

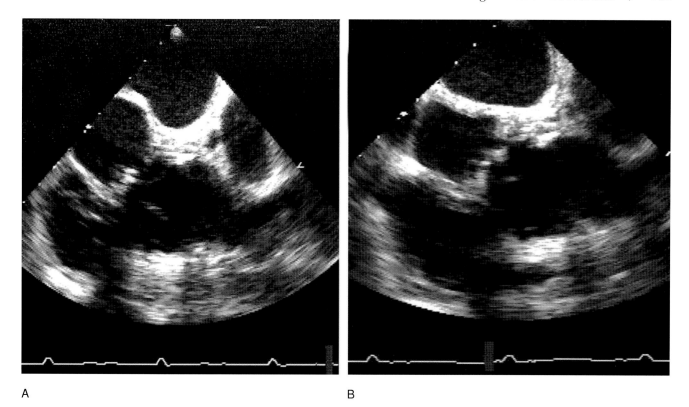

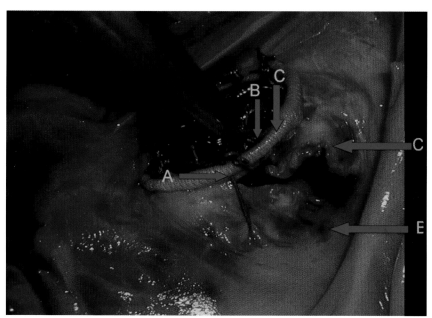

FIGURE 6.5. (A, B) Transesophageal echo from a patient with aortic root abscess in the form of a cavity adjacent to the sinuses that changes shape during different phases of the cardiac cycle. (C) Abscess cavity around a xenograft. (arrows)

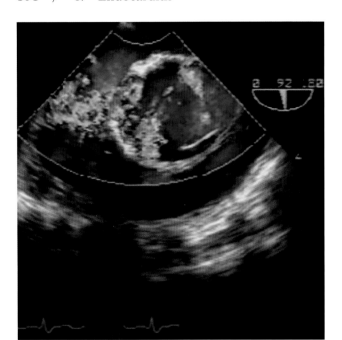

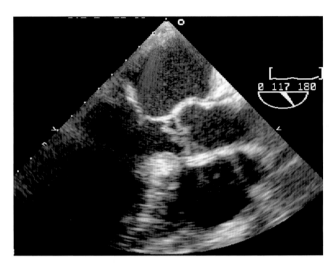

FIGURE 6.7. Transesophageal views of the aortic valve and root showing vegetations attached to the leaflets.

FIGURE 6.6. Transesophageal images of the aortic root from a patient with endocarditis showing a fistula formation between the aortic root and the right atrium.

Finally, endocarditis may affect other congenital heart lesions. The most commonly seen in adults other than valves is the ventricular septal defect. When present, vegetations are usually seen at the low-pressure side of the shunt.

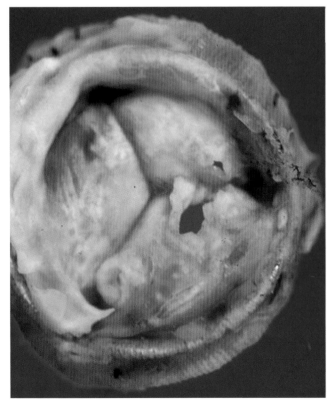

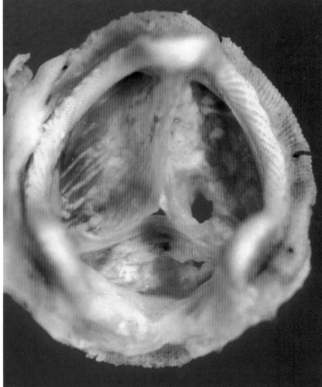

FIGURE 6.8. Pathologic picture of a xenograft from the aortic position demonstrating a tear in one of the leaflets caused by infective endocarditis.

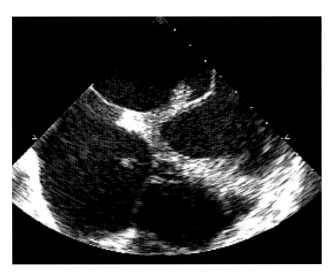

FIGURE 6.9. A four-chamber view from a patient with infective endocarditis involving the mitral and tricuspid valve.

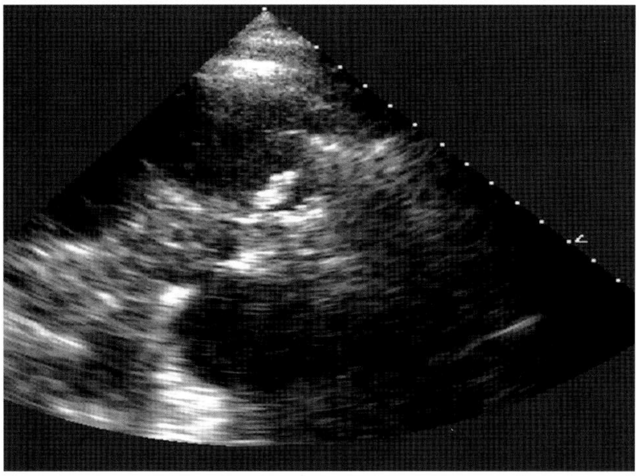

FIGURE 6.10. Short-axis view of the aortic valve showing a small mass (vegetation attached to the pulmonary valve leaflet and moving freely with it).

REFERENCES

1. Mintz GS, Kotler MN, Segal BL, et al. Comparison of two-dimensional and M-mode echocardiography in the evaluation of patients with infective endocarditis. *Am J Cardiol* 1979; 43:738–744.
2. Wann LS, Hallam CC, Dillon JC, et al. Comparison of M-mode and cross-sectional echocardiography in infective endocarditis. *Circulation* 1979;60:728–733.
3. Mintz GS, Kotler MN. Clinical value and limitations of echocardiography. Its use in the study of patients with infectious endocarditis. *Arch Intern Med* 1980;140:1022–1027.
4. Ellis SG, Goldstein J, Popp RL. Detection of endocarditis-associated perivalvular abscesses by two-dimensional echocardiography. *J Am Coll Cardiol* 1985;5:647–653.
5. Martin RP, Meltzer RS, Chia BL, et al. Clinical utility of two dimensional echocardiography in infective endocarditis. *Am J Cardiol* 1980;46:379–385.
6. Daniel WG, Mugge A, Martin RP, et al. Improvement in the diagnosis of abscesses associated with endocarditis by transesophageal echocardiography. *N Engl J Med* 1991;324: 795–800.
7. Mugge A, Daniel WG, Frank G, et al. Echocardiography in infective endocarditis: reassessment of prognostic implications of vegetation size determined by the transthoracic and the transesophageal approach. *J Am Coll Cardiol* 1989;14: 631–638.
8. Buda AJ, Zotz RJ, Gallagher KP. Characterization of the functional border zone around regionally ischemic myocardium using circumferential flow-function maps. *J Am Coll Cardiol* 1986;8:150–158.
9. Jaffe WM, Morgan DE, Pearlman AS, et al. Infective endocarditis, 1983–1988: echocardiographic findings and factors influencing morbidity and mortality. *J Am Coll Cardiol* 1990; 15:1227–1233.
10. Steckelberg JM, Murphy JG, Ballard D, et al. Emboli in infective endocarditis: the prognostic value of echocardiography. *Ann Intern Med* 1991;114:635–640.
11. Boucher CA, Fallon JT, Myers GS, et al. The value and limitations of echocardiography in recording mitral valve vegetations. *Am Heart J* 1977;94:37–43.
12. Chandraratna PA, Langevin E. Limitations of the echocardiogram in diagnosing valvular vegetations in patients with mitral valve prolapse. *Circulation* 1977;56:436–438.
13. Kunis RL, Sherrid MV, Mccabe JB, et al. Successful medical therapy of mitral anular abscess complicating infective endocarditis. *J Am Coll Cardiol* 1986;7:953–955.
14. Mintz GS, Kotler MN, Segal BL, et al. Survival of patients with aortic valve endocarditis. The prognostic implications of the echocardiogram. *Arch Intern Med* 1979;139:862–866.
15. Hirschfeld DS, Schiller N. Localization of aortic valve vegetations by echocardiography. *Circulation* 1976;53: 280–285.
16. Fox S, Kotler MN, Segal BL, et al. Echocardiographic diagnosis of acute aortic valve endocarditis and its complications. *Arch Intern Med* 1977;137:85–89.
17. Pollak SJ, Felner JM. Echocardiographic identification of an aortic valve ring abscess. *J Am Coll Cardiol* 1986;7: 1167–1173.
18. Karalis DG, Bansal RC, Hauck AJ, et al. Transesophageal echocardiographic recognition of subaortic complications in aortic valve endocarditis. Clinical and surgical implications. *Circulation* 1992;86:353–362.
19. Saner HE, Asinger RW, Homans DC, et al. Two-dimensional echocardiographic identification of complicated aortic root endocarditis: implications for surgery. *J Am Coll Cardiol* 1987;10:859–868.
20. Kim JH, Wiseman A, Kisslo J, et al. Echocardiographic detection and clinical significance of left atrial vegetations in active infective endocarditis. *Am J Cardiol* 1989;64:950–952.
21. Panidis IP, Kotler MN, Mintz GS, et al. Right heart endocarditis: clinical and echocardiographic features. *Am Heart J* 1984;107:759–764.
22. Cassling RS, Rogler WC, Mcmanus BM. Isolated pulmonic valve infective endocarditis: a diagnostically elusive entity. *Am Heart J* 1985;109(Pt 1):558–567.

23. Berger M, Delfin LA, Jelveh M, et al. Two-dimensional echocardiographic findings in right-sided infective endocarditis. *Circulation* 1980;61:855–861.

24. Nakamura K, Satomi G, Sakai T, et al. Clinical and echocardiographic features of pulmonary valve endocarditis. *Circulation* 1983;67:198–204.

25. Panidis IP, Kotler MN, Mintz GS, et al. Clinical and echocardiographic correlations in right heart endocarditis. *Int J Cardiol* 1984;6:17–34.

26. Shapiro SM, Young E, Ginzton LE, et al. Pulmonic valve endocarditis as an underdiagnosed disease: role of transesophageal echocardiography. *J Am Soc Echocardiogr* 1992; 5:48–51.

Pulmonary Hypertension

Pulmonary hypertension describes raised pulmonary circulatory pressure, venous or arterial.

Pulmonary venous hypertension is caused by increased left atrial pressure due to left heart disease[1,2]:

1. Mitral valve disease stenosis or regurgitation.[3,4]

2. Aortic valve disease, stenosis, or regurgitation, particularly in the presence of left ventricular disease.[5]

3. Severe left ventricular disease due to an incompliant cavity, irrespective of its size or systolic function. Ventricular disease can be either idiopathic or secondary to coronary artery disease, systemic hypertension, valvular disease, or infiltrative myocardial disease.[6,7]

4. Incompliant left atrium. Long-standing raised left atrial pressure may result in increased wall stress, atrial dilatation, and loss of systolic function. In this case the atrium behaves as a conduit for blood to pass through, from the pulmonary veins to the left ventricle, in early diastole.[8,9]

PATHOPHYSIOLOGY

Increased left atrial pressure either due to volume or pressure overload will eventually affect passive and active atrial function. The raised atrial pressure will propagate retrogradely to the pulmonary venous system, resulting in pulmonary hypertension.[10,11] Atrial contraction in late diastole against a stenosed mitral valve or raised left ventricular end-diastolic pressure will accentuate the reversed flow into the pulmonary veins. With severe ventricular disease, the long axis of the ventricle loses its systolic function and the ventricle becomes more spherical. Atrial longitudinal function also becomes very limited; consequently, the systolic component of the pulmonary venous flow is compromised.[12,13] Patients with significant mitral regurgitation, whether functional or organic, demonstrate systolic flow reversal in the pulmonary veins caused by mitral regurgitation jet and increased pressure in the left atrium during systole.[14]

Pulmonary Arterial Hypertension

Pulmonary arterial hypertension is caused by

1. *Raised pulmonary venous pressure* that is reflected on the right heart and the pulmonary circulation. Long-standing high pulmonary venous pressure will result in right ventricular hypertrophy followed by dilatation. Acute or rapidly developing pulmonary hypertension may be associated with completely normal right heart size and function, disproportionate to the degree of symptoms (e.g., acute mitral regurgitation or obstructed mitral prosthesis).

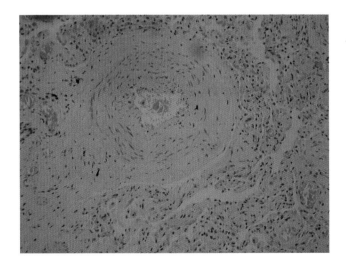

FIGURE 7.1. Histologic section from a patient with primary pulmonary hypertension showing medial hypertrophy of the muscular layer of the pulmonary artery.

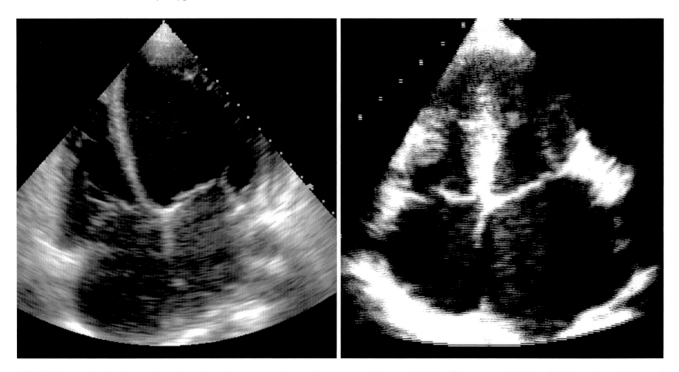

FIGURE 7.2. Apical four-chamber view from a patient with severe left ventricular disease and dilated left atrium (left), and another with restrictive cardiomyopathy, normal size but significantly stiff left ventricle causing left atrial dilatation (right).

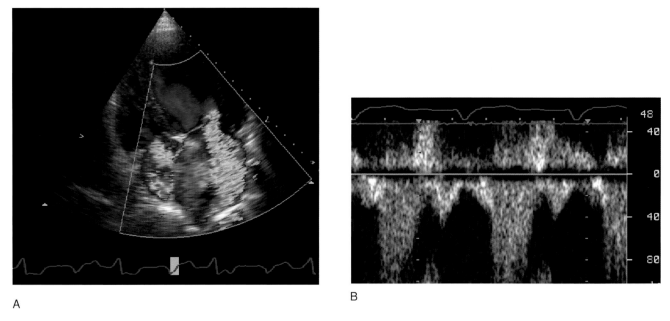

A

B

FIGURE 7.3. (A) Apical four-chamber view from a patient with severe mitral regurgitation. Note the mitral regurgitation jet on color flow Doppler that flushes most of the atrium until the pulmonary veins. (B) the equivalent pulsed-wave Doppler flow of the pulmonary veins demonstrating systolic flow reversal due to mitral regurgitation and late diastolic flow reversal consistent with raised end-diastolic pressure.

2. *Parenchymal pulmonary hypertension*. Although it is not usually the normal course of events, pulmonary hypertension may develop in patients with parenchymal or alveolar lung disease (e.g., systemic sclerosis, fibrosing aveolitis, emphysema). In such patients the left heart may be completely normal, but the pulmonary artery and the right heart may show signs of raised pulmonary pressures, so-called "cor pulmonale."[15]

3. *Idiopathic pulmonary arterial hypertension*. This is the most common cause of pulmonary arterial hyper-

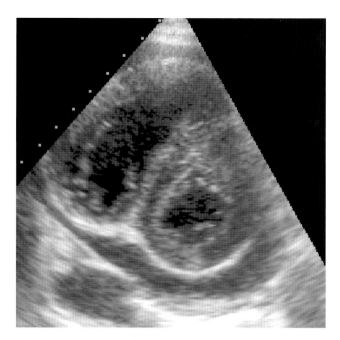

FIGURE 7.4. Short axis view from a patient with systemic sclerosis involving the lung. Notice the normal-sized left ventricle and the disproportionate enlargement of the right ventricle, consistent with pulmonary hypertention.

tension in the absence of left heart disease. Patients may present with unexplained exertional breathlessness that may progress to breathlessness at rest as disease severity worsens. Pulmonary hypertension is generally a slowly progressing disease, and when severe it may affect left heart size and function.

Doppler Echocardiography and Pulmonary Hypertension

Doppler echocardiography is used in assessing the following markers of pulmonary hypertension:

1. ***Peak tricuspid regurgitation pressure drop***: The most reliable marker of pulmonary hypertension in clinical practice is the peak retrograde pressure drop across the tricuspid valve. The higher the pressure drop, the more severe is the pulmonary hypertension. Peak retrograde transtricuspid pressure drop added to right atrial pressure (5–10 mmHg) provides a good noninvasive estimate of pulmonary artery pressure, although it tends to underestimate its absolute value.[16]

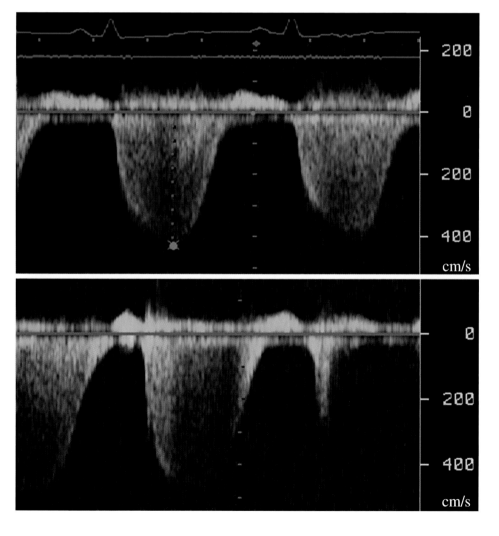

FIGURE 7.5. Continuous-wave Doppler from a patient who developed progressive pulmonary hypertension over 2 years. Note the significant increase of transtricuspid pressure drop from 60 mmHg (top) to 100 mmHg (bottom).

2. ***Delayed onset of right ventricular filling***: In patients with pulmonary hypertension the high retrograde pressure drop across the tricuspid valve (on the continuous-wave Doppler velocity recording) has a long and slow decline rate in early and mid diastole. This causes significant delay in the onset of right ventricular filling with respect to end of ejection (pulmonary component of the second heart sound–P2). The normal delay in the onset of right ventricular filling is up to 80 ms with respect to end ejection or P2.[17] In patients in whom tricuspid regurgitation cannot be detected by continuous-wave Doppler, a delayed onset of right ventricular filling with respect to the second heart sound, wrongly named right ventricular isovolumic relaxation time, can be taken as a surrogate marker for raised pulmonary artery pressure. Delayed onset of right ventricular filling due to incoordinate free-wall relaxation, as seen in coronary artery disease, should not be taken as a sign of pulmonary hypertension.

3. ***Short pulmonary acceleration time***: The increase in pulmonary vascular resistance is reflected in the pattern of the pulmonary valve flow. In a normal subject right ventricular ejection occupies all of systole until the second heart sound. By contrast, in pulmonary hypertension, pulmonary flow is made of two components: a dominant early systolic component with a very short acceleration time followed by a smaller late systolic component. In general, the shorter the acceleration time of the early component, the higher the pulmonary vascular resistance and hence the pulmonary artery pressure.[18,19]

The mid-systolic notch on the pulmonary flow in pulmonary hypertension corresponds to the mid-systolic closure of the pulmonary valve itself. This is caused by the sudden cessation of pulmonary flow in mid systole because of the raised pulmonary vascular resistance.[20,21]

4. ***Pulmonary artery to right ventricular pressure drop***: Most patients with pulmonary hypertension demonstrate some degree of functional pulmonary regurgitation on color Doppler images of the pulmonary valve.

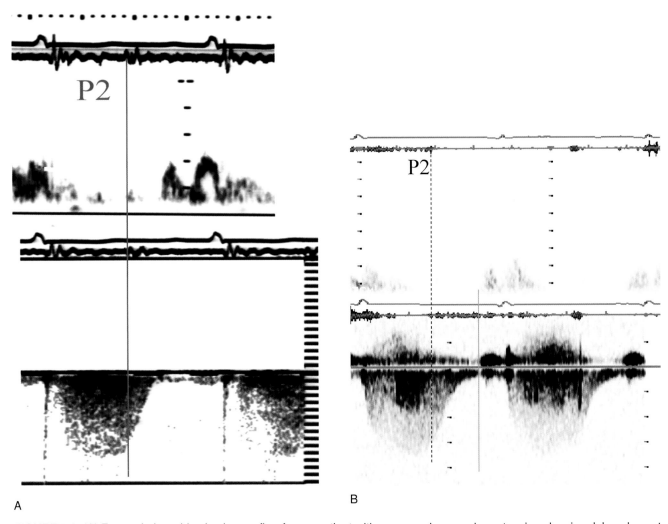

A

B

FIGURE 7.6. (A) Forward tricuspid pulsed-wave flow from a patient with severe pulmonary hypertension showing delayed onset of right ventricular filling due to significantly long tricuspid regurgitation. (B) Similar recordings from a patient with isolated late diastolic right ventricular filling due to long tricuspid regurgitation.

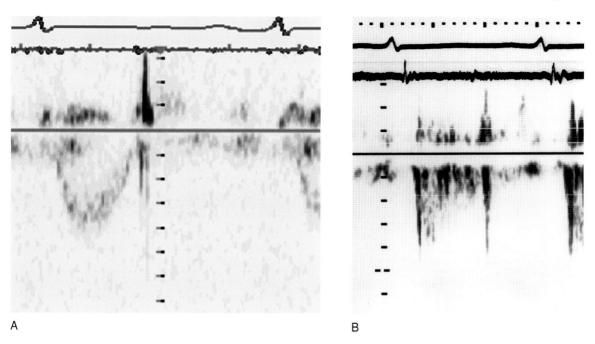

A   B

FIGURE 7.7. Pulmonary forward flow from two patients; normal (left) and pulmonary hypertension (right). Note the short acceleration time in the latter.

The peak early diastolic continuous-wave Doppler pressure drop of the pulmonary regurgitation provides a good estimate of mean pulmonary artery pressure in such patients.

With slowly progressing pulmonary hypertension, all the preceding markers may be present. Rapidly developing pulmonary hypertension (e.g., thromboembolic disease) may only demonstrate raised retrograde pressure drop across the tricuspid valve in the presence of completely normal right heart size and function.

Pulmonary Hypertension and Right Ventricular Function

Right ventricular disease: Severe long-standing pulmonary hypertension eventually affects right ventricular function, which with time becomes significantly impaired. Right ventricular function can objectively be monitored by recording the free-wall long-axis amplitude of movement (normally 25 mm) and velocities by tissue Doppler technique, if available. Assessment of right ventricular function in this way has a strong predictive value for exercise tolerance[22] and clinical outcome in different cardiac conditions.[23] Inability of the right ventricle to generate enough pressure to support right ventricular ejection contributes to the deterioration of patient's clinical condition. Furthermore, the retrograde pressure drop across the tricuspid valve that is usually taken as a measure of pulmonary artery pressure falls because of the right ventricular failure and the increased right atrial pressure. Therefore the retrograde transtricuspid pressure drop should not be taken in isolation as a sole measure of pulmonary artery pressure. With severe right ventricular disease and raised right atrial pressure, patients may develop restrictive right ventricular physiology, which itself adds to the deterioration of the condition and the poor outcome.

Significant tricuspid regurgitation: Severe right ventricular disease represents a late stage in pulmonary hypertension. It is often associated with tricuspid ring dilatation and significant tricuspid regurgitation. This may cause right-sided heart failure and systemic congestion. Tricuspid regurgitation can be assessed by color and continuous-wave Doppler[24] as discussed in Chapter 3.

Pulmonary artery aneurysm: the pulmonary artery can dilate in patients with significant pulmonary hypertension. In most cases, pulmonary artery dilatation is proportional to that of the right ventricle. However, an aneurysm may rarely develop, which adds to the risk of potential rupture.[25]

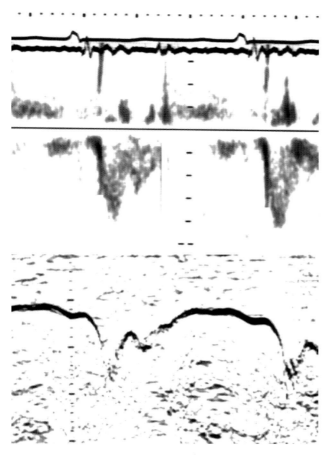

The Effect of Primary Pulmonary Hypertension on the Left Heart

In primary pulmonary hypertension, the right heart is frequently dilated and the left is normal in size. Raised right-sided ventricular pressure results in reversed septal movement, thus making the septum seem to function as part of the right ventricle rather than the left ventricle. This is clearly demonstrated on two-dimensional and M-mode recordings of the left ventricular minor axis from the parasternal long-axis view.[25,26]

With progressive increase in right-sided pressure, the left ventricle becomes increasingly squashed and the septum flat, the so-called D-shaped ventricle. This is a characteristic echocardiographic feature of pulmonary hypertension.

The reversed septal movement in systole is followed by a septal bounce toward the left ventricular cavity in

FIGURE 7.8. Pulmonary flow and pulmonary valve M-mode from a patient with pulmonary hypertension showing mid-systolic valve closure and cessation of flow.

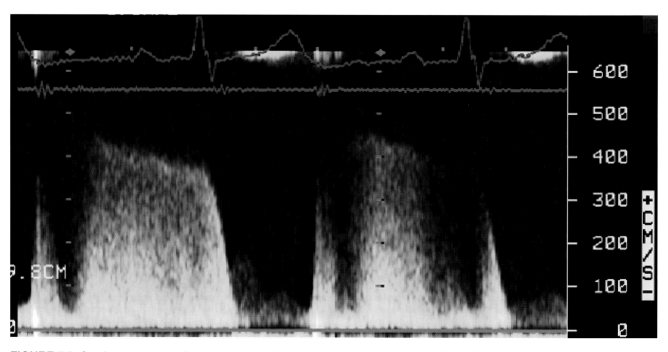

FIGURE 7.9. Continuous-wave pulmonary regurgitation Doppler velocities from a patient with pulmonary hypertension showing a peak early diastolic value of 80 mmHg.

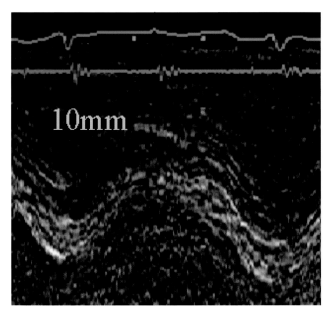
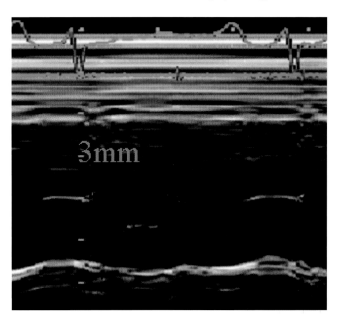

FIGURE 7.10. Right ventricular long-axis function from a patient with pulmonary hypertension before (left) and after (right) development of right ventricular disease. Note the significant drop in right ventricular free-wall amplitude of movement over time.

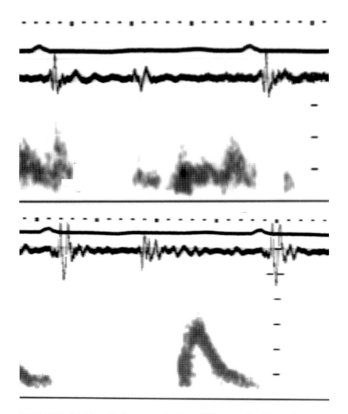

FIGURE 7.11. Right ventricular filling velocities from a patient with pulmonary hypertension while the right ventricular function was maintained (top) showing delayed filling and after it deteriorated (bottom) showing restrictive filling pattern consistent with raised right atrial pressure.

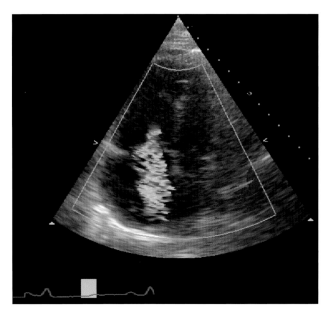

FIGURE 7.12. A four-chamber view from a patient with severe pulmonary hypertension who developed right ventricular failure, dilatation of the tricuspid valve ring, and severe tricuspid regurgitation on color Doppler. Note the extent of regurgitation, to the rear of the right atrium.

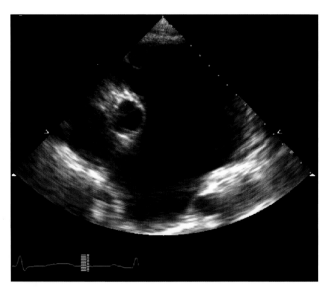

FIGURE 7.13. Parasternal short-axis view from a patient with pulmonary hypertension and aneurysmal pulmonary artery that involves the left branch. Note the diameter of the main pulmonary artery is 8 cm.

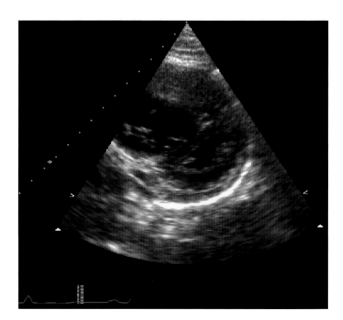

FIGURE 7.15. Parasternal short-axis view of the left ventricle from a patient with pulmonary hypertension showing D-shaped cavity and dilated right ventricle.

early diastole. This is caused by the relative increase in right ventricular early diastolic pressure being greater than that of the left ventricle. The inward movement of the septum in early diastole reduces left ventricular minor axis and compromises early left ventricular filling which consequently becomes predominantly late diastolic.

With severe pulmonary hypertension, the left ventricular shape becomes a deformed "banana shape." Consequently, the filling of the left ventricle becomes exclusively late diastolic.

Patients with pulmonary hypertension and long-standing systemic hypertension frequently develop left

ventricular hypertrophy. The contribution of deformation of septal function and the left ventricular hypertrophy in these patients may cause left ventricular outflow tract obstruction, systolic anterior movement of the mitral valve, and high-pressure drop (gradient) across the outflow tract with fast heart rate. This is usually associ-

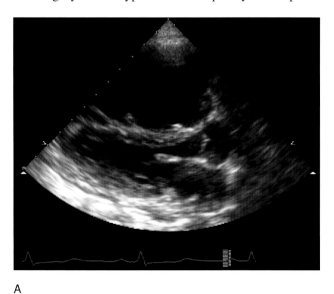

A

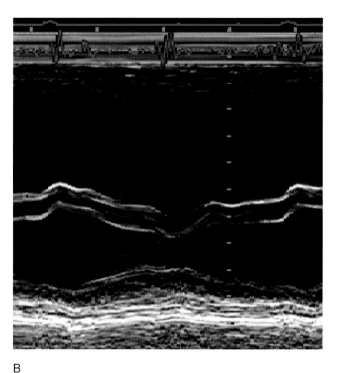

B

FIGURE 7.14. Two dimensional images and M-mode recordings of left and right ventricular cavities from a patient with advanced pulmonary hypertension demonstrating large right ventricle and abnormal septal movement.

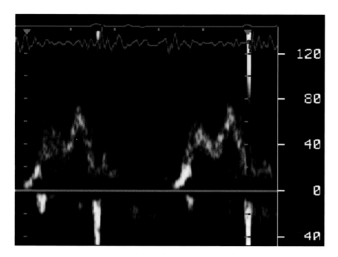

FIGURE 7.16. Left ventricular filling velocities from a patient with pulmonary hypertension showing a dominant A wave. Notice the suppressed early diastolic filling.

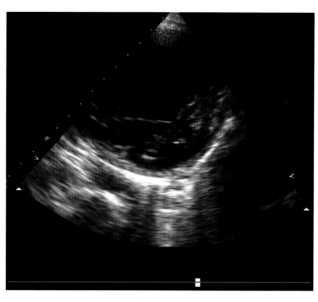

FIGURE 7.17. Parasternal short-axis view from a patient with advanced pulmonary hypertension showing banana-shaped left ventricular cavity and large right ventricular cavity.

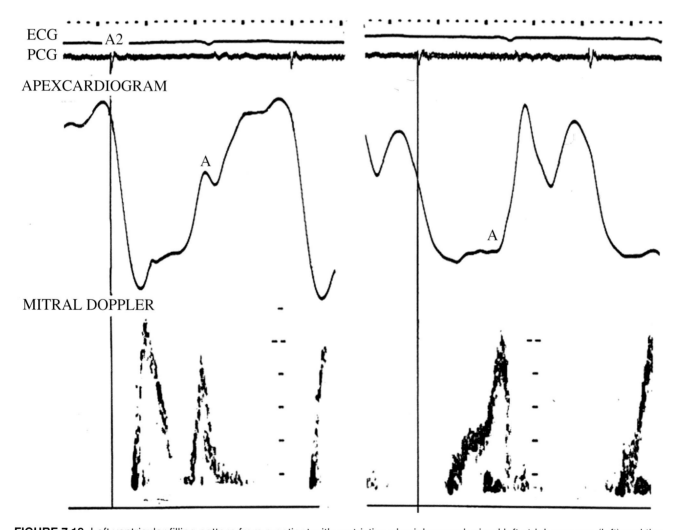

FIGURE 7.18. Left ventricular filling pattern from a patient with restrictive physiology and raised left atrial pressure (left) and the patient 3 weeks after commencing angiotensin-converting enzyme inhibitors (right). Note the significant change in left ventricular physiology from the restrictive to the late diastolic filling pattern that resulted in significant drop in retrograde tricuspid valve pressure drop and improvement of symptoms.

ated with a drop in systolic blood pressure and presyncopal attacks.

MANAGEMENT

Pulmonary venous hypertension due to left-sided organic valvular heart disease is eminently treatable by correcting the underlying anatomic abnormality. Raised left atrial pressure due to severe left ventricular disease may respond to angiotensin-converting enzyme inhibitors; consequently, the secondary pulmonary hypertension may regress.[27] Patients with an incompliant left atrium may be symptomatically controlled by diuretics, although a mild degree of mitral regurgitation may increase left atrial pressure and cause significantly limiting symptoms.

Vasodilators in patients with primary pulmonary hypertension are given routinely.[28] However, the evidence behind their effect on symptoms and functional improvement remains controversial. Patients with concurrent left ventricular hypertrophy who develop signs of outflow tract obstruction with stress may have worsening symptoms with vasodilators because of the accentuated pressure gradient across the outflow tract. In them, a small dose of beta blocker, with appropriate monitoring, may control the heart rate and the outflow tract obstruction, and may improve symptoms.

REFERENCES

1. Hofmann T, Keck A, van Ingen G, et al. Simultaneous measurement of pulmonary venous flow by intravascular catheter Doppler velocimetry and transesophageal Doppler echocardiography: relation to left atrial pressure and left atrial and left ventricular function. *J Am Coll Cardiol* 1995;26:239–249.
2. Mahmud E, Raisinghani A, Hassankhani A, et al. Correlation of left ventricular diastolic filling characteristics with right ventricular overload and pulmonary artery pressure in chronic thromboembolic pulmonary hypertension. *J Am Coll Cardiol* 2002;40:318–324.
3. Sajja LR, Mannam GC. Role of closed mitral commissurotomy in mitral stenosis with severe pulmonary hypertension. *J Heart Valve Dis* 2001;10:288–293.
4. Vincens JJ, Temizer D, Post JR, et al. Long-term outcome of cardiac surgery in patients with mitral stenosis and severe pulmonary hypertension. *Circulation* 1995;92(9 Suppl):II137–II142.
5. Snopek G, Pogorzelska H, Zielinski T, et al. Valve replacement for aortic stenosis with severe congestive heart failure and pulmonary hypertension. *J Heart Valve Dis* 1996;5: 268–272.
6. Lanzarini L, Fontana A, Lucca E, et al. Noninvasive estimation of both systolic and diastolic pulmonary artery pressure from Doppler analysis of tricuspid regurgitant velocity spectrum in patients with chronic heart failure. *Am Heart J* 2002; 144:1087–1094.
7. Spinelli L, Petretta M, Vicario ML, et al. Losartan treatment and left ventricular filling during volume loading in patients with dilated cardiomyopathy. *Am Heart J* 2002;143:433–440.
8. Ko YG, Ha JW, Chung N, et al. Effects of left atrial compliance on left atrial pressure in pure mitral stenosis. *Catheter Cardiovasc Interv* 2001;52:328–333.
9. Schwammenthal E, Vered Z, Agranat O, et al. Impact of atrioventricular compliance on pulmonary artery pressure in mitral stenosis: an exercise echocardiographic study. *Circulation* 2000;102:2378–2384.
10. Nishimura RA, Abel MD, Hatle LK, et al. Relation of pulmonary vein to mitral flow velocities by transesophageal Doppler echocardiography. Effect of different loading conditions. *Circulation* 1990;81:1488–1497.
11. Rossvoll O, Hatle LK. Pulmonary venous flow velocities recorded by transthoracic Doppler ultrasound: relation to left ventricular diastolic pressures. *J Am Coll Cardiol* 1993;21: 1687–1696.
12. Eren M, Bolca O, Dagdeviren B, et al. The determinants of systolic pulmonary venous flow reversal by transthoracic pulsed Doppler in mitral regurgitation: its value in determining the severity of regurgitation. *Acta Cardiol* 2001;56:83–89.
13. Barbier P, Solomon S, Schiller NB, et al. Determinants of forward pulmonary vein flow: an open pericardium pig model. *J Am Coll Cardiol* 2000;35:1947–1959.
14. Yang H, Jones M, Shiota T, et al. Pulmonary venous flow determinants of left atrial pressure under different loading conditions in a chronic animal model with mitral regurgitation. *J Am Soc Echocardiogr* 2002;15(10 Pt 2):1181–1188.
15. Kawut SM, Taichman DB, Archer-Chicko CL, et al. Hemodynamics and survival in patients with pulmonary arterial hypertension related to systemic sclerosis. *Chest* 2003; 123:344–350.
16. Yock PG, Popp RL. Noninvasive estimation of right ventricular systolic pressure by Doppler ultrasound in patients with tricuspid regurgitation. *Circulation* 1984;70:657–662.
17. Yu CM, Sanderson JE, Chan S, et al. Right ventricular diastolic dysfunction in heart failure. *Circulation* 1996;93: 1509–1514.
18. Shivkumar K, Ravi K, Henry JW, et al. Right ventricular dilatation, right ventricular wall thickening, and Doppler evidence of pulmonary hypertension in patients with a pure restrictive ventilatory impairment. *Chest* 1994;106: 1649–1653.
19. van Dijk AP, Hopman JC, Klaessens JH, et al. Is noninvasive determination of pulmonary artery pressure feasible using deceleration phase Doppler flow velocity characteristics in mechanically ventilated children with congenital heart disease? *Am J Cardiol* 1996;78:1394–1399.
20. Lew W, Karliner JS. Assessment of pulmonary valve echogram in normal subjects and in patients with pulmonary arterial hypertension. *Br Heart J* 1979;42:147–161.
21. Scarpini S, Brambilla R, Mazza P, et al. [Specificity and sensitivity of pulmonary valve motion in echocardiographic examination as an index of pulmonary hypertension]. *G Ital Cardiol* 1980;10:1349–1355.
22. Webb-Peploe KM, Henein MY, Coats AJ, et al. Echo derived variables predicting exercise tolerance in patients with dilated and poorly functioning left ventricle. *Heart* 1998;80:565–569.
23. Faris R, Coats AJ, Henein MY. Echocardiography-derived variables predict outcome in patients with nonischemic dilated cardiomyopathy with or without a restrictive filling pattern. *Am Heart J* 2002;144:343–350.
24. Vaturi M, Shapira Y, Vaknin-Assa H, et al. Echocardiographic markers of severe tricuspid regurgitation associated with right-

sided congestive heart failure. *J Heart Valve Dis* 2003;12: 197–201.

25. Sonmez B, Tansal S, Unal M, et al. A left pulmonary artery aneurysm secondary to pulmonary hypertension. *J Cardiovasc Surg (Torino)* 2001;42:629–632.

26. Moustapha A, Kaushik V, Diaz S, et al. Echocardiographic evaluation of left-ventricular diastolic function in patients with chronic pulmonary hypertension. *Cardiology* 2001;95: 96–100.

27. Henein MY, Amadi A, O'Sullivan C, et al. ACE inhibitors unmask incoordinate diastolic wall motion in restrictive left ventricular disease. *Heart* 1996;76:326–331.

28. Kao PN, Faul JL. Emerging therapies for pulmonary hypertension: striving for efficacy and safety. *J Am Coll Cardiol* 2003;41:2126–2129.

Coronary Artery Disease

CONGENITAL CORONARY ARTERY DISEASE

Anomalous origin of the left coronary artery from the pulmonary trunk usually presents in early infancy with congestive cardiac failure due to ischemic myocardial dysfunction. The diagnosis can usually be made by parasternal short-axis sections of the great arteries. The most characteristic finding is reversed flow in the left coronary artery demonstrated by color flow Doppler. Usually, the anomalous coronary artery connects to the pulmonary trunk at one of the sinuses, but in some cases the connection may be to the more distal pulmonary arteries. A less common presentation of this condition is in late childhood or early adult life, usually with left ventricular dysfunction and mitral regurgitation. There is almost always reversed blood flow in the left coronary artery, representing a left-to-right shunt from the right coronary artery into the pulmonary trunk.

Congenital anomalies of the coronary arteries are also found in various types of congenital heart disease. The most important of these is complete transposition of the great arteries. Abnormalities such as an intramural course, single coronary artery, or abnormal origin add an incremental risk factor for the arterial switch operation performed in early life.

Fistula communications from the coronaries may connect to the left or right ventricle, the right atrium, or the pulmonary trunk. They are almost always associated with marked dilatation of the proximal coronary arteries. Color flow Doppler is extremely helpful in the diagnosis showing at the site of the fistulous communication the characteristic continuous-flow profile demonstrated with pulse or continuous-wave Doppler.

ACQUIRED CORONARY ARTERY DISEASE

Kawasaki's disease is the most common cause of acquired coronary artery anomalies in infants and children. Coronary artery aneurysms are characteristic, often leading to coronary artery stenosis and features of ischemic heart disease. Coronary artery aneurysms usually occur in the proximal left and right coronary arteries and are readily demonstrated from parasternal sections of the aortic valve. Aneurysms may be more difficult to define by echocardiography when they persist into adult life. It is important to be aware, however, that Kawasaki's disease in childhood can present with evidence of ischemic heart disease in young adults.[1]

CORONARY ARTERY ANATOMY

Two main coronary arteries arise from two of the three sinuses of Valsalva, the right coronary and left coronary sinuses, respectively. The two coronary arteries have major differences in their branching patterns once they have emerged from their sinuses.

After arising from its sinus, the right coronary artery runs around the orifice of the tricuspid valve in the interventricular groove. In this initial course it usually gives off the sinus nodal artery into the atrial musculature and the infundibular (or conal) artery into the right ventricular muscle mass. The conal/infundibular branch commonly anastomoses with a small branch of the left coronary artery to form the anastomotic ring (of Vieussens). These branches and the ring are sometimes considerably enlarged when there is distal atherosclerotic disease in the right coronary artery. The artery then runs

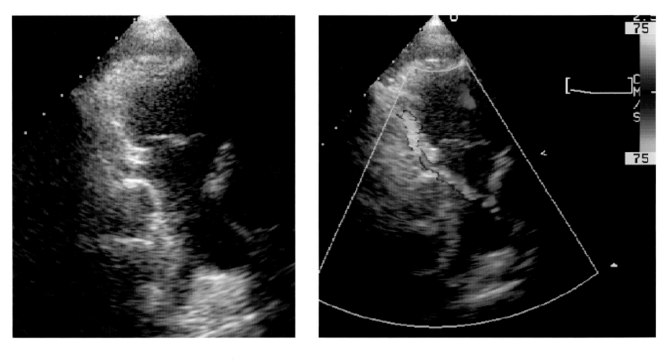

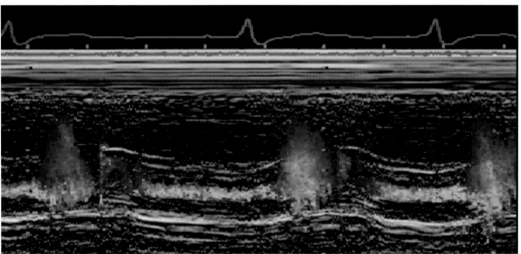

FIGURE 8.1. Parasternal short-axis view from a patient with anomalous left coronary artery origin, arising from the pulmonary artery. Notice the continuous retrograde flow in the coronary artery shown on the color M-mode picture.

to the acute margin of the heart, where it gives rise to the acute marginal artery of the right ventricle and usually a lateral atrial artery. Continuing around the tricuspid orifice, the right coronary artery gives off various smaller ventricular branches before, in the majority of hearts, it merges into the posterior interventricular artery. The area of the junction of the posterior interventricular and the atrioventricular grooves is generally called the *crux of the heart*. Before it forms the posterior descending branch, the right coronary artery itself makes a U turn into the area of atrioventricular muscular septum and gives off the artery to the atrioventricular node from the apex of the U angle. The foregoing describes the anatomy of the majority of people (i.e. that the artery supplying the posterior descending branch is the right coronary artery). This arrangement is called *right coronary dominance*. Although the left coronary artery always supplies a greater mass of muscle than the right coronary artery, echocardiography only visualizes the left main stem and the proximal left anterior descending artery. Although its sensitivity in detecting significant lesions is debatable, it can detect proximal lumen calcification.[1-3] Transesophageal echo with color flow Doppler provides an ideal noninvasive tool for studying the proximal seg-

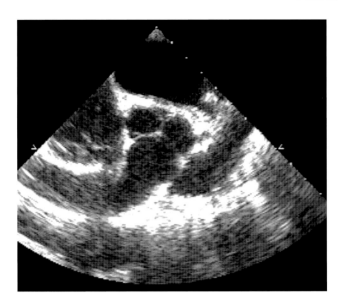

FIGURE 8.2. Short-axis view of the aortic valve leaflets and root demonstrating a right coronary fistula opening into the right ventricle.

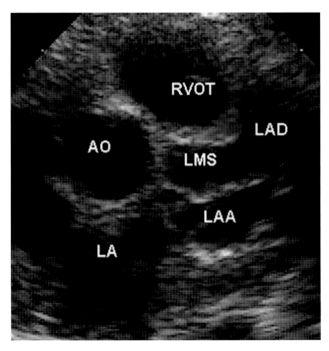

FIGURE 8.3. Short-axis view of the aortic root and origin of the coronary arteries from a patient with Kawasaki disease. Note the aneurysmal (beaded) appearance of the left coronary artery that measured 12 mm in diameter and its branches.

ments of the right and left coronary artery. Left dominance (posterior descending branch arising from the circumflex) is found in only about 15% of people.

The left coronary artery originates in the left (anterolateral) aortic sinus and passes undivided for up to 2.5 cm as the left main coronary artery between the aorta and the left atrial appendage. It generally bifurcates into anterior

descending and circumflex branches, but in about a third of individuals it trifurcates. The branch between the anterior descending and circumflex branches is called the *intermediate branch.* The anterior descending branch passes in the anterior interventricular sulcus toward the apex. During its course it gives a variable number of branches (diagonal branches) to the left ventricle. These, together with their parent branch, are important for arterial and vein grafting. Septal branches, known as septal perforators, arise from proximal left anterior descending artery and penetrate into septal myocardium. The first perforator is usually the largest and is used in alcohol septal ablation in patients with hypertrophic cardiomyopathy. The course of the circumflex artery is more variable than the other coronary arteries. In some hearts, it terminates almost immediately and often gives off the atrial circumflex artery, which runs in the atrial myocardium around the mitral orifice. More commonly, the circumflex artery continues to the obtuse margin of the left ventricle and breaks up into the obtuse marginal arteries, which are often embedded within the muscle of the left ventricle. The circumflex artery runs in the left atrioventricular groove, and the obtuse marginal branches are often sites for vein grafts. The circumflex artery itself may not be graftable because of its inaccessibility in the left atrioventricular groove.

ECHOCARDIOGRAPHIC IMAGING OF THE CORONARY ARTERIES

Transthoracic echocardiography allows visualization of the proximal segments of the left coronary artery, in

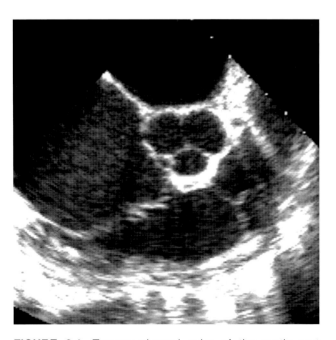

FIGURE 8.4. Transesophageal echo of the aortic root showing the proximal segments of the right and left coronary arteries.

particular. The addition of pulsed-wave Doppler assesses coronary flow velocities and may serve as an indirect means to confirm flow-limiting narrowings, particularly after coronary bypass surgery.[4–6]

Intravascular ultrasound (IVUS) is the commonly used echocardiographic technique for studying coronary luminal disease. It permits direct visualization of the arterial lumen; the luminal surface of the vessel, protruding atherosclerotic plaques, intraluminal thrombi, and intimal flaps can all be assessed by the fiberoptic angioscopy.[7] During coronary angioplasty, intravascular ultrasound has been used to guide the operator for optimal stent deployment and management of related complications (e.g., intimal dissection).[8] When combined with Doppler facilities, intravascular ultrasound scanning may offer detailed assessment of the site and extent of luminal narrowing. It may also assist in optimizing stent positioning. However, intravascular ultrasound imaging has recognized shortcomings. For clear visualization of the arterial wall, coronary flow should be interrupted and replaced with a clear and transparent fluid. Applying this technique is clearly undesirable, particularly in multisite lesions that require lengthy study time due to unavoidable vessel movement, especially in patients with critical coronary disease. Difficulty in accurate calibration of the measurements and inability to assess arterial structures below the vessel wall adds to the limitation of IVUS for routine use. Like conventional angiography IVUS is unable to assess wall thickness, accurate plaque size, nature of its contents or plaque stability.[9] Despite these limitations, intravascular angioscopy has greater sensitivity in identifying nonstenotic atherosclerotic arterial disease compared with conventional angiography. Conceptually, this advantage can be used for the follow-up of nonstenotic coronary disease, as is the case in post-transplant coronary artery disease and its response to pharmacologic therapy. Finally, intravascular ultrasound imaging provides a unique means for assessing arterial atherosclerotic "stiffness" as well as endothelial function and its response to different pharmacologic agents. Ideal intravascular ultrasound scanning seems to be the three-dimensional reconstruction on-line imaging that determines the spatial relationship in the areas of interest. Whereas the two-dimensional images define the circumferential extent of the plaque, the three-dimensional images both define the longitudinal extent and provide accurate assessment before coronary intervention.

Epicardial coronary artery scanning with high-frequency ultrasound transducers has been used intraoperatively to assess coronary artery stenosis, and the results have been compared with angiography. This way of coronary scanning is able to differentiate post-stenotic flow patterns in patients with varying degrees of coronary artery disease, but until now this technique has been restricted to research purposes only.

MYOCARDIAL INFARCTION

Left Ventricular Infarction

Resting two-dimensional images combined with M-mode recordings can demonstrate signs of myocardial infarction. In acute infarction, an asynchronous segment in the affected territory corresponding to the electrical changes

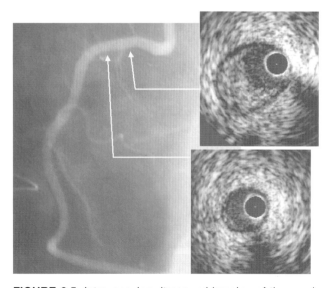

FIGURE 8.5. Intravascular ultrasound imaging of the proximal segment of the right coronary artery demonstrating plaque formation.

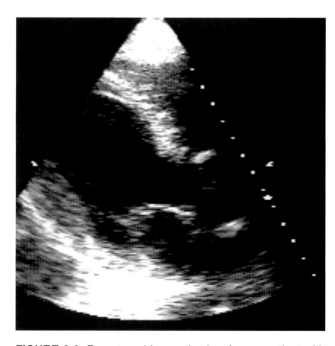

FIGURE 8.6. Parasternal long-axis view from a patient with anterior myocardial infarction. Note the extent of anterior wall scarring that has spared the proximal anterior segment.

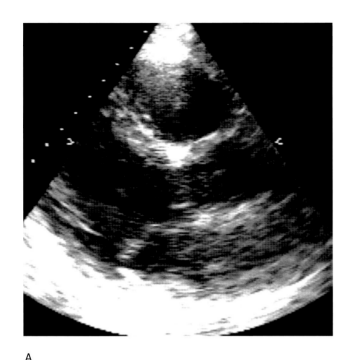

A

FIGURE 8.7. (A) Parasternal long-axis view from a patient with posterior wall infarction showing scarred and akinetic segment. (B) Left ventricular long-axis recordings of the three segments: left, septal, and posterior demonstrating global incoordination (postejection shortening) in the patient with inferior MI compared with isolated septal incoordination from a patient with anterior MI.

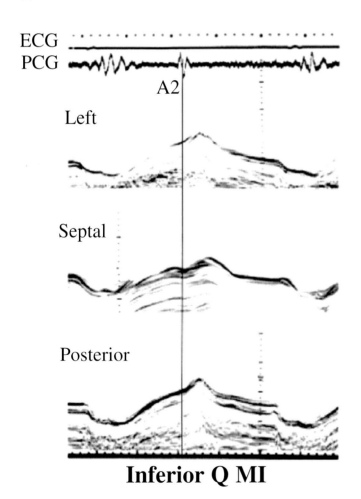

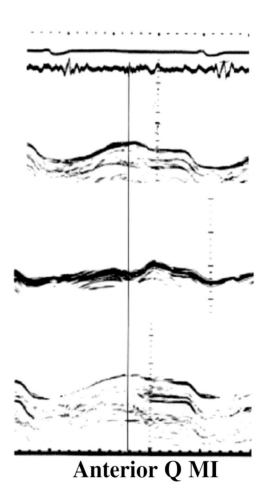

B

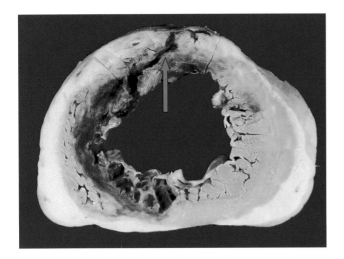

A

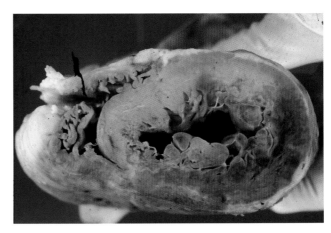

B

FIGURE 8.8. Pathologic specimen from two patients (A) with anteroseptal infarct with myocardial rupture and (B) posterolateral infarct extending into posterior aspect of the right ventricle.

on the surface ECG supports the diagnosis.[10,11] In patients with limited views, the use of left ventricular cavity contrast during the acute presentation has been shown to clearly delineate the endocardium of the dysfunctioning areas.[12] Echocardiography can also be used in the follow-up of these patients, providing important data on the segmental response to thrombolytic therapy and thereby identifying patients who may need rescue angioplasty. In addition, Doppler velocities provide evidence for physiologic disturbances, which may contribute to delayed recovery (e.g., raised left atrial pressure or significant mitral regurgitation). Scarred segments are the commonest presentation of old myocardial infarction, particularly with Q-wave infarction irrespective of its location. The extent of segmental involvement can also predict the site of coronary artery blockage, to some degree, particularly left anterior descending artery disease in anterior infarction. The combination of mid and apical anteroseptal wall infarct and absence of bundle branch block suggests spared proximal left anterior descending artery, with the site of the lesion distal to the first septal branch.[13] The same applies to the posterior wall. Conversely, the extent of fibrosis and scarring is minimal with non–Q-wave infarction, and the most common presentation is hypokinesia combined with ventricular long-axis dysfunction. Frequent long axis incoordination in inferior infarction suggests papillary muscle involvement. With an old infarction, the affected segment may appear akinetic with poor thickening fraction.

Right Ventricular Infarction

Right ventricular infarction should be excluded in patients presenting with low cardiac output and maintained left ventricular systolic function. It occurs in 30% of patients with inferior myocardial infarction who present with hypotension.[14] When present, depressed right ventricular free-wall long-axis amplitude and the presence of significant incoordination represent sensitive diagnostic criteria for right ventricular infarction, particularly in patients who have not previously undergone cardiac surgery. Assessment of right ventricular free-wall amplitude of motion and incoordination with M-mode and tissue Doppler imaging as well as ventricular filling pattern is crucial for confirming the diagnosis. A short early diastolic deceleration time in such cases, particularly in the presence of raised systemic venous pressure that also demonstrates early diastolic steep descent, suggests restrictive right ventricular physiology and associated raised right atrial pressure. A degree of tricuspid regurgitation is usually present in these patients that may vary in severity according to the extent of tricuspid ring dilatation. Management of such patients is critical, since a considerable degree of raised right atrial pressure is required to secure left ventricular filling and hence cardiac output.

Complications

Complications of myocardial infarction are readily studied by echo-Doppler technique.

1. *Ventricular aneurysms:* An aneurysm represents segmental full-thickness fibrosis of ventricular wall with loss of function. Aneurysmal formation occurs in 8% to 15% of patients within 3 months of acute infarction.[15] The common site for aneurysm formation is at the apical and anteroapical segments and rarely at the basal posterior wall.[16] The hinge point or the apical end of the healthy proximal segment determines the edge and the size of the aneurysm.[17] The outward movement of the aneurysm

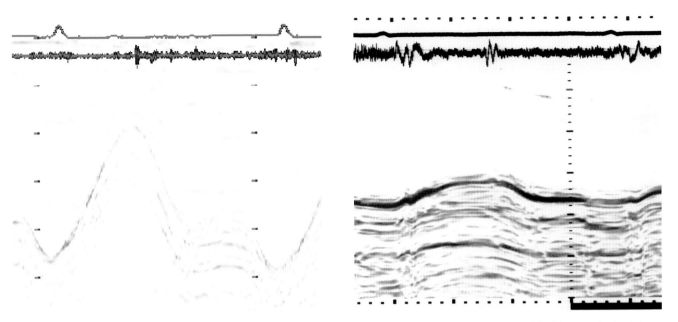

FIGURE 8.9. Right ventricular free-wall longitudinal motion from a normal subject (left) and a patient with right ventricular infarction (right). Note the marked reduction in the free-wall amplitude of motion in the patient as well as the reduced lengthening velocity.

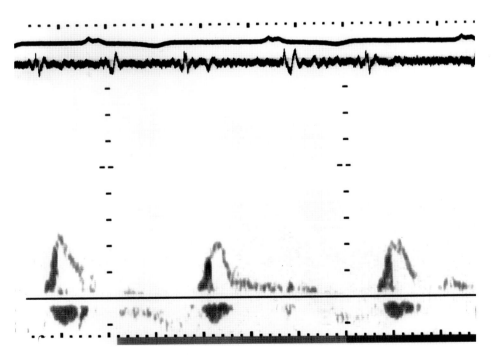

FIGURE 8.10. Right ventricular filling velocities from a patient with prior infarction. Note the dominant early diastolic component of filling with short deceleration time consistent with raised right atrial pressure along with a third heart sound on the phonocardiogram.

commonly described as "dyskinesia" represents passive movement of the dysfunctioning segment in response to the increased ventricular pressure generated by the rest of the myocardium during systole. The size of the aneurysm depends on the extent of the area affected by the blocked artery. A subjective assessment of relative aneurysm size with respect to that of the ventricle has been shown to determine mortality and surgical recovery after aneurysmectomy.[18,19] In general, the more basal ventricular function that is maintained, the better the prognosis. The same applies to the number of coronary arteries involved in the ischemic ventricular process. From a prognostic point of view, a massive anterior infarct with anteroapical aneurysm formation carries a worse prognosis than a localized akinetic segment.[19] Aneurysms also represent a substrate for thrombus formation and hence thromboembolic complications.[20] The more rapid the development of a ventricular aneurysm after acute infarction, the worse the prognosis.[19] An aneurysm that is noted after 5 days of infarction carries an 80% 1-year mortality. Finally, a true ventricular aneurysm should be differentiated from a false aneurysm that represents a localized myocardial rupture

that is sealed by the surrounding parietal pericardium. False aneurysms are usually small and carry a better prognosis than a true aneurysm.[21] Two-dimensional echo images are ideal for differentiation between true and false aneurysms.

2. ***Ventricular septal defect:*** This is a rare complication of acute myocardial infarction. When it occurs, it tends to affect the apical third of the anteroseptal segment in anterior myocardial infarction and the proximal part of the posterior septum in inferior infarction. Color flow Doppler is ideal for demonstrating the presence of any left-to-right shunt, and transvenous echo contrast usually confirms the site of the septal defect and the exact direction of the shunt.[22,23] A small apical septal defect is usually protected by the muscle bulk surrounding it. A septal defect associated with hemodynamic disturbances may require either device or surgical closure at the time of revascularization. A sizeable mid-septal defect is usually associated with clinical and hemodynamic instability, and surgical closure is mandatory. Associated LV disease and mitral regurgitation should also be assessed.

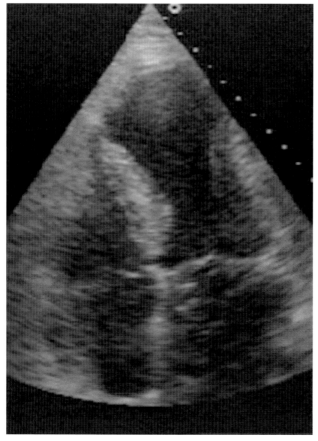

A

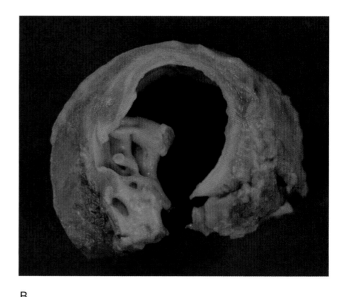

B

FIGURE 8.11. (A) Apical four-chamber view from a patient with anterior infarction complicated by apical aneurysm. Note the site of the aneurysm and the hinge point that marks the edge of the aneurysm. (B) Pathologic section from a patient with an apical aneurysm.

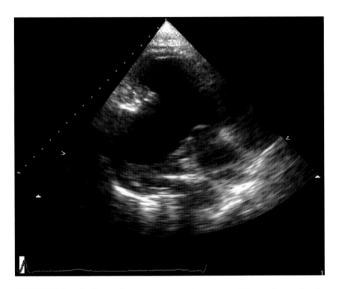

FIGURE 8.12. Parasternal long-axis view of the left ventricle from a patient with posterior wall aneurysm and clot.

3. *Papillary muscle rupture:* This is a rare complication of myocardial infarction. Patients present with acute severe mitral regurgitation and pulmonary edema. A mitral regurgitation murmur may not be heard, and if present, may be even difficult to differentiate from that caused by a ventricular septal defect. Echocardiography, particularly transesophageal echo, is the initial investigation to determine the exact cause of the valve regurgitation. Urgent surgical repair in this condition is life saving.[24–26]

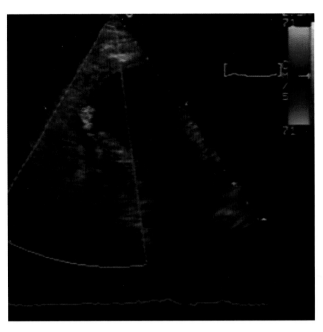

FIGURE 8.13. Apical four-chamber view from a patient with apical ventricular septal defect complicating anterior infarction. Note the left-to-right shunt on color flow Doppler at the apical level.

4. *Mitral regurgitation:* Mild mitral regurgitation is a common finding in patients with ventricular disease, particularly secondary to coronary artery disease.[27] Functional (secondary) mitral regurgitation may be caused by papillary muscle dysfunction or asynergy of the free wall

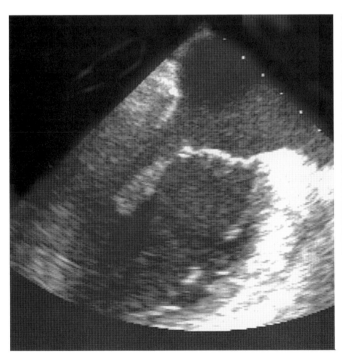

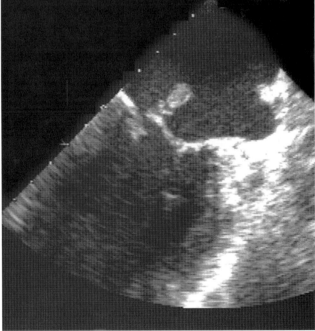

FIGURE 8.14. Transesophageal echocardiogram from a patient with ruptured posterolateral papillary muscle. Note the free movement of the detached segment with the mural mitral valve leaflet.

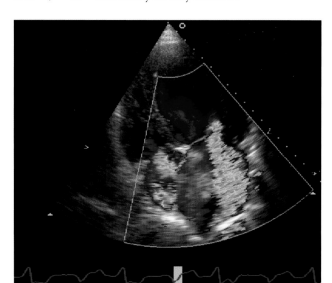

FIGURE 8.15. Apical four-chamber view from a patient with free-wall infarction and posterior mitral valve leaflet prolapse. Note the resulting severe regurgitation on the color flow Doppler.

supporting the papillary muscle.[28] Significant mitral regurgitation may develop either in association with free-wall infarction and posterior mitral valve leaflet prolapse caused by papillary muscle dysfunction or as a consequence of progressive deterioration of ventricular function and mitral ring dilatation. Whereas the management of the papillary muscle dysfunction is surgical repair, the appropriate management of ventricular ischemic dysfunction is revascularization and insertion of a mitral ring in selected cases.[29]

Stress echocardiography may be needed not only to assess myocardial viability, but to provide information on severity of the mitral regurgitation, particularly in patients with moderate regurgitation. Patients in whom mitral regurgitation volume drops at peak stress suggest myocardial dysfunction that may respond to revascularization.

5. *Ischemic left ventricular disease:* Long-standing coronary artery disease, with or without infarction, may result in progressive deterioration of ventricular function and an increase in left atrial pressure. This is one of the most common causes of breathlessness in these patients. A restrictive ventricular filling pattern is diagnostic of raised left atrial pressure.[30] It is characterized by a short isovolumic relaxation time, dominant early diastolic ventricular filling, and short deceleration time. Atrial contraction in late diastole results in retrograde blood flow into the pulmonary veins, thereby exaggerating pulmonary congestion. A longer retrograde "a" wave in the pulmonary veins with respect to the forward transmitral "A" is consistent with raised LV end-diastolic pressure.[31] Furthermore, patients with this degree of ischemic LV disease almost always have some degree of functional

mitral regurgitation that adds to the increase in left atrial pressure. A consequence of raised left atrial pressure is the development of secondary pulmonary hypertension.

ANGINA

Stable Angina

This is an exertional symptom due to the mismatch of supply and demand of oxygen to the myocardium. The most common cause is coronary artery disease. Resting echocardiography is frequently normal in patients with uncomplicated coronary artery disease. Therefore stress echo is recommended to induce possible wall motion disturbances during symptom provocation. Exercise or pharmacologic stress using adenosine, dipyridamole, or dobutamine are the most common stressors for echocardiographic studies. Conventional wall motion analysis is based on scoring 16 individual myocardial segments according to their response to stress (normal, hypokinetic, akinetic, or dyskinetic).[32;33] A normal response to stress is demonstrated by increased segmental thickness and hence amplitude of endocardial inward movement. Segments are analyzed from the parasternal long-axis, short-axis, apical four-chamber, and apical two-chamber views. The currently available digital storage system in most echocardiographic systems has made multiple image acquisition easy, and hence deduction of segmental response at different stages of stress can be assessed. A subjective assessment of the diseased coronary artery can be made according to the distribution of the developed segmental abnormalities.[34] A technical limitation in demonstrating a complete endocardial display at rest and peak stress may limit the use of this test in certain patients. Harmonic imaging technique and echo contrast agents (e.g., Optison, Levovist and Sonoview) have proved to have a significant impact in increasing the definition of the endocardial border throughout the ventricular cavity by opacifying the whole cavity.[35] Recently, intravenous myocardial echo contrast has also added to the importance of assessing coronary flow reserve as well as segmental reversible opacification with stress.[36]

To determine the overall ischemic burden, a global score index is obtained from the relative sum of the segmental scores with respect to the number of the segments visualized. This has been shown to be 80% sensitive and 90% specific for diagnosing coronary artery disease.[37] The accuracy of this technique in diagnosing multivessel coronary disease is significantly higher than that for single-vessel disease.[38] The sensitivity of wall motion scoring has proved comparable to that of thallium scanning, whereas specificity is significantly higher.[39] Stress echo has also been shown to predict outcome in patients with ischemic ventricular disease.[40]

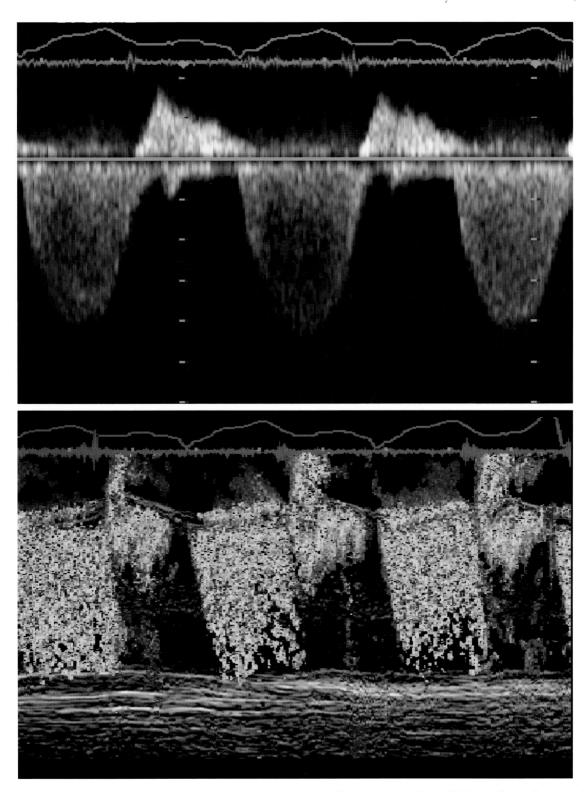

FIGURE 8.16. Continuous-wave Doppler and color flow M-mode recordings from a patient with ischemic cardiomyopathy and dilated mitral ring showing severe mitral regurgitation.

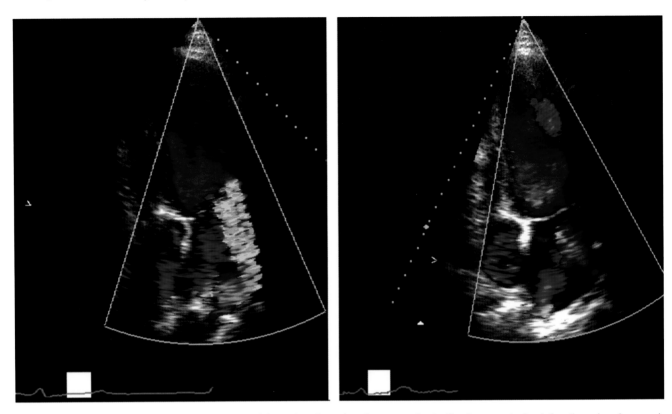

FIGURE 8.17. Stress echo images of the apical four-chamber view from a patient after large anterior infarction showing moderate mitral regurgitation at rest that becomes mild at peak stress.

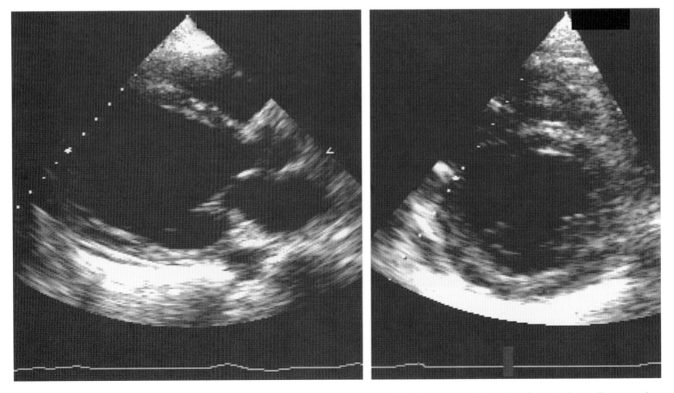

FIGURE 8.18. Left ventricular 2D recording from a patient with posterior wall infarction and hypokinetic anterior wall presenting with breathlessness. Note the cavity dilatation and poor overall systolic function (fractional shortening 10%).

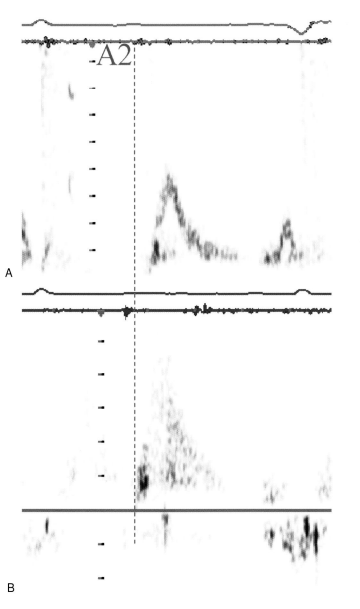

A

B

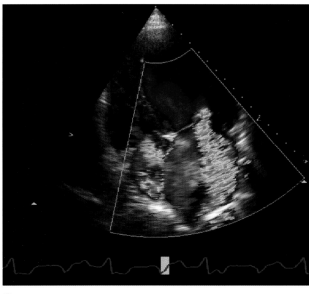

C

FIGURE 8.19. (A) Transmitral Doppler flow velocities from a patient demonstrating typical restrictive left ventricular filling pattern with short isovolumic relaxation time and E wave deceleration time. (B) Pulmonary venous Doppler flow velocities showing retrograde flow in late diastole of a significantly longer period compared with that of transmitral Doppler. (C) Apical four-chamber view from the same patient showing severe mitral regurgitation.

Although this method of analyzing wall motion behavior with stress is widely used, inherent limitations are present:

1. Analysis of wall motion is subjective in nature and depends on technical experience.

2. Lack of objective quantitation, which makes its reproducibility vary between observers and different centers.

3. Wall motion scores are based on the inward movement of the segments in systole that is determined by the function of the circumferential muscle layer. This method ignores the subendocardial component of the myocardium, which is longitudinally orientated.

4. The technique is unable to register segmental diastolic dysfunction that may be present before systolic dysfunction.

5. The test terminates when the most significant lesion has caused ischemia. This raises the possibility of underestimating other important coronary disease that may remain undiagnosed.

Stress Long Axis

Stress ventricular long axis demonstrates the mechanical behavior of the subendocardial layer of the myocardium. The myocardial fibers of this layer are longitudinal in orientation. They originate from the ventricular apex and insert around the circumference of the mitral and tricuspid valve rings. In systole, as they contract they bring the insertion site (mitral and tricuspid annulus) toward their origin (the apex), and in diastole they move in the opposite direction, bringing the annuli back toward the atria in early diastole and again in late diastole, during

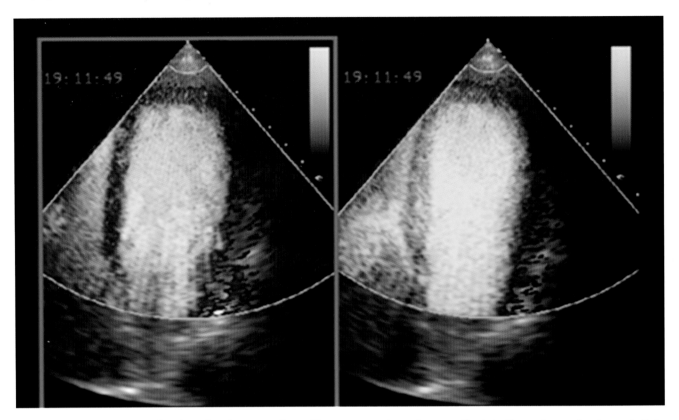

FIGURE 8.20. Apical four-chamber view from a patient with coronary artery disease after injecting echo contrast agent. Note the full opacification of the cavity and the clear delineation of the endocardium.

atrial contraction.[41] These two components of diastolic movement correspond to the "E" and "A" wave of ventricular filling velocities, in early and late diastole. Having the ability to record the long-axis function from the valve annulus movement (fibrous landmark) makes the technique highly reproducible. Long-axis function can be studied at different segments–anterior, posterior, left, and septal sites–and at other levels of the ventricle, particularly when using tissue Doppler techniques.[42] The same principle can be used for studying the free-wall function of the right ventricle, which cannot be assessed by other stress techniques. Finally, measurements of long-axis function, including amplitude, velocities, timing, and incoordination, can be obtained, and thus a comprehensive assessment of systolic and diastolic function of each of the five longitudinal segments can be performed. Disturbances of the anterior and septal segments usually represent left anterior descending coronary artery disease. The left segment represents the circumflex artery disease, and the posterior and right ventricular free wall represent the right coronary disease.[43]

Stress long-axis technique has shown a significantly higher sensitivity and specificity for diagnosing coronary artery disease when compared with conventional wall motion score index.[44] Its sensitivity to single-vessel

disease, particularly that of the right coronary artery, is higher than that of thallium scanning, probably due to its ability to assess right ventricular behavior during stress. Furthermore, combining ventricular long-axis analysis and simultaneous 12-lead electrocardiogram at rest and peak stress demonstrates the close relationship between the two, probably based on the anatomic fact that the conduction system runs in the subendocardium.[45] The fall in long-axis amplitude with stress correlates with the delayed ventricular depolarization, or "QRS broadening," seen in patients with coronary artery disease. In addition, detailed analysis of different long-axis phases differentiates between the effect of inotropy and conduction disturbances themselves. The delay in the onset of segmental long-axis shortening (inward movement) correlates closely with the extent of the delay in ventricular depolarization.[46] The latter also correlates with the delay in early diastolic long-axis lengthening, resulting in delayed early filling. Finally, the exaggerated incoordination seen at peak stress results in very long isovolumic periods that correlate with the drop in cardiac output in patients with ischemic cardiomyopathy.[47] Thus ventricular long-axis analysis not only confirms the presence of coronary artery disease, but distinguishes the global ventricular response to stress.

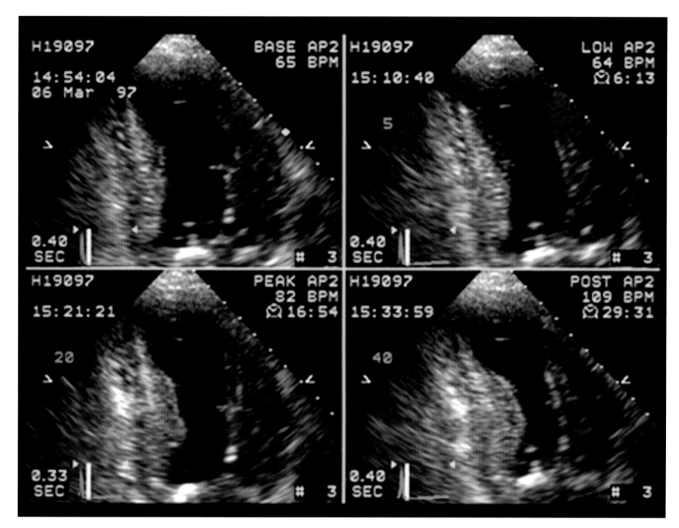

FIGURE 8.21. Apical views from a patient with exertional angina at rest (top-left) and peak dobutamine stress (bottom-right). Note the significant development of akinesia of the apex with stress consistent with left anterior descending artery disease.

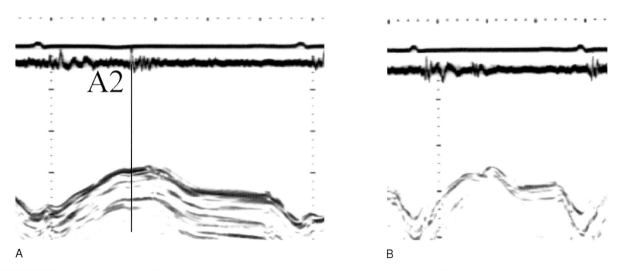

A   B

FIGURE 8.22. Septal long axis function at rest and peak stress from a normal subject. Note the normal increase in amplitude and shortening and lengthening velocities with stress.

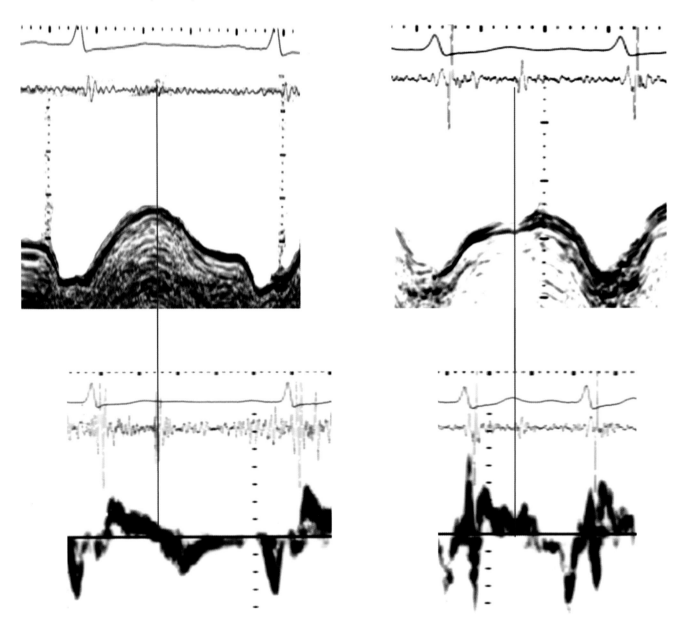

FIGURE 8.23. Septal long-axis recording from a patient with coronary artery disease at rest (left) and peak stress (right). Note the fall in amplitude (top) and velocities (bottom) and the development of incoordination in early diastole with stress.

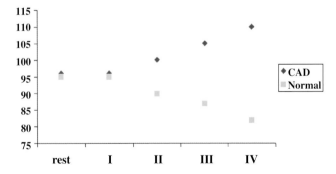

FIGURE 8.24. Graph demonstrating the incremental change in QRS duration in normals and in patients with coronary artery disease. Note the progressive broadening of QRS duration in the latter compared with the former.

Unstable Angina

In patients presenting with unstable angina in whom the coronary arteries prove to be anatomically normal, the resting echocardiography is generally normal. In those with coronary disease, no specific pattern on two-dimensional images has been identified. However, analysis of ventricular long-axis function may demonstrate an exaggerated incoordination pattern (post-ejection shortening) in more than one segment.[48] The extent of this incoordination in early diastole may itself have a mechanical effect in compromising coronary flow, thus perpetuating progression of myocardial ischemia at rest.

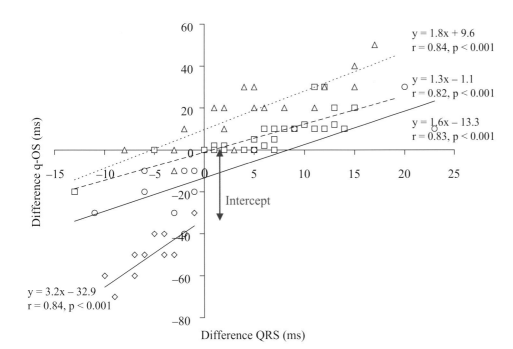

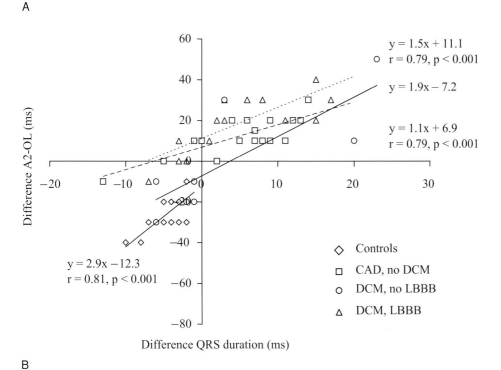

FIGURE 8.25. Graph demonstrating a close relationship between QRS broadening and delay in septal onset of shortening and lengthening.

A

B

ISCHEMIC CARDIOMYOPATHY

The question of revascularization often arises in patients with ischemic cardiomyopathy and previous myocardial infarction who are not medically controlled. The evidence for ischemic myocardium can be demonstrated by various techniques, including exercise electrocardiogram, stress echo, or myocardial perfusion scanning. Surgical decision making depends on the extent of the viable myocardium whose function is likely to improve with revascularization. This is often referred to as hibernating myocardium. These areas may be hypokinetic at rest, so that stress

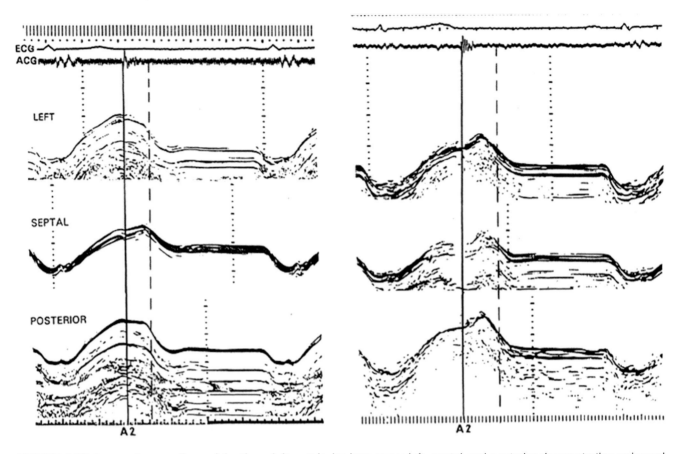

FIGURE 8.26. Long-axis recordings of the three left ventricular long axes; left, septal and posterior demonstrating universal incoordination pattern, from a patient with unstable angina (right).

echo, thallium perfusion, or positron emission tomography scanning are necessary to define such regions.[49,50] Hibernating myocardium has been defined as a state of persistently impaired myocardial and LV function at rest as a result of reduced coronary blood flow that can be partially or completely restored to normal if the myocardial oxygen supply/demand ratio is corrected. Its presence can be demonstrated by a number of techniques. Altered thallium or technetium uptake is the current routinely used technique to assess the degree of myocardial hibernation. Conventional stress echo and wall motion scoring have shown significant accuracy for identifying viable myocardium in different segments with potential implications for selecting suitable patients for surgery and predicting revascularization outcome.[50] Again, the sensitivity of stress echo is significantly improved when using echo contrast agents for delineating clear endocardial border and segmental thickening.[51] Viable segments characteristically show a biphasic response to stress. At low-dose stress, local amplitude increases, but at higher doses it falls again. This biphasic response has been widely used as a marker of viable myocardium in patients with ischemic cardiomyopathy.[52]

In addition to the other limitations of wall motion scoring, patients with ischemic cardiomyopathy commonly present with secondary complications, which may influence the overall pattern of ventricular function. Functional mitral regurgitation, frequently seen in ischemic cardiomyopathy, may overestimate wall motion activity, whereas high left atrial pressure (restrictive physiology) may suppress wall motion. Left bundle branch block is known to affect wall motion behavior even in the absence of coronary disease and is expected therefore to affect wall motion score. The severity of mitral regurgitation with stress reduces as the ring diameter falls with the increase in heart rate during stress echo in patients with viable myocardium, particularly at the basal ventricular level.

Ventricular Long-Axis Function in Ischemic Cardiomyopathy

An increase in long-axis amplitude with stress (a normal response) is a reliable sign of viability irrespective of the appearance of additional markers of ischemic dysfunction such as incoordination. A cutoff value of 6-mm amplitude at rest has been shown to be 90% sensitive and 95% specific in predicting surgical recovery. An incremental increase in long-axis amplitude with stress by 1.5 mm has proved a more sensitive predictor of the pres-

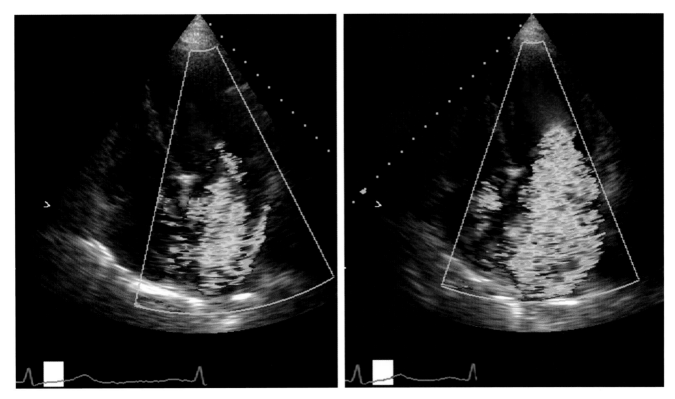

FIGURE 8.27. Apical four-chamber view from a patient with ischemic cardiomyopathy and significant functional mitral regurgitation at rest (left) and peak stress (right). Note the increase in mitral regurgitation severity with stress, suggesting development of severe ischaemic dysfunction with stress.

ence of coronary artery disease in patients with dilated cardiomyopathy than the increase in tissue Doppler lengthening velocity or wall motion score index.[53]

Long-axis measurements may also provide an opportunity for detailed analysis of ventricular segmental and global function in patients with ischemic cardiomyopathy. With a superimposed ECG, segmental electromechanical behavior can be studied in different phases of the cardiac cycle. In addition to the preceding markers of ischemic dysfunction, timing with respect to onset of ventricular depolarization and repolarization has been shown to determine the overall performance of the ventricle (stroke volume and cardiac output).[54] In these patients, stress long axis can also demonstrate characteristic incoordination patterns such as early systolic outward movement or post-ejection shortening (in early diastole) that cannot be visualized by wall motion scoring. Finally, long-axis disturbances can affect the overall pattern of ventricular filling. The delayed onset of long-axis lengthening with respect to end-ejection is associated with a delay of the peak early diastolic filling,[54] the consequences of which are increased early diastolic acceleration and compromised filling time. LV filling pattern during stress may be therefore taken as a surrogate marker of segmental long-axis behavior in diastole.

The overall effect of delayed long-axis shortening and lengthening and the exaggerated incoordination is significant compromise of LV filling and hence cardiac output with stress.

Similar findings can be demonstrated in the right ventricular free-wall behavior, which are difficult to study using other stress techniques.

MANAGEMENT OF CORONARY ARTERY DISEASE

Medical Follow-up

Echocardiography aims at following up segmental as well as overall ventricular function. Transmitral Doppler velocities provide revalidated noninvasive markers of filling pressures.

● Optimal use of vasodilators [angiotensin-converting enzyme (ACE) inhibitors] as well as others can be monitored.

● Adequate response to ACE inhibition in patients with restrictive filling results in normalization of filling velocities and left atrial size.[55]

● The direct cause of patients' symptoms can be derived from echocardiographic assessment of LV filling

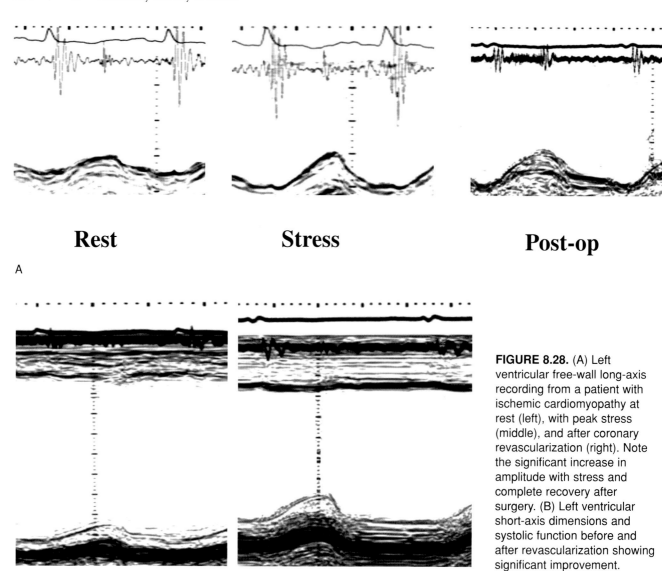

Rest   **Stress**   **Post-op**

A

B

FIGURE 8.28. (A) Left ventricular free-wall long-axis recording from a patient with ischemic cardiomyopathy at rest (left), with peak stress (middle), and after coronary revascularization (right). Note the significant increase in amplitude with stress and complete recovery after surgery. (B) Left ventricular short-axis dimensions and systolic function before and after revascularization showing significant improvement.

time and mitral regurgitation length. Prolonged mitral regurgitation with pre-systatic component in patients with ischemic cardiomyopathy may cause breathlessness by limiting filling time and stroke volume. This condition, particularly with QRS of more than 150 ms, usually responds favorably to dual chamber pacing and optimized atrioventricular delay.[56]

Coronary Angioplasty

Echocardiography is not routinely essential during coronary angioplasty. However, it may be necessary in exceptional cases following related complications (e.g., in patients with hypotension to exclude pericardial tamponade). Ventricular long-axis ischemic dysfunction shows early recovery following successful revascularization. The reverse of these findings can be regarded as markers of vessel occlusion.[57]

Coronary Artery Bypass Surgery

Intraoperative Echocardiography

Intraoperative echocardiograophy aims at monitoring global and segmental ventricular function during and after a revascularization procedure. The preoperative study provides a baseline assessment against which postoperative studies can be compared. Transesophageal echocardiography plays an important role for monitoring these patients, particularly those with ischemic cardiomyopathy. The four-chamber view is the most commonly used image, although a transgastric short-axis view also provides a satisfactory assessment of LV minor-axis function by monitoring segmental thickening as assessed on two-dimensional images and M-mode recordings. Viable segments that remain dysfunctioning after complete revascularization are considered stunned. For academic interest, obtaining a LV pressure recording

Non-ischemic

Ischemic

5cm/s

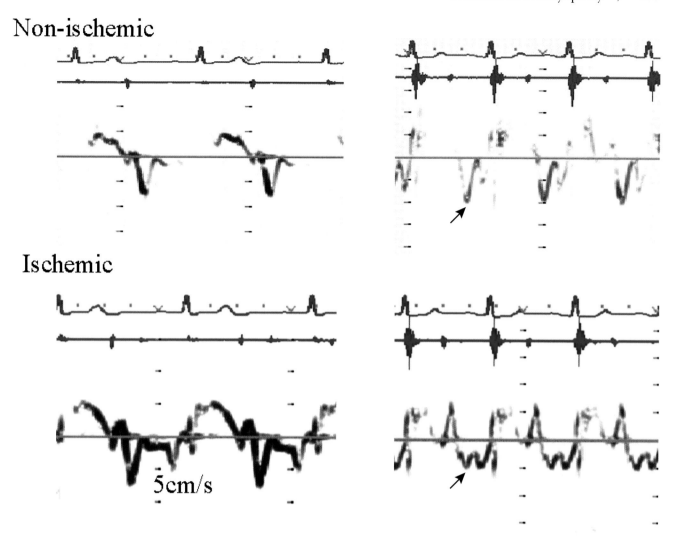

FIGURE 8.29. Myocardial tissue Doppler recordings from two patients with dilated cardiomyopathy; nonischemic (top) and ischemic (bottom) at rest (left) and peak stress (right). Note the normal increase in early diastolic velocities in the absence of coronary artery disease and the fall of velocities and appearance of incoordination in coronary disease (arrows).

superimposed on the M-mode trace using an intraventricular catheter tip manometer provides a wealth of information on segmental as well as global power production and cycle efficiency. This technique has shown significant early segmental recovery after revascularization with nonbypass (octopus) procedure when compared with traditional bypass procedure.[58]

Direct visualization of the origin of the coronary artery as well as graft insertion sites may be important in determining the cause of the delay in weaning a patient from the bypass circulation. A blocked or kinked graft supplying a vital segment may be the direct cause of such complication. Color flow as well as pulsed-wave Doppler showing high velocities at branch origin or graft insertion along with segmental hypokinesia suggests the presence of significant occlusion that needs urgent attention and possible reintervention.

Finally, intraoperative transesophageal echo provides evidence for additional abnormalities that could be dealt with in the same setting (e.g., significant mitral regurgitation that needs leaflet repair or ring insertion, small patent foramen ovale, or left atrial appendage clot as a possible cause of transient ischemic attacks).

Intensive Care Unit Echocardiography

Patients with normal ventricular systolic function before surgery usually have an uneventful recovery. Those with poor ventricular function may progress more slowly and may require balloon pump insertion. Echocardiographic studies may be requested when recovery is delayed and in those who are ventilator dependent. The transthoracic window is usually limited in such patients, so that transesophageal echo is essential for an

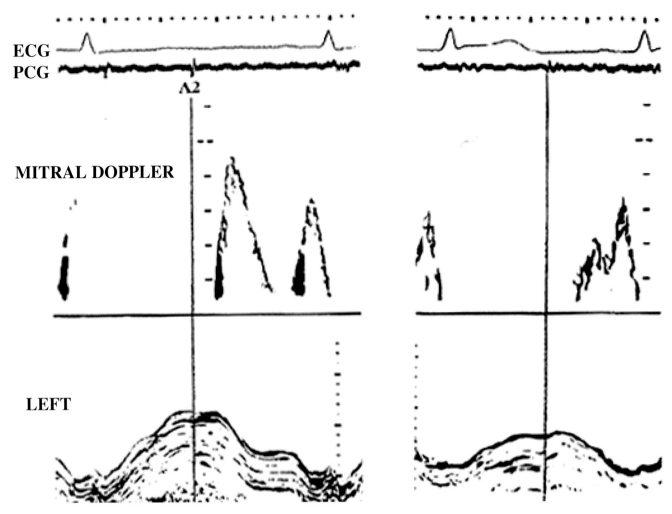

ECG

PCG

MITRAL DOPPLER

LEFT

FIGURE 8.30. Left ventricular septal long-axis recording (bottom) from a patient with ischemic cardiomyopathy along with transmitral filling velocities (top) at rest (left) and peak stress (right). Note the marked development of incoordination that compromised early ventricular filling.

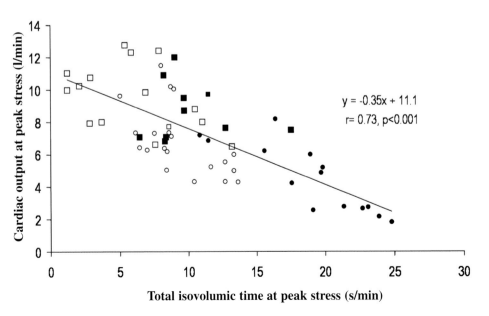

$$y = -0.35x + 11.1$$
$$r = 0.73, p < 0.001$$

FIGURE 8.31. A graph demonstrating the close relationship between stress isovolumic time and peak cardiac output in patients with ischemic cardiomyopathy.

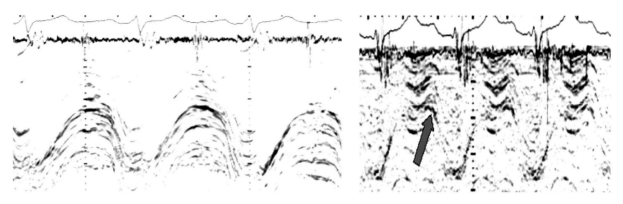

FIGURE 8.32. Right ventricular free-wall long-axis recording from a patient with biventricular ischemic myopathy at rest (left) and peak stress (right). Note the significantly reduced amplitude at rest that becomes more depressed with stress. Also note the appearance of exaggerated incoordination consistent with ischemic dysfunction (arrow).

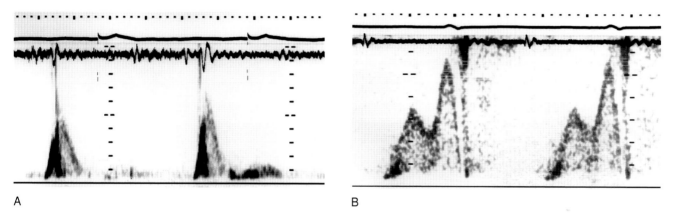

A

B

FIGURE 8.33. Transmitral Doppler flow velocities from a patient with ischemic cardiomyopathy and limiting dyspnoea. Note the restrictive filling pattern (A) and third heart sound on the phonocardiogram consistent with raised left atrial pressure and the effect of angiotensin-converting enzyme inhibition (B).

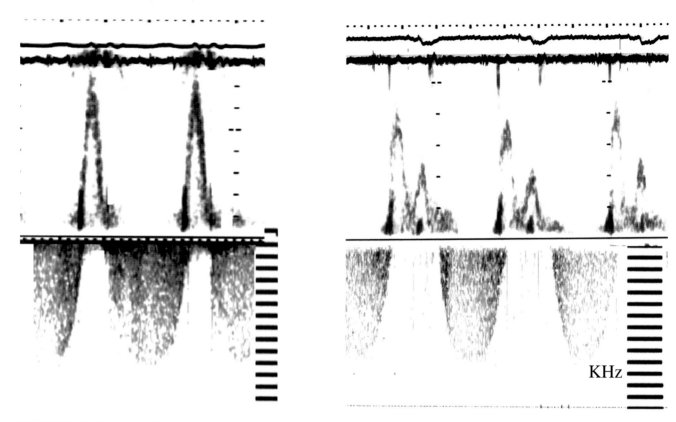

FIGURE 8.34. Transmitral Doppler flow velocities from a patient with ischemic cardiomyopathy and resistant dyspnea. Note the short filling time caused by the long mitral regurgitation (left) and the beneficial effect of dual chamber pacing and atrioventricular delay optimization (right).

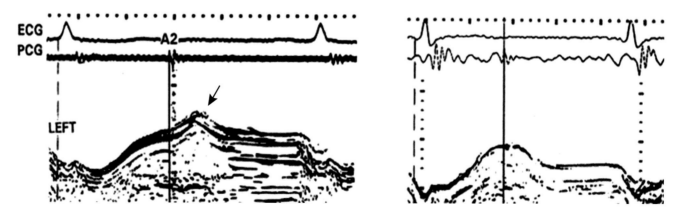

FIGURE 8.35. Left ventricular free-wall long-axis recording from a patient with coronary artery disease before (left) and after (right) coronary angioplasty. Note the remarkable normalization of the incoordinate pattern (arrow) after procedure.

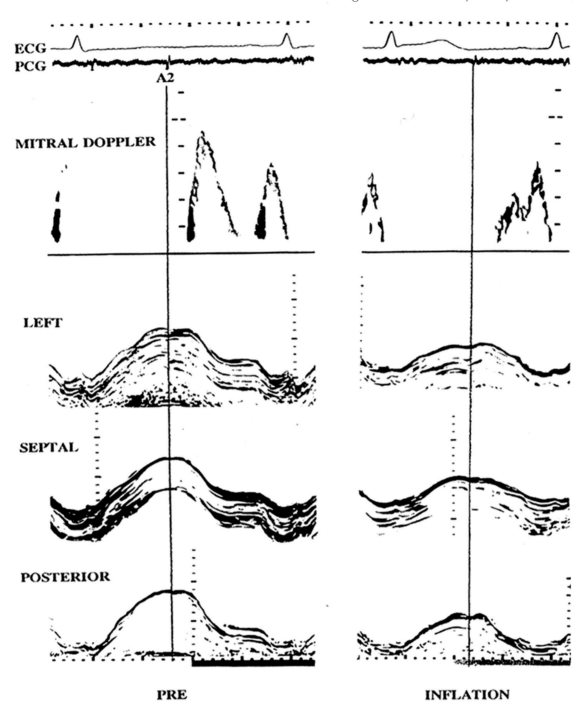

FIGURE 8.36. Left ventricular free wall and septal long axis from a patient during balloon inflation in the proximal left anterior descending artery. Note the significant fall in long-axis amplitude and lengthening velocities.

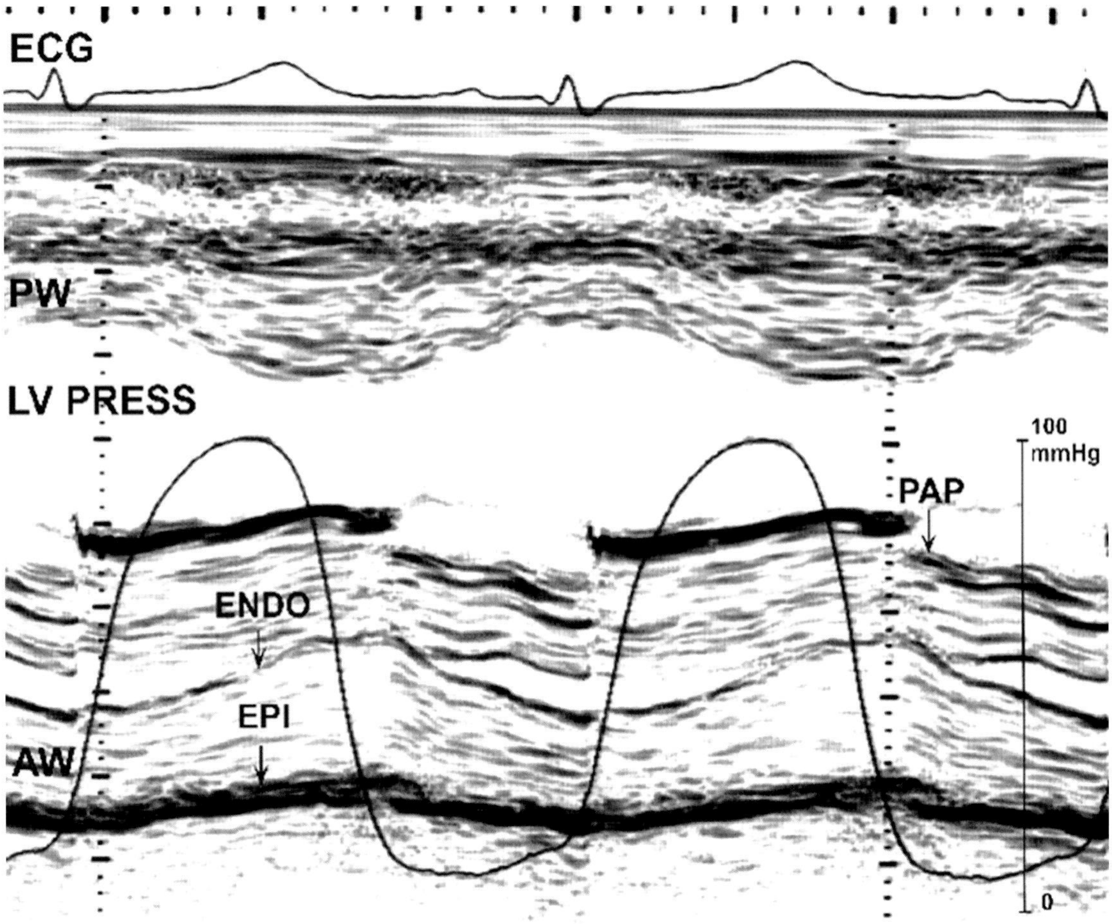

FIGURE 8.37. Transgastric left ventricular M-mode recording of the minor axis before establishing the bypass circulation with superimposed left ventricular pressure.

adequate evaluation. The objective of the TOE in this setting is to assess

- Regional LV wall motion and estimation of systolic function (ejection fraction).

- LV filling pattern as a marker of left atrial pressure.

- Evidence for pulmonary hypertension as an indirect marker of raised left atrial pressure.

- Right ventricular systolic function as a less common cause of an underfilled and hence poorly functioning left ventricle by two-dimensional imaging and long axis.

- Presence of pericardial effusion – a small, localized collection, particularly posterior to the left atrium–may have its deleterious effect on ventricular recovery.

Patients with resistant segmental disturbances may demonstrate clear evidence for ischemic dysfunction with dobutamine stress. Simultaneous documentation of deterioration of segmental wall motion function and ischemic ECG changes at peak stress usually confirms an underlying ischemic cause for the delayed recovery. Emergency coronary angiography and possible reintervention may be life-saving procedures in such patients.

Postoperative Echocardiography

Postoperative echocardiography aims at providing baseline data on ventricular function after complete revascularization. It is also helpful for assessing right ventricular function, which is known to deteriorate after cardiopulmonary bypass circulation. In addition, any pericardial or left-sided pleural effusion can be assessed. Recurrence of angina-like symptoms can be evaluated using stress echo techniques as discussed earlier, particularly in patients with conduction disturbance as a possible cause of angina, in whom information provided by other stress techniques may be inconclusive.

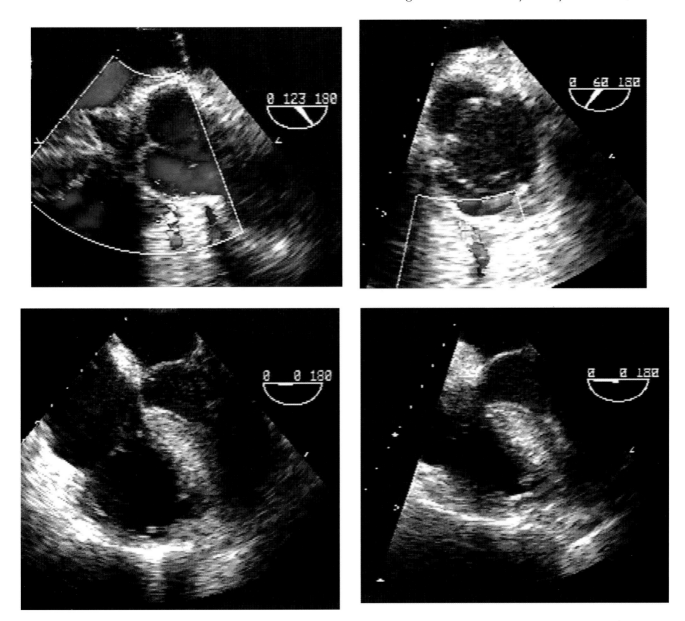

FIGURE 8.38. Intraoperative transesophageal echocardiogram demonstrating high right coronary artery velocities on color flow Doppler (aliasing) after grafting, suggesting graft occlusion or kinking (top left) and apical four-chamber view showing reduced right ventricular free-wall movement (bottom left). Equivalent pictures after releasing the coronary graft obstruction (right). Note the significant fall in the right coronary artery aliasing along with improvement of right ventricular free well function afterwards.

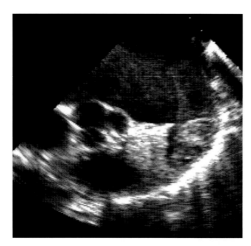

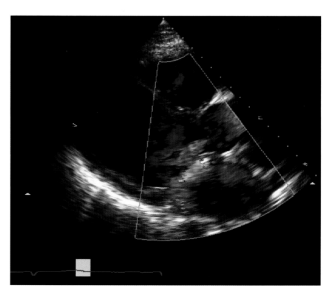

FIGURE 8.39. Intraoperative transesophageal echocardiography from a patient before coronary artery bypass graft surgery showing additional left atrial appendage clot, probably complicating long-standing atrial fibrillation.

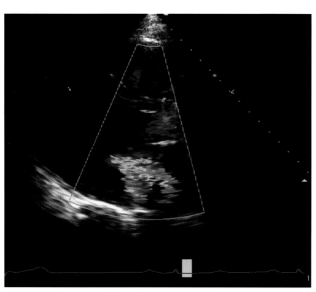

A

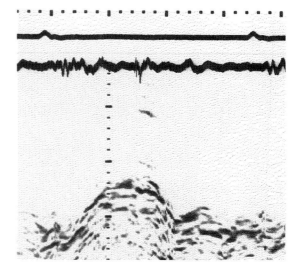

B

FIGURE 8.40. Parasternal views from a patient with ischemic cardiomyopathy and functional mitral regurgitation before (A) and after (B) coronary artery bypass graft surgery and mitral valve repair. Note the disappearance of mitral regurgitation.

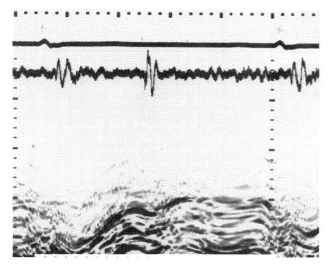

FIGURE 8.41. Left ventricular long-axis recording from the free wall before and after CABG surgery demonstrating significant normalization of function and regression of incoordination.

REFERENCES

1. Douglas PS, Fiolkoski J, Berko B, et al. Echocardiographic visualization of coronary artery anatomy in the adult. *J Am Coll Cardiol* 1988;11:565–571.
2. Block PJ, Popp RL. Detecting and excluding significant left main coronary artery narrowing by echocardiography. *Am J Cardiol* 1985;55:937–940.
3. Vered Z, Katz M, Rath S, et al. Two-dimensional echocardiographic analysis of proximal left main coronary artery in humans. *Am Heart J* 1986;112:972–976.
4. Iliceto S, Marangelli V, Memmola C, et al. Transesophageal Doppler echocardiography evaluation of coronary blood flow velocity in baseline conditions and during dipyridamole-induced coronary vasodilation. *Circulation* 1991;83:61–69.
5. Yamagishi M, Miyatake K, Beppu S, et al. Assessment of coronary blood flow by transesophageal two-dimensional pulsed Doppler echocardiography. *Am J Cardiol* 1988;62:641–644.
6. Yoshida K, Yoshikawa J, Hozumi T, et al. Detection of left main coronary artery stenosis by transesophageal color Doppler and two-dimensional echocardiography. *Circulation* 1990;81:1271–1276.
7. Waller BF, Pinkerton CA, Slack JD. Intravascular ultrasound: a histological study of vessels during life. The new "gold standard" for vascular imaging. *Circulation* 1992;85:2305–2310.
8. Yock PG, Fitzgerald PJ, Linker DT, et al. Intravascular ultrasound guidance for catheter-based coronary interventions. *J Am Coll Cardiol* 1991;17(6 Suppl B):39B–45B.
9. Nissen SE, Gurley JC, Grines CL, et al. Intravascular ultrasound assessment of lumen size and wall morphology in normal subjects and patients with coronary artery disease. *Circulation* 1991;84:1087–1099.
10. Buda AJ, Zotz RJ, Gallagher KP. Characterization of the functional border zone around regionally ischemic myocardium using circumferential flow-function maps. *J Am Coll Cardiol* 1986;8:150–158.
11. Horowitz RS, Morganroth J, Parrotto C, et al. Immediate diagnosis of acute myocardial infarction by two-dimensional echocardiography. *Circulation* 1982;65:323–329.
12. Kaul S, Pandian NG, Gillam LD, et al. Contrast echocardiography in acute myocardial ischemia. III. An in vivo comparison of the extent of abnormal wall motion with the area at risk for necrosis. *J Am Coll Cardiol* 1986;7:383–392.
13. Engelsen DJ, Gorgels AP, Cheriex EC, et al. Value of the electrocardiogram in localising the occlusion site in the left anterior descending coronary artery in acute anterior myocardial infarction. *J Am Coll Cardiol* 1999;34:389–395.
14. D'Arcy B, Nanda NC. Two-dimensional echocardiographic features of right ventricular infarction. *Circulation* 1982;65:167–173.
15. Pasternack RC, Braunwald E, Sobel BE. Acute myocardial infarction. In: Braunwald E, ed. *Heart disease.* Philadelphia: WB Saunders, 1992:1255–1260.
16. Visser CA, Kan G, David GK, et al. Echocardiographic-cineangiographic correlation in detecting left ventricular aneurysm: a prospective study of 422 patients. *Am J Cardiol* 1982;50:337–341.
17. Catherwood E, Mintz GS, Kotler MN, et al. Two-dimensional echocardiographic recognition of left ventricular pseudoaneurysm. *Circulation* 1980;62:294–303.
18. Barrett MJ, Charuzi Y, Corday E. Ventricular aneurysm: cross-sectional echocardiographic approach. *Am J Cardiol* 1980;46:1133–1137.
19. Matsumoto M, Watanabe F, Goto A, et al. Left ventricular aneurysm and the prediction of left ventricular enlargement studied by two-dimensional echocardiography: quantitative assessment of aneurysm size in relation to clinical course. *Circulation* 1985;72:280–286.
20. Jordan RA, Miller RD, Edwards JE, et al. Thromboembolism in acute and healed myocardial infarction: intracardiac mural thrombosis. *Circulation* 1952;6:1–6.
21. Rueda B, Panidis IP, Gonzales R, et al. Left ventricular pseudoaneurysm: detection and postoperative follow-up by color Doppler echocardiography. *Am Heart J* 1990;120:990–992.
22. Drobac M, Gilbert B, Howard R, et al. Ventricular septal defect after myocardial infarction: diagnosis by two-dimensional contrast echocardiography. *Circulation* 1983;67:335–341.
23. Smyllie JH, Sutherland GR, Geuskens R, et al. Doppler color flow mapping in the diagnosis of ventricular septal rupture and acute mitral regurgitation after myocardial infarction. *J Am Coll Cardiol* 1990;15:1449–1455.
24. Chirillo F, Totis O, Cavarzerani A, et al. Transesophageal echocardiographic findings in partial and complete papillary muscle rupture complicating acute myocardial infarction. *Cardiology* 1992;81:54–58.
25. Koenig K, Kasper W, Hofmann T, et al. Transesophageal echocardiography for diagnosis of rupture of the ventricular septum or left ventricular papillary muscle during acute myocardial infarction. *Am J Cardiol* 1987;59:362.
26. Stoddard MF, Keedy DL, Kupersmith J. Transesophageal echocardiographic diagnosis of papillary muscle rupture complicating acute myocardial infarction. *Am Heart J* 1990;120:690–692.
27. Barzilai B, Gessler C, Jr., Perez JE, et al. Significance of Doppler-detected mitral regurgitation in acute myocardial infarction. *Am J Cardiol* 1988;61:220–223.
28. Alam M, Thorstrand C, Rosenhamer G. Mitral regurgitation following first-time acute myocardial infarction–early and late findings by Doppler echocardiography. *Clin Cardiol* 1993;16:30–34.
29. Izumi S, Miyatake K, Beppu S, et al. Mechanism of mitral regurgitation in patients with myocardial infarction: a study using real-time two-dimensional Doppler flow imaging and echocardiography. *Circulation* 1987;76:777–785.
30. Appleton CP, Hatle LK, Popp RL. Relation of transmitral flow velocity patterns to left ventricular diastolic function: new insights from a combined hemodynamic and Doppler echocardiographic study. *J Am Coll Cardiol* 1988;12:426–440.
31. Rossvoll O, Hatle LK. Pulmonary venous flow velocities recorded by transthoracic Doppler ultrasound: relation to left ventricular diastolic pressures. *J Am Coll Cardiol* 1993;21:1687–1696.
32. Bolognese L, Sarasso G, Bongo AS, et al. Dipyridamole echocardiography test. A new tool for detecting jeopardized myocardium after thrombolytic therapy. *Circulation* 1991;84:1100–1106.
33. Jaarsma W, Visser CA, Kupper AJ, et al. Usefulness of two-dimensional exercise echocardiography shortly after myocardial infarction. *Am J Cardiol* 1986;57:86–90.

34. Berthe C, Pierard LA, Hiernaux M, et al. Predicting the extent and location of coronary artery disease in acute myocardial infarction by echocardiography during dobutamine infusion. *Am J Cardiol* 1986;58(13):1167–1172.

35. Keller MW, Glasheen W, Smucker ML, et al. Myocardial contrast echocardiography in humans. II. Assessment of coronary blood flow reserve. *J Am Coll Cardiol* 1988; 12:925–934.

36. Sakata Y, Kodama K, Adachi T, et al. Comparison of myocardial contrast echocardiography and coronary angiography for assessing the acute protective effects of collateral recruitment during occlusion of the left anterior descending coronary artery at the time of elective angioplasty. *Am J Cardiol* 1997; 79:1329–1333.

37. Picano E. Stress echocardiography. From pathophysiological toy to diagnostic tool. *Circulation* 1992;85:1604–1612.

38. Marwick TH, Nemec JJ, Pashkow FJ, et al. Accuracy and limitations of exercise echocardiography in a routine clinical setting. *J Am Coll Cardiol* 1992;19:74–81.

39. Picano E, Parodi O, Lattanzi F. Comparison of dipyridamole-echocardiography test and exercise thallium-201 for diagnosis of coronary artery disease. *Am J Noninvas Cardiol* 1989;3: 85–92.

40. Sawada SG, Ryan T, Conley MJ, et al. Prognostic value of a normal exercise echocardiogram. *Am Heart J* 1990;120: 49–55.

41. Henein MY, Gibson DG. Normal long axis function. *Heart* 1999;81:111–113.

42. Henein M, Lindqvist P, Francis D, et al. Tissue Doppler analysis of age-dependency in diastolic ventricular behaviour and filling: a cross-sectional study of healthy hearts (the Umea General Population Heart Study). *Eur Heart J* 2002;23: 162–171.

43. Henein MY, Gibson DG. Long axis function in disease. *Heart* 1999;81:229–231.

44. Mishra MB, Lythall DA, Chambers JB. A comparison of wall motion analysis and systolic left ventricular long axis function during dobutamine stress echocardiography. *Eur Heart J* 2002;23:579–585.

45. O'Sullivan CA, Henein MY, Sutton R, et al. Abnormal ventricular activation and repolarisation during dobutamine stress echocardiography in coronary artery disease. *Heart* 1998;79: 468–473.

46. Duncan AM, O'Sullivan CA, Carr-White GS, et al. Long axis electromechanics during dobutamine stress in patients with coronary artery disease and left ventricular dysfunction. *Heart* 2001;86:397–404.

47. Duncan AM, Francis DP, Henein MY, et al. Limitation of cardiac output by total isovolumic time during pharmacologic stress in patients with dilated cardiomyopathy: activation-mediated effects of left bundle branch block and coronary artery disease. *J Am Coll Cardiol* 2003;41:121–128.

48. Henein MY, Patel DJ, Fox KM, et al. Asynchronous left ventricular wall motion in unstable angina. *Int J Cardiol* 1997;59: 37–45.

49. Pierard LA, De Landsheere CM, Berthe C, et al. Identification of viable myocardium by echocardiography during dobutamine infusion in patients with myocardial infarction after thrombolytic therapy: comparison with positron emission tomography. *J Am Coll Cardiol* 1990;15:1021–1031.

50. Senior R, Lahiri A. Role of dobutamine echocardiography in detection of myocardial viability for predicting outcome after revascularization in ischemic cardiomyopathy. *J Am Soc Echocardiogr* 2001;14:240–248.

51. Senior R. Role of contrast echocardiography for the assessment of left ventricular function. *Echocardiography* 1999; 16(7, Pt 2):747–752.

52. Meza MF, Ramee S, Collins T, et al. Knowledge of perfusion and contractile reserve improves the predictive value of recovery of regional myocardial function postrevascularization: a study using the combination of myocardial contrast echocardiography and dobutamine echocardiography. *Circulation* 1997;96:3459–3465.

53. Duncan AM, Francis DP, Gibson DG, et al. Differentiation of ischemic from nonischemic cardiomyopathy during dobutamine stress by left ventricular long-axis function. Additional effect of left bundle-branch block. *Circulation* 2003;108:1214–1220.

54. Duncan AM, O'Sullivan C, Gibson DG, et al. The effect of dobutamine stress on left ventricular long axis and early diastolic filling in patients with coronary artery disease. *J Am Coll Cardiol* 2001;37:433A.

55. Henein MY, Amadi A, O'Sullivan C, et al. ACE inhibitors unmask incoordinate diastolic wall motion in restrictive left ventricular disease. *Heart* 1996;76:326–331.

56. Brecker SJ, Xiao HB, Sparrow J, et al. Effects of dual-chamber pacing with short atrioventricular delay in dilated cardiomyopathy. *Lancet* 1992;340:1308–1312.

57. Henein MY, Priestley K, Davarashvili T, et al. Early changes in left ventricular subendocardial function after successful coronary angioplasty. *Br Heart J* 1993;69:501–506.

58. Koh TW, Carr-White GS, DeSouza AC, et al. Effect of coronary occlusion on left ventricular function with and without collateral supply during beating heart coronary artery surgery. *Heart* 1999;81:285–291.

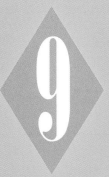

9   Dilated Cardiomyopathy

Dilated cardiomyopathy is characterized by left ventricular (LV) dilatation, increased end-diastolic volume, and reduced systolic function (typically, ejection fraction less than 40%).[1,2]

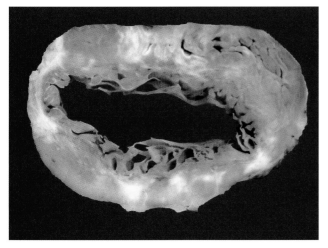

A

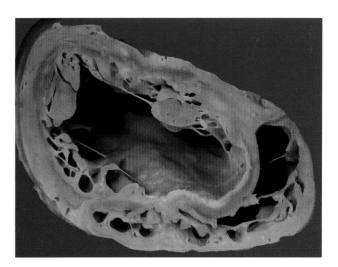

B

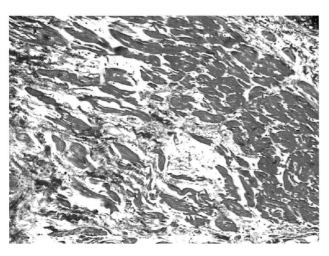

C

FIGURE 9.1. (A) Transverse section showing end-stage dilated cardiomyopathy with thin walls and extensive scarring. (B) Universal thinning of the left ventricular wall with endocardial thickening. (C) Trichrome stain showing myocytes in red and collagen in blue replacing the myocytes.

149

ETIOLOGY

Most cases of dilated cardiomyopathy are idiopathic, although a number of etiologies have been identified.

1. *Ischemic cardiomyopathy.* Long-standing coronary artery disease may remain silent until patients present with dilated left ventricle and signs of heart failure.

2. *Familial X-linked cardiomyopathy.* This is a familial condition in which the abnormality is in the centromeric half of the dystrophic genome region in the heart. This explains its link to Duchenne muscular dystrophy gene locus.[3]

3. *Peripartum cardiomyopathy.* This occurs during pregnancy, usually manifests late in the last trimester, and has a prognosis that is much better than idiopathic cardiomyopathy.[4,5]

4. *Viral cardiomyopathy.* This form commonly occurs following viral upper respiratory tract infection in adults or gastrointestinal infection in children. Children with viral cardiomyopathy may achieve complete recovery and have a better prognosis than adults.[6,7]

5. *Alcoholic cardiomyopathy.* This complicates excessive alcohol intake. Despite the severity of impairment of ventricular systolic function, the disease tends to recover gradually after abstinence from alcohol.

6. *Less common causes.* Auto-organ antibodies to x and b myosin heavy-chain isoform and complicating Acquired Immuno Deficiency Syndrome (AIDS).[8,9]

7. *Metabolic disorders.* Metabolic disorders that cause dilated cardiomyopathy are rare and present in early infancy. The cardiac condition in dilated cardiomyopathy may be silent for a while until it is accidentally discovered on a routine checkup or identified following clinical presentation with congestive heart failure.[10]

VENTRICULAR FUNCTION

Transthoracic echocardiography demonstrates a dilated left ventricle with increased systolic and diastolic dimensions and reduced systolic function (ejection fraction or fractional shortening). There is no definitive echocardiographic picture that depicts different clinical stages of the disease apart from the difference in cavity size.[11] The LV cavity shows globally impaired segmental function with reduced wall thickness and thickening fraction. Patients with dilated cardiomyopathy may demonstrate localized segmental dysfunction, making a definitive differentiation between idiopathic and ischemic etiology difficult.[12–14] As the disease progresses, the left ventricle further dilates, resulting in increased wall stress (Laplace's law), increased myocardial oxygen consump-

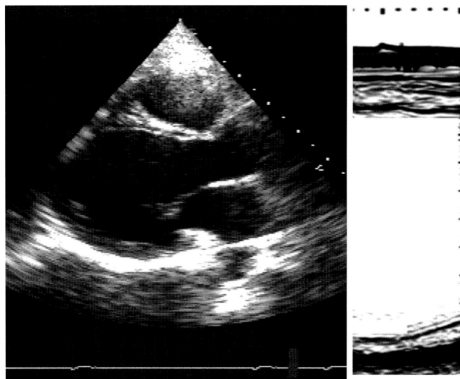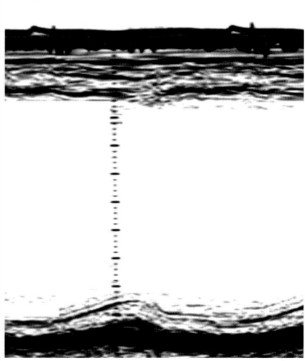

FIGURE 9.2. Parasternal long-axis view from a patient with dilated cardiomyopathy (left). Corresponding M-mode recording of the basal ventricular region (right).

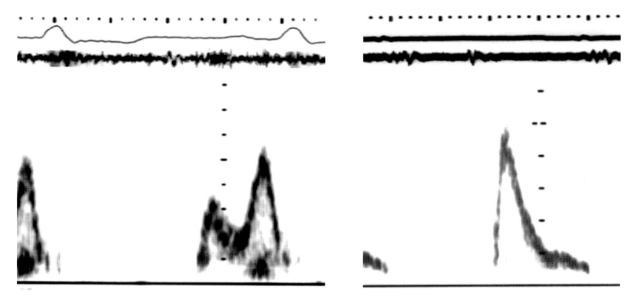

FIGURE 9.3. Left ventricular filling pattern from two patients with DCM, slow relaxation (left), and restrictive high filling pressures (right).

tion, reduced systolic function, and altered myocardial architecture. In late stages, the ventricle becomes spherical rather than ellipsoid, adding to the reduction in the overall ventricular systolic performance.[15]

VENTRICULAR FILLING

There is no characteristic filling pattern in dilated cardiomyopathy.[16] In early stages ventricular filling may be normal for age or show a slow ventricular relaxation pattern, characterized by long isovolumic relaxation time and predominant LV filling in late diastole. In later stages as the ventricle becomes stiff and incompliant, the end-diastolic pressure rises, LV filling becomes of the restrictive pattern, short isovolumic relaxation time and dominant early diastole filling component with short deceleration time.[17,18] This is often associated with some degree of mitral regurgitation. In early diastole, restrictive LV filling is characterized by a raised atrioventricular pressure gradient, resulting in a delay or complete suppression of early diastolic right ventricular filling through pressure transfers across the ventricular septum (ventricular interaction effect).[19]

COMPLICATIONS

Mitral Regurgitation

The mitral ring dilates as the left ventricle dilates, causing failure of mitral valve leaflets to coapt. In late stages of the disease when the ventricle becomes spherical, the papillary muscles are displaced laterally, causing significant chordal tension. This results in disturbed leaflet movement, incomplete valve closure, and valvular incompetence.[20]

Mitral regurgitation varies in severity, from mild in the early disease to severe in late stages. The retrograde pressure drop across the mitral valve aids in estimating left atrial pressure, when the left atrial pressure is raised and the pressure drop across the mitral valve is low.

Raised Left Atrial Pressure

Raised left atrial pressure is manifest late in the disease as the LV diastolic pressure rises, resulting in left atrial dilatation, impairment of function, and tendency to arrhythmia. Even in patients with maintained sinus rhythm, atrial contraction is resisted by ventricular stiffness and high LV end-diastolic pressure. This causes backward flow in the pulmonary veins that adds to the pulmonary congestion. Retrograde flow in the pulmonary veins occurring during atrial systole that is more than 30 ms longer than the duration of the transmitral A wave suggests raised LV end-diastolic pressure.[21–23] Patients with severe LV disease and raised left atrial pressure often present with a poor systolic component of the pulmonary venous flow consistent with depressed movement of the ventricular long axis in systole and consequently limited atrial enlargement in systole.

Pulmonary Hypertension

Raised left atrial pressure, complicating LV disease and mitral regurgitation, may cause pulmonary hypertension.

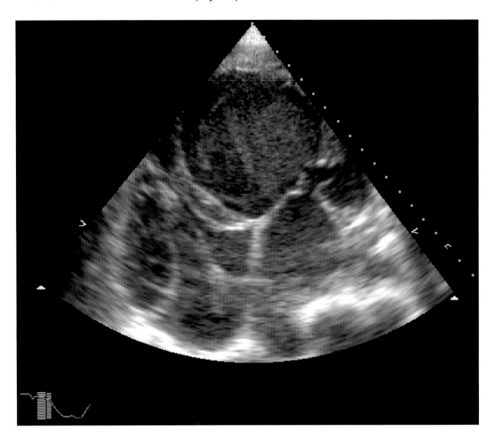

FIGURE 9.4. Apical four-chamber view from a patient with late-stage DCM showing spherical left ventricular cavity and spontaneous contrast.

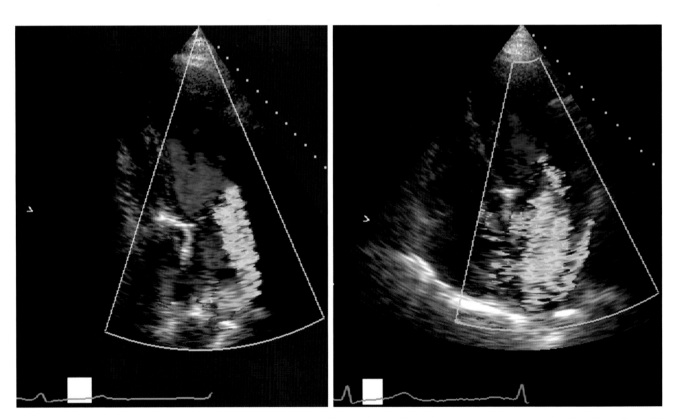

FIGURE 9.5. Apical four-chamber views from two patients with DCM showing mitral regurgitation on color flow Doppler, mild (left) and severe (right).

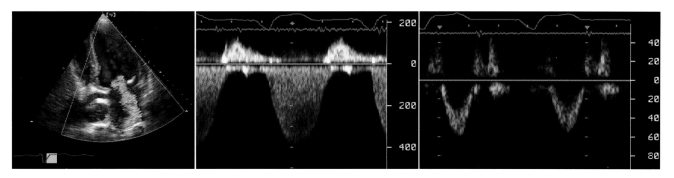

FIGURE 9.6. Apical four-chamber image of a DCM patient with severe mitral regurgitation on color Doppler (left) and continuous-wave Doppler (middle). Note the peak left ventricular-left atrial pressure drop is 60 mmHg, suggesting severely raised left atrial pressure and low cardiac output state (low aortic velocity) (right).

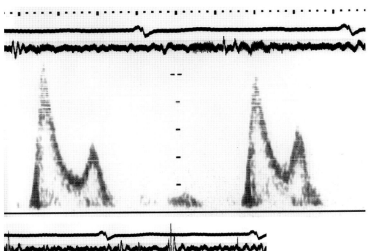

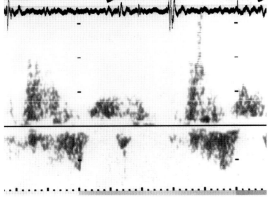

FIGURE 9.7. Transmitral flow from a patient with restrictive left ventricular filling and raised left atrial pressures (top) and corresponding pulmonary venous flow (bottom). Note the longer duration of the pulmonary venous flow compared with the forward mitral flow.

Pulmonary venous hypertension is difficult to diagnose echocardiographically. A short E-wave deceleration time is a good marker of raised pulmonary wedge pressure. The progressively developing pulmonary arterial hypertension affects the size and function of the right heart. The right ventricle becomes hypertrophied, its function becomes impaired, and the cavity itself dilates. The right atrium also dilates. Pulmonary artery pressure can be estimated from peak tricuspid regurgitation pressure drop added to the right atrial pressure. Although this equation tends to underestimate peak pulmonary artery pressure, it helps in assessing disease progression in symptomatic patients and in monitoring their response to treatment.[24]

Tricuspid Regurgitation

As is the case with other causes of right ventricular dilatation and enlargement of tricuspid annulus, tricuspid regurgitation is common and varies in severity in dilated cardiomyopathy.[20] Severe tricuspid regurgitation may be present in late disease or if the primary pathology involves the right ventricle. In this case the right atrium

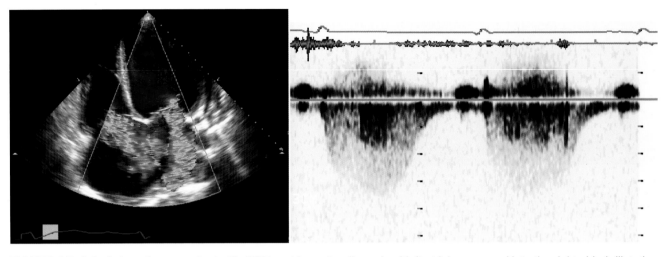

FIGURE 9.8. Apical views from a patient with DCM and long-standing raised left atrial pressure. Note the right-sided dilatation and raised right ventricular-right atrial pressure drop on the tricuspid regurgitation continuous-wave Doppler.

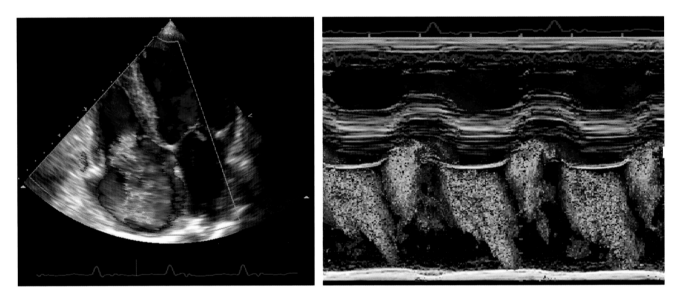

FIGURE 9.9. Apical views from a patient with DCM and dilated right heart. Note the severity of tricuspid regurgitation on color Doppler (left) and color M-mode Doppler (right).

and ventricle are both dilated, the right atrial pressure is increased, and the peak right ventricular–right atrial pressure drop falls. This fall in pressure drop should not be taken as a sign of reduction of pulmonary artery pressure, particularly in patients who show clinical deterioration, but as a sign of increasing right atrial pressure.

Left Ventricular Thrombus

Late stages of dilated cardiomyopathy and increased ventricular diastolic pressure are characterized by slow intraventricular circulation. Spontaneous intracavitary echo contrast may be seen. With significantly high early diastolic atrioventricular pressure gradient and intraventricular flow acceleration, the mitral leaflet opening is disturbed

and the valve behaves as if functionally stenosed, thus adding to the disturbed cavity function in diastole. This degree of ventricular disease may be associated with apical stagnation of blood and potential thrombus formation, suggesting the need for prophylactic anticoagulation.[25,26]

Extracardiac Fluid Compression

Late stages of DCM with biventricular failure, pulmonary hypertension, and systemic congestion may be complicated by pericardial and/or pleural effusion. Large fluid collection increases the intrathoracic pressure and frequently exacerbates the patient's breathlessness. The consequences of the increased intrathoracic pressure on right heart phys-

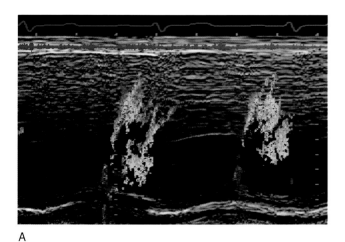

A

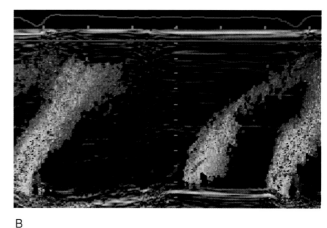

B

FIGURE 9.10. Apical views showing large left ventricular cavity and fast flow acceleration on color M-mode recording of left ventricular filling (left) compared with normal pattern (right).

iology are assessed by studying the vena caval, tricuspid, and pulmonary flows during different phases of the respiratory cycle. Right-sided filling and ejection that increase significantly during inspiration (>20% of that during expiration) suggest increased intrathoracic pressures.

Pulsus Alternans

With severe deterioration of ventricular function and absence of extracardiac fluid collection, pulsus alternans

may develop. This can easily be confirmed on pulsed Doppler velocities of LV filling and ejection as well as wall motion pattern. The exact mechanism of pulsus alternans is not clearly understood.

Activation-Induced Left Ventricular Dysfunction

Severe LV disease is almost always associated with delayed depolarization (i.e., broad QRS complex).[27]

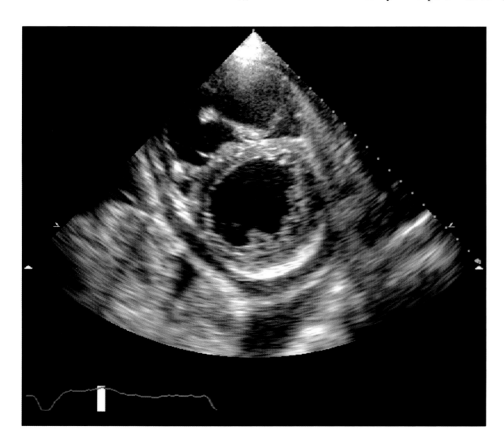

FIGURE 9.11. Parasternal short-axis view from a patient with DCM showing pericardial and left pleural effusion.

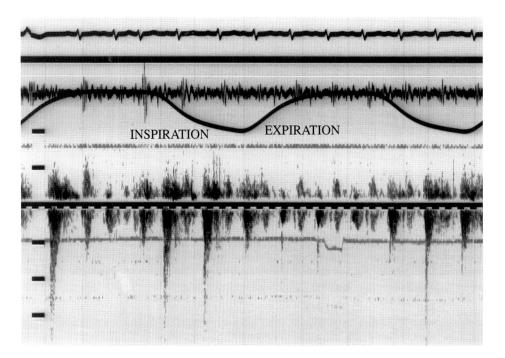

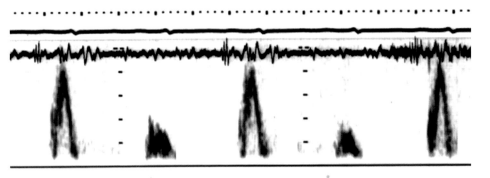

FIGURE 9.12. Inferior vena caval flow from a patient with DCM and severe breathlessness showing predominant inspiratory flow consistent with significantly raised intrathoracic pressure.

INSPIRATION   EXPIRATION

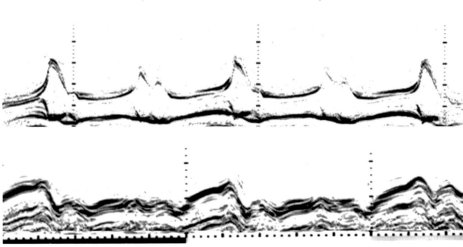

FIGURE 9.13. Transmitral forward-flow velocities, mitral valve echogram, and ventricular long-axis movement demonstrating alternating normal and compromised left ventricular filling along with failure of long-axis movement in the compromised cycles patient presented with pulsus alternans.

Progressive prolongation of ventricular depolarization has been shown to be associated with poor clinical outcome. This electrical disturbance is closely related to the delayed and prolonged ventricular shortening and lengthening and hence incoordination. The latter contributes to raised diastolic segmental wall tension resulting in presystolic mitral regurgitation. Such long mitral regurgitation can limit ventricular filling time, particularly at fast heart rate in patients with poor LV function, and consequently can reduce the stroke volume.[28]

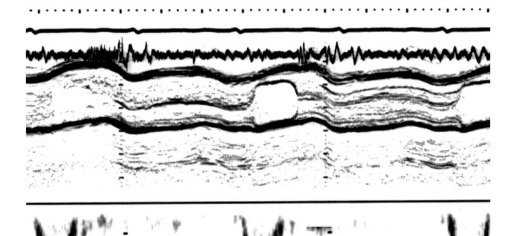

FIGURE 9.14. Aortic flow velocities and valve echogram from the same patient with pulsus alternans demonstrating alternating complete cessation of aortic flow and valve opening.

Although most of these ventricles fill with a single-component "summation filling pattern," the long mitral regurgitation adds to the raised left atrial pressure and pulmonary pressures.

FOLLOW-UP OF DCM

Patients with moderate or severe degree of LV impairment should be followed up regularly by Doppler echocardiography for the assessment of LV function, pressure, and complications, as well as for response to management. Although there are no current guidelines to suggest how frequently patients should be assessed, markers of increased filling pressure, pulmonary hypertension, and mitral regurgitation can provide an accurate indication for deterioration of ventricular function or beneficial response to therapy.

TREATMENT

Conventional management of dilated cardiomyopathy is with diuretics and Angiotensin-converting enzyme (ACE) inhibitors. The aim of this policy is to keep the filling pressures low and to protect against further deterioration of ventricular function. ACE inhibitors in particular have shown a significant effect on mortality reduction and improvement of clinical outcome in patients with dilated cardiomyopathy.[29] Doppler echocardiography assesses patient response to ACE inhibitors, particularly those

with raised left atrial pressure (restrictive filling pattern). Successful unloading of the atrium and the ventricle with ACE inhibition reverses the restrictive filling pattern to the dominant late diastolic filling pattern and unmasks LV incoordination.[30] This is usually associated with the disappearance of mitral regurgitation, a fall in left atrial size, and significant improvement of symptoms. As the LV early diastolic pressure gradient drops and its filling becomes nonrestrictive, the delay in the right ventricular filling regresses, overall right ventricular filling time increases, and the degree of pulmonary hypertension decreases.[19] β blockers have also been shown to improve outcome in patients with dilated cardiomyopathy and to reduce mortality.[31] In patients with poor LV function and tachycardia, small doses of β blockers (e.g., carvedilol) slow the heart rate and increase LV filling time and consequently stroke volume.[31] However, not all patients with dilated cardiomyopathy can tolerate β blockers. Those with late-stage ventricular disease and very short isovolumic relaxation time, in particular, seem to prefer a faster heart rate in order to sustain LV filling and cardiac output and therefore tolerate β blockers poorly.

Pacing

Patients presenting with a broad QRS complex (>150 ms) and long mitral regurgitation with a presystolic component that limits total LV filling time respond to Dual chamber pacing with optimized atrioventricular (A-V)

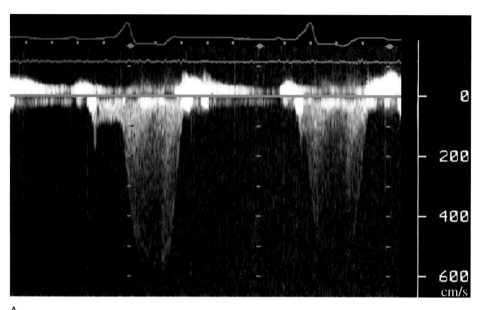

A

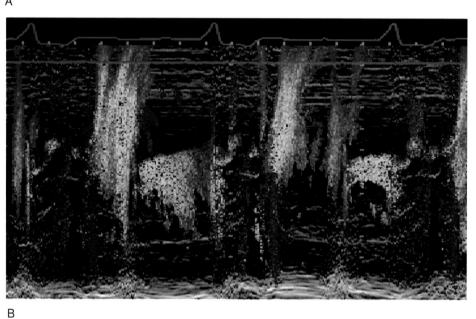

B

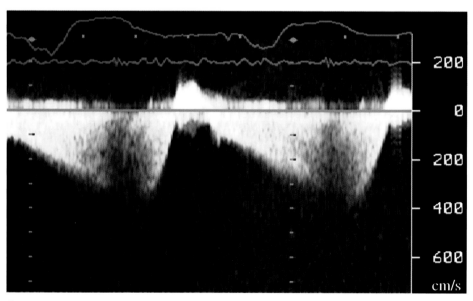

C

FIGURE 9.15. Continuous-wave Doppler recording demonstrating long mitral regurgitation in a patient with severe DCM. Note (A) the presystolic component on continuous-wave Doppler recording and (B) its corresponding velocities on color flow Doppler. (C) an extreme example of long mitral regurgitation.

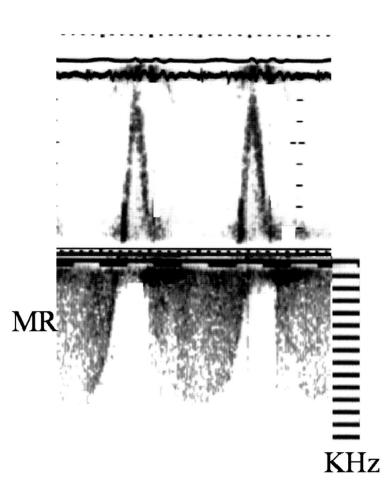

MR

KHz

FIGURE 9.16. Continuous-wave Doppler from a patient with late DCM and long mitral regurgitation that is limiting ventricular filling time.

delay. Short A-V delay results in immediate increase in filling time and stroke volume and improvement of overall cardiac performance.[30]

Long-term outcome of this intervention in individual patients is very satisfactory. Those who show significant early diastolic asynchrony, particularly of the LV free wall, that causes prolonged tension development and compromised early filling may benefit from biventricular pacing. The procedure aims at optimizing the time of LV free-wall stimulation that results in regression of asynchonous wall motion, and an increase in the overall ventricular filling time.[32] Long-term assessment of biventricular pacing mode needs further evaluation.

Assist Devices

Failure to control patient's symptoms by the preceding methods suggests the need for a ventricular assist device. The rationale behind the use of the assist device is a bridge to either recovery of ventricular function or transplantation. In a minority of patients, ventricular function recovers within weeks or months of the device insertion. The pump sucks from the ventricle and ejects directly into the aorta, thus reducing wall stress and allowing the myocardium to recover. The currently available assist devices are either phasic or continuous. The phasic Heart Mate functions independently of the cardiac cycle and carries the risk of significant interference with valve function and of clot formation.[33] The continuous pump is not without limitation, since at fast speed the suction force may cause mid-cavity obliteration, potential free-wall collapse, and high intracavity pressure difference between ventricular regions.[34]

Transplantation

Cardiac transplantation is now a well-established treatment, but because of the severe shortage of adequate donor organs this form of treatment is only available for a small number of patients. In general terms the most favorable recipients are young, highly motivated people with disease confined to their heart and with excellent renal, hepatic, and pulmonary function. The operation is an orthotopic heart transplant whereby the dilated heart is removed and a new donor heart is inserted with anastomoses at the left atrium, pulmonary artery, aorta, and caval orifices. Over the last 10 years the use of caval orifice anastomosis has become more usual, as this is found to result in a lower incidence of tricuspid regurgitation and improved right ventricular function. The main problems related to the management of these patients postoperatively are infection and the control of

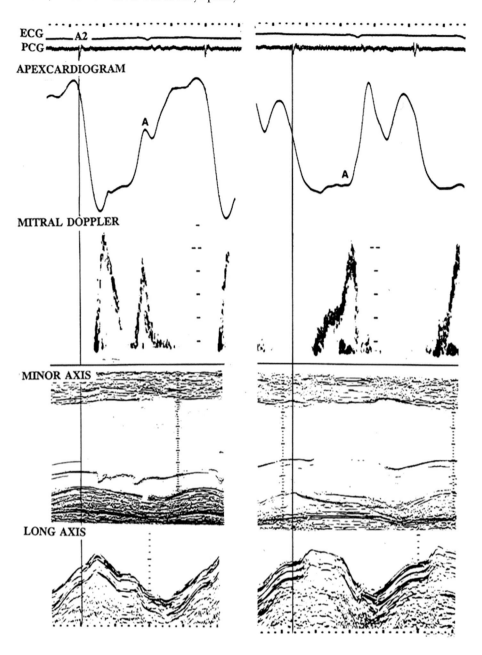

ECG
A2
PCG
APEXCARDIOGRAM
A
MITRAL DOPPLER
MINOR AXIS
LONG AXIS

FIGURE 9.17. Left ventricular filling and apex cardiogram from a patient with DCM and raised left atrial pressure (left) and its response to ACE inhibition (right). Note the significant fall in end-diastolic pressure with treatment and reversal of left ventricular filling pattern.

rejection. Modern immunosuppressive therapy with cyclosporin, mycophenolate mofetil, and a short course of steroids has resulted in significantly improved results. The 1-year survival after heart transplantation is of the order of 80%, and the 5-year survival is 70%. These patients require careful lifelong surveillance, largely because of the complications arising from immunosuppression. These complications comprise hypertension, which is extremely frequent and usually can be controlled by calcium channel blocker, renal impairment, slowly progressive LV fibrosis, B-cell hyperplasias, and tumors. Nevertheless, the quality of life from a good heart transplant is excellent, and more than 80% of these patients return to an active life for at least 10 years. This is a considerable achievement, given that the majority had a prognosis of less than 6 months at the time they were placed on the transplant waiting list.

PROGNOSIS

The prognosis of dilated cardiomyopathy differs significantly between patients. Although alcoholic cardiomyopathy tends to recover with abstinence from alcohol, other forms continue to cause deterioration over time. With medical therapy, patients may respond to ACE inhibitors, showing a reduction in left atrial pressure and improvement in overall cardiac function as well as symptoms. Patients who retain high left atrial pressure are considered unstable and are at risk of developing pulmonary hypertension, subendocardial ischemia, and arrhythmia. Long-standing high pulmonary wedge pressure is reflected on right ventricular function, which deteriorates irreversibly, with subsequent poor outcome. Right ventricular long-axis amplitude of less than 14 mm predicts poorer outcome than an amplitude of more than 14 mm.[35] Addi-

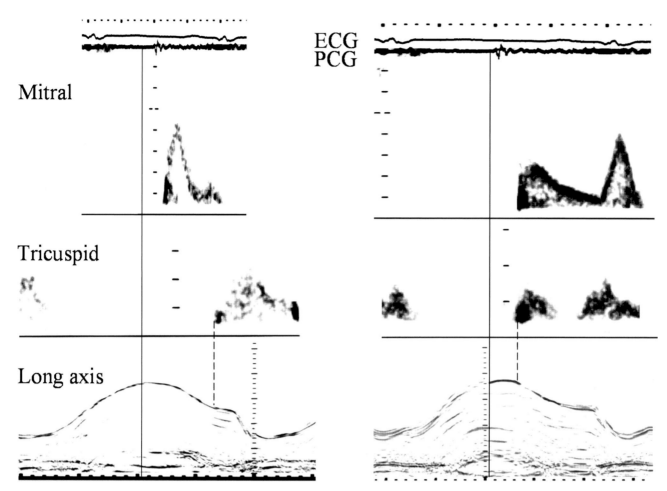

FIGURE 9.18. Left and right ventricular (RV) filling from a patient with restrictive filling before (left) and with angiotensin-converting enzyme inhibition (right). Note the normalization of the RV filling with off-loading of the left atrium.

tional right ventricular disease with a restrictive filling pattern makes the outcome poorer still. Although DDD pacing with A-V optimized delay has offered great assistance to overall ventricular performance in patients with dilated cardiomyopathy, no trials are available to support its beneficial use on a broader scale. Furthermore, although optimistic results with the use of biventricular pacing in patients with QRS of more than 150 ms were published in two different trials (MUSTIC & MIRACLE),[36,37] a number of resistant cases remain. This supports the need for stringent criteria regarding patient selection for different pacing modes in accordance with the underlying ventricular disturbances.

Signs of Disease Progression and Functional Deterioration

Signs of the progression of disease and functional deterioration include the following:

1. Development of restrictive LV filling with very short isovolumic relaxation time, which is resistant to off-loading by medication. Patients with this degree of disease cannot tolerate β blockers, and pacing seems unable to offer any functional assistance.

2. Right ventricular deterioration of function, particularly with raised right atrial pressures.

3. Severe mitral regurgitation or tricuspid regurgitation.

4. Progressive broadening of QRS associated with worsening of symptoms, ventricular function, and clinical outcome.

OTHER FORMS OF DILATED CARDIOMYOPATHY

Chagas Cardiomyopathy

Late-stage ventricular dysfunction may be indistinguishable from idiopathic dilated cardiomyopathy. Early stages of the disease can only be detected in seropositive subjects to *Trypanosoma cruzi,* commonly seen in South America. Although patients may be completely asymptomatic, some may present with conduction

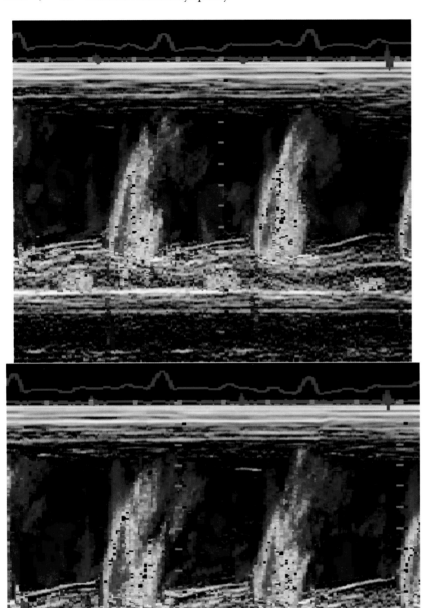

FIGURE 9.19. Colour M-mode of transmitral forward-flow velocities from a DCM patient with long mitral regurgitation before (top) and after (bottom) dual chamber pacing. Note the significant increase in LU filling time.

disturbances (right or left bundle branch block). Echocardiographically variable degrees of localized myocardial involvement may also be present (e.g., aneurysmal apex, hypokinetic basal septum, or incoordinate relaxation pattern). Late disease manifests as congestive heart failure with the two ventricles grossly dilated, high filling pressures, and A-V valve regurgitation.[38]

Right Ventricular Dysplasia

Right ventricular dysplasia is a rare condition that presents with either serious arrhythmia or sudden death. The right ventricle is selectively dilated, particularly at the apex that looks aneurysmal, with a significant increase in myocardial echo intensity. The right ventricular inlet and

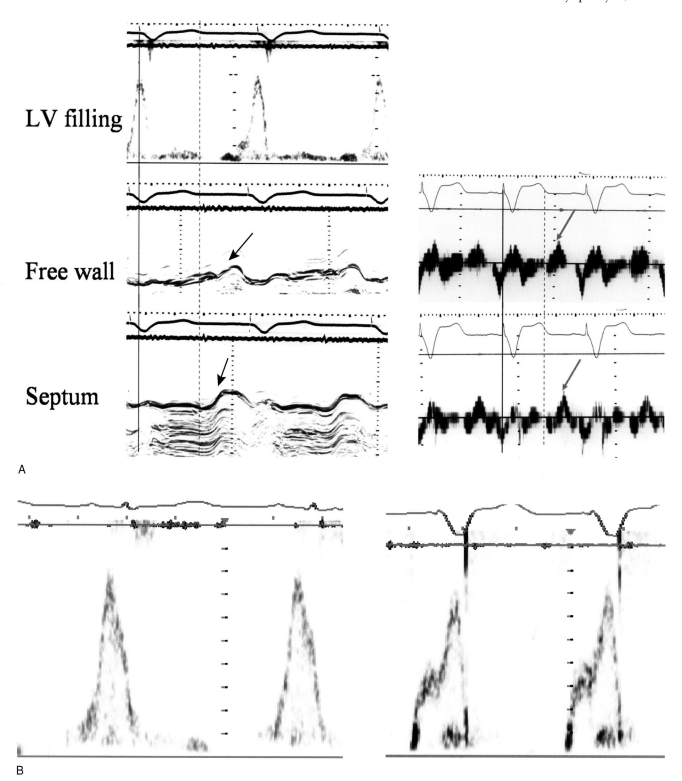

FIGURE 9.20. (A) Patient with DCM and early diastolic asynchrony (on M-mode and tissue Doppler velocities) (arrows) and limited filling to late diastole. (B) Left ventricular filling from a patient with DCM before (left) and after (right) biventricular pacing showing increased filling time.

LVAD   LVAD
S1 S2   eject   fill

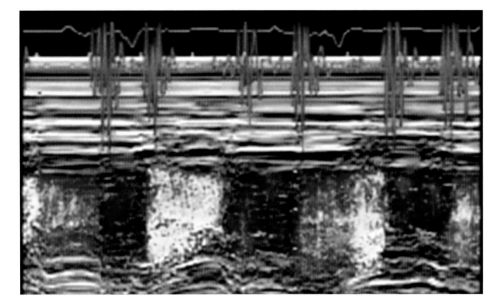

FIGURE 9.21. Color M-mode of left ventricular filling from a patient with DCM and phasic assist device. Note the independent pump filling and ejection with respect to the cardiac cycle.

Apex

Base

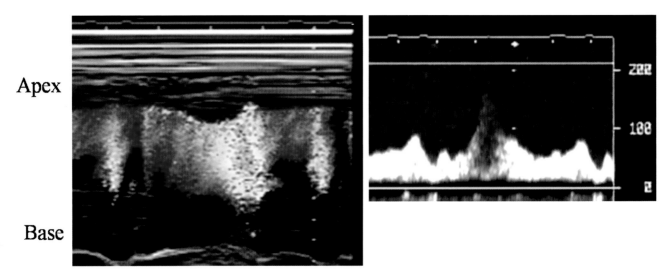

FIGURE 9.22. Color M-mode from a patient with DCM and continuous assist device. Note the high mid-cavity velocities with fast speed (right) and mid-cavity obliteration (left).

exit are also dilated. Right ventricular myocardium is replaced by fibrolipomatous material, as shown in the pathology specimens.[39]

Pharmacologic Cardiomyopathy

Cardiotoxic pharmacologic agents used for treating malignancy may have a damaging effect on the myocardium. Doxorubicin and cyclophosphamide in therapeutic doses may cause severe myocardial dys-function and deterioration of ventricular function, although end-diastolic volume may remain within normal limits. Doxorubicin toxicity is particularly dose-related but tends to recover after reducing the drug dosage or its rate. Cyclophosphamide given as an immunosuppressive agent may cause rapid onset of interstitial myocardial hemorrhage and suppression of ventricular systolic function. Chloroquine has also been documented to have a significant cardiotoxic effect.[40]

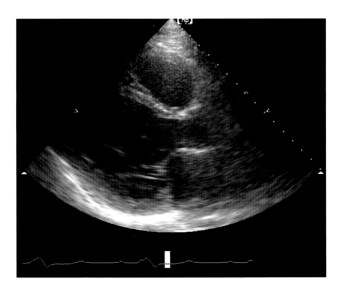

FIGURE 9.23. Left ventricular minor axis recording from a patient with late Chagas disease showing dilated cavity and poor systolic function.

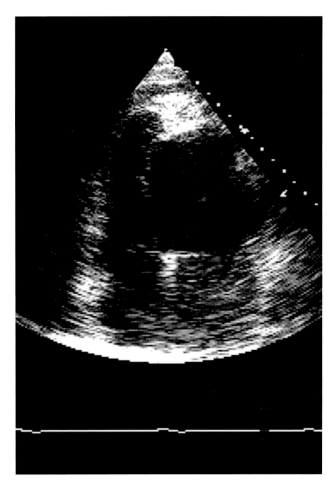

FIGURE 9.25. Apical four-chamber view from a patient with right ventricular (RV) dysplasia showing aneurysmal RV apex.

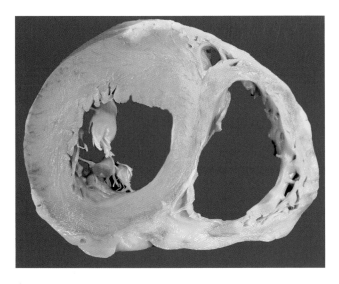

A

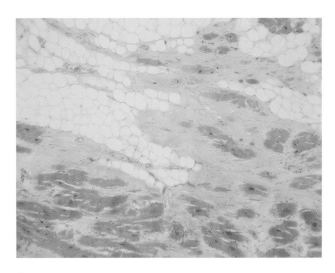

B

FIGURE 9.24. (A) Transverse section of the heart showing transmural fatty replacement of the right ventricle that extends to the anterior wall of the left ventricle with fibrous scarring from a patient with right ventricular dysplasia. (B) Histologic section showing distorted myocytes surrounded by pale fibrous tissue and fatty infiltration.

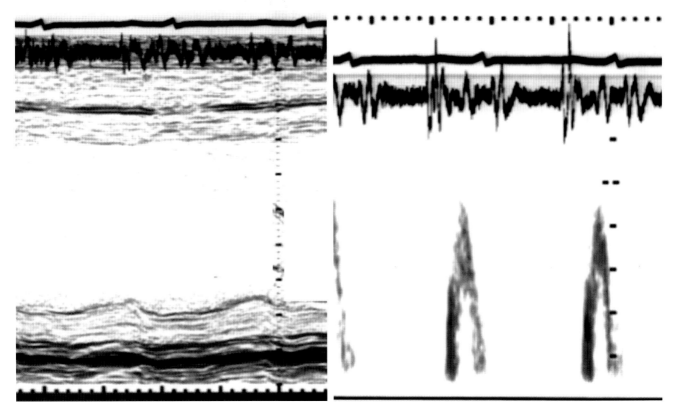

FIGURE 9.26. Left ventricular minor-axis recording from a patient presenting with breathlessness after doxorubicin treatment. Note the poor systolic function and the limited filling time.

Neurologic Cardiomyopathy

Ventricular involvement in neurologic disorders is related to individual conditions. Friedreich's ataxia is associated with ventricular hypertrophy, and Nemaline myopathy is associated with biventricular dilatation that is indistinguishable from dilated cardiomyopathy. Duchenne muscle dystrophy and Becker's disease both present with segmental ventricular dysfunction caused by localized fibrosis. Finally, dystrophia myotonia is associated with conduction disturbances and localized segmental ventricular dysfunction.[41]

REFERENCES

1. Goodwin JF. Congestive and hypertrophic cardiomyopathies. A decade of study. *Lancet* 1970;1:732–739.
2. Corya B, Feigenbaum H, Rasmussen S, et al. Echocardiographic features of congestive cardiomyopathy compared with normal subjects and patients with coronary artery disease. *Circulation* 1974;49:1153–1159.
3. Towbin JA, Hejtmancik JF, Brink P, et al. X-linked dilated cardiomyopathy. Molecular genetic evidence of linkage to the Duchenne muscular dystrophy (dystrophin) gene at the Xp21 locus. *Circulation* 1993;87:1854–1865.
4. Hadjimiltiades S, Panidis IP, Segal BL, et al. Recovery of left ventricular function in peripartum cardiomyopathy. *Am Heart J* 1986;112:1097–1099.
5. Sutton MS, Cole P, Plappert M, et al. Effects of subsequent pregnancy on left ventricular function in peripartum cardiomyopathy. *Am Heart J* 1991;121(6 Pt 1):1776–1778.
6. Cambridge G, MacArthur CG, Waterson AP, et al. Antibodies to Coxsackie B viruses in congestive cardiomyopathy. *Br Heart J* 1979;41:692–696.
7. Obeyesekere I, Hermon Y. Arbovirus heart disease: myocarditis and cardiomyopathy following dengue and chikungunya fever–a follow-up study. *Am Heart J* 1973;85:186–194.
8. Corallo S, Mutinelli MR, Moroni M, et al. Echocardiography detects myocardial damage in AIDS: prospective study in 102 patients. *Eur Heart J* 1988;9:887–892.
9. Herskowitz A, Vlahov D, Willoughby S, et al. Prevalence and incidence of left ventricular dysfunction in patients with human immunodeficiency virus infection. *Am J Cardiol* 1993;71:955–958.
10. Abelmann WH, Lorell BH. The challenge of cardiomyopathy. *J Am Coll Cardiol* 1989;13:1219–1239.
11. DeMaria AN, Bommer W, Lee G, et al. Value and limitations of two dimensional echocardiography in assessment of cardiomyopathy. *Am J Cardiol* 1980;46:1224–1231.
12. Medina R, Panidis IP, Morganroth J, et al. The value of echocardiographic regional wall motion abnormalities in detecting coronary artery disease in patients with or without a dilated left ventricle. *Am Heart J* 1985;109:799–803.
13. Wallis DE, O'Connell JB, Henkin RE, et al. Segmental wall motion abnormalities in dilated cardiomyopathy: a common finding and good prognostic sign. *J Am Coll Cardiol* 1984;4:674–679.

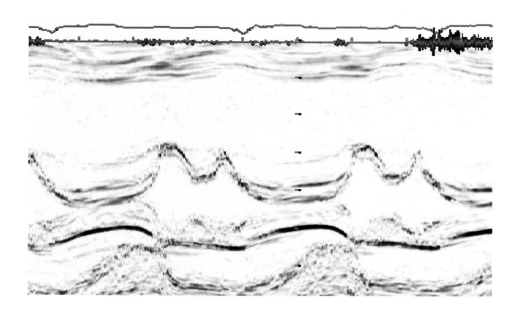

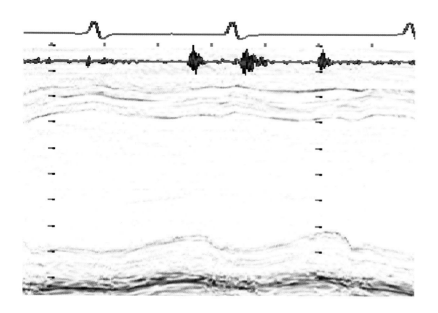

FIGURE 9.27. M-mode recording from a patient with Duchenne muscle dystrophy showing enlarged left ventricular cavity and zero isovolumic relaxation time consistent with left atrial pressure of 30 mmHg.

14. Yazawa Y, Hayashi S, Hosokawa O, et al. [Regional wall motion of the left ventricle in congestive cardiomyopathy: in comparison with progressive muscular dystrophy of Duchenne type (author's transl)]. *J Cardiogr* 1981;11:1233–1239.

15. Laskey WK, Sutton MS, Zeevi G, et al. Left ventricular mechanics in dilated cardiomyopathy. *Am J Cardiol* 1984;54:620–625.

16. Takenaka K, Dabestani A, Gardin JM, et al. Pulsed Doppler echocardiographic study of left ventricular filling in dilated cardiomyopathy. *Am J Cardiol* 1986;58:143–147.

17. Appleton CP, Hatle LK, Popp RL. Demonstration of restrictive ventricular physiology by Doppler echocardiography. *J Am Coll Cardiol* 1988;11:757–768.

18. Henein MY, Gibson DG. Abnormal subendocardial function in restrictive left ventricular disease. *Br Heart J* 1994;72:237–242.

19. Henein MY, O'Sullivan CA, Coats AJ, et al. Angiotensin-converting enzyme (ACE) inhibitors revert abnormal right ventricular filling in patients with restrictive left ventricular disease. *J Am Coll Cardiol* 1998;32:1187–1193.

20. Dickerman SA, Rubler S. Mitral and tricuspid valve regurgitation in dilated cardiomyopathy. *Am J Cardiol* 1989;63:629–631.

21. Nishimura RA, Abel MD, Hatle LK, et al. Relation of pulmonary vein to mitral flow velocities by transesophageal Doppler echocardiography. Effect of different loading conditions. *Circulation* 1990;81:1488–1497.

22. Pinamonti B, Di Lenarda A, Sinagra G, et al. Restrictive left ventricular filling pattern in dilated cardiomyopathy assessed by Doppler echocardiography: clinical, echocardiographic and hemodynamic correlations and prognostic implications. *J Am Coll Cardiol* 1993;22:808–815.

23. Rossvoll O, Hatle LK. Pulmonary venous flow velocities recorded by transthoracic Doppler ultrasound: relation to left ventricular diastolic pressures. *J Am Coll Cardiol* 1993;21:1687–1696.

24. Yock PG, Popp RL. Noninvasive estimation of right ventricular systolic pressure by Doppler ultrasound in patients with tricuspid regurgitation. *Circulation* 1984;70:657–662.

25. Gottdiener JS, Gay JA, Van Voorhees L, et al. Frequency and embolic potential of left ventricular thrombus in dilated cardiomyopathy: assessment by 2-dimensional echocardiography. *Am J Cardiol* 1983;52:1281–1285.

26. Asinger RW, Mikell FL, Sharma B, et al. Observations on detecting left ventricular thrombus with two dimensional echocardiography: emphasis on avoidance of false positive diagnoses. *Am J Cardiol* 1981;47:145–156.

27. Shamim W, Yousufuddin M, Cicoria M, et al. Incremental changes in QRS duration in serial ECGs over time identify high risk elderly patients with heart failure. *Heart* 2002;88:47–51.

28. Brecker SJ, Xiao HB, Sparrow J, et al. Effects of dual-chamber pacing with short atrioventricular delay in dilated cardiomyopathy. *Lancet* 1992;340:1308–1312.

29. Effects of enalapril on mortality in severe congestive heart failure. Results of the Cooperative North Scandinavian Enalapril Survival Study (CONSENSUS). *N Engl J Med* 1987;316:1429–1435.

30. Henein MY, Amadi A, O'Sullivan C, et al. ACE inhibitors unmask incoordinate diastolic wall motion in restrictive left ventricular disease. *Heart* 1996;76:326–331.

31. Hjalmarson A, Goldstein S, Fagerberg B, et al. Effects of controlled-release metoprolol on total mortality, hospitalizations, and well-being in patients with heart failure: the Metoprolol CR/XL Randomized Intervention Trial in congestive heart failure (MERIT-HF). *JAMA* 2000;283:1295–1302.

32. Yu CM, Lin H, Fung WH, et al. Comparison of acute changes in left ventricular volume, systolic and diastolic functions, and intraventricular synchronicity after biventricular and right ventricular pacing for heart failure. *Am Heart J* 2003;145:E18.

33. Dalby MC, Banner NR, Tansley P, et al. Left ventricular function during support with an asynchronous pulsatile left ventricular assist device. *J Heart Lung Transplant* 2003;22:292–300.

34. Henein M, Birks EJ, Tansley PD, et al. Images in cardiovascular medicine. Temporal and spatial changes in left ventricular pattern of flow during continuous assist device "HeartMate II." *Circulation* 2002;105:2324–2325.

35. Ghio S, Recusani F, Klersy C, et al. Prognostic usefulness of the tricuspid annular plane systolic excursion in patients with congestive heart failure secondary to idiopathic or ischemic dilated cardiomyopathy. *Am J Cardiol* 2000;85:837–842.

36. Linde C, Leclercq C, Rex S, et al. Long-term benefits of biventricular pacing in congestive heart failure: results from the MUltisite STimulation in cardiomyopathy (MUSTIC) study. *J Am Coll Cardiol* 2002;40:111–118.

37. Abraham WT, Fisher WG, Smith AL, et al. Cardiac resynchronization in chronic heart failure. *N Engl J Med* 2002;346:1845–1853.

38. Patel AR, Lima C, Parro A, et al. Echocardiographic analysis of regional and global left ventricular shape in Chagas' cardiomyopathy. *Am J Cardiol* 1998;82:197–202.

39. Kisslo J. Two-dimensional echocardiography in arrhythmogenic right ventricular dysplasia. *Eur Heart J* 1989;10(Suppl D):22–26.

40. Nousiainen T, Jantunen E, Vanninen E, et al. Early decline in left ventricular ejection fraction predicts doxorubicin cardiotoxicity in lymphoma patients. *Br J Cancer* 2002;86:1697–1700.

41. de Kermadec JM, Becane HM, Chenard A, et al. Prevalence of left ventricular systolic dysfunction in Duchenne muscular dystrophy: an echocardiographic study. *Am Heart J* 1994;127:618–623.

10 Hypertrophic Cardiomyopathy

Hypertrophic cardiomyopathy (HCM) is a primary cardiac disorder with unique pathophysiology, heterogeneous expression, and diverse clinical presentations. It is probably the most common genetically transmitted heart disease. HCM is often familial, is transmitted by autosomal dominant means, and has a high degree of penetrance. The latter is age related, with typical features developing during adolescence. The disease is characterized by mutations in the DNA encoding β cardiac myosin heavy chain (chromosome 14), a tropomyosin (chromosome 15), and cardiac troponin T (chromosome 1), in addition to a locus on chromosome 11.[1–6] Despite dramatic improvements in understanding HCM, challenges and controversies regarding its diagnosis, etiology, natural history, and management still exist. Terminology is likewise difficult, but HCM is generally preferred,

avoiding the term *idiopathic subaortic stenosis* or *hypertrophic obstructive cardiomyopathy,* which implies left ventricular (LV) outflow tract obstruction. It also excludes secondary causes of LV hypertrophy.[7,8]

CLINICAL PICTURE

Patients with HCM may be asymptomatic and may be discovered accidentally during family screening for sudden death or medical check-up that reveals LV hypertrophy and T-wave changes on resting ECG. Others may rarely present with arrhythmias, shortness of breath, or chest pain. Postmortem diagnosis of HCM may be the first presentation in patients with sudden cardiac death.

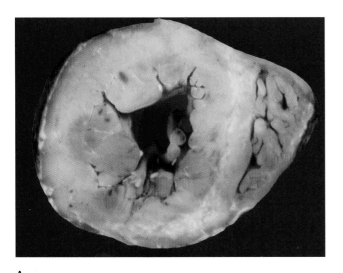

A

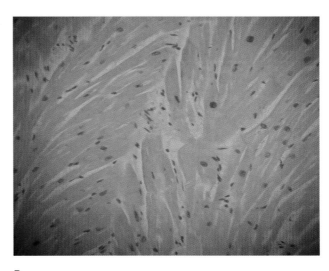

B

FIGURE 10.1. (A) Transverse section of the left and right ventricles of a hypertrophic cardiomyopathy patient showing concentric hypertrophy of the left ventricle with scarring involving the subendocardium interventricular septum and posterior wall. (B) Histologic section showing disarrayed and hypertrophied myocytes at abnormal angles to each other.

PATHOLOGY

The distribution of myocardial hypertrophy in HCM may be generalized (symmetric)[9,10] or localized (asymmetric).[11,12] The localized hypertrophy tends to affect predominantly the anteroseptal wall of the left ventricle, but it may involve other regions (i.e., posterior wall, ventricular apex, the right ventricle, or rarely, isolated thickened muscle trabeculae in the ventricular cavity).[13] The degree of segmental hypertrophy varies and may be extensive, with a septal thickness up to 40 mm.

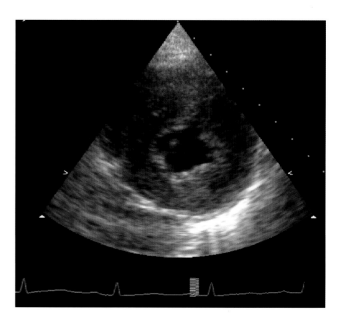

FIGURE 10.2. Left ventricular minor axis view in diastole showing concentric myocardial hypertrophy.

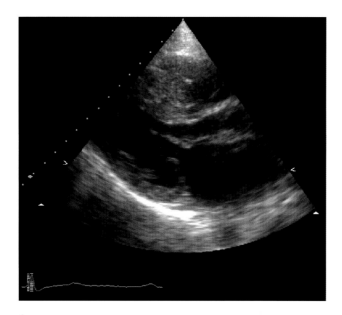

FIGURE 10.3. Parasternal long-axis two-dimensional view (A) from a patient with localized septal hypertrophic cardiomyopathy and (B) corresponding M-mode recording.

A

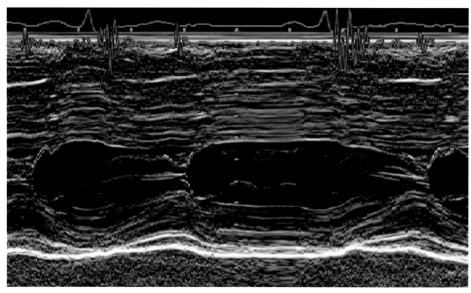

B

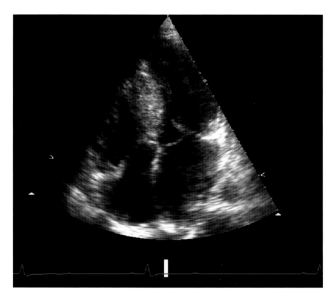
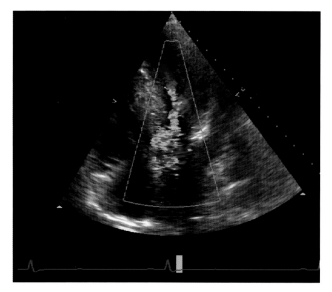

A   B

FIGURE 10.4. Apical four-chamber view from a patient with hypertrophic candiomyopathy. Note (A) the systolic anterior move-ment (SAM) of the mitral valve and (B) the resulting high-outflow tract velocities by color Doppler.

PHYSIOLOGY

It is generally believed that LV hypertrophy is subject to dynamic changes as part of the HCM disease process, through the consistent narrowing of the outflow tract by approximation of anterior mitral valve leaflet to the prox-imal interventricular septum in systole, possibly as a result of a "Venturi effect."[14] This systolic anterior move-ment (SAM) of the mitral valve is a characteristic echocardiographic feature of the LV outflow tract nar-rowing or obstruction, and results in significant high velocities (equivalent to a pressure drop) with an increase in heart rate. In a number of patients with this condition the main site of myocardial bulk is the mid cavity, which results in mid-cavity obliteration rather than outflow tract obstruction.[15–17] The apical form of HCM is commonly seen in Japan with characteristic ECG presentation of giant negative T waves.[18]

Systolic anterior movement of the mitral valve is always associated with some degree of LV outflow tract obstruction (pressure drop or high velocities) at rest. In symptomatic patients with morphologic ventricular fea-tures of HCM but no signs of outflow tract obstruction, a form of stress test (Valsalva or dobutamine) often helps in demonstrating signs of dynamic outflow tract obstruction and high pressure drop (gradient) that may coincide with development of symptoms.

Raised outflow tract velocities in HCM must be distin-guished from benign intracavitary gradients that have no significant hemodynamic effect and are not usually asso-ciated with symptoms.[19] What confirms the direct rela-tionship between SAM of the mitral valve and outflow tract velocities is the disappearance of SAM when the

systolic outflow tract gradient is abolished either by myotomy–myectomy, alcohol septal ablation, or mitral valve plication.

Systolic anterior movement of the valve may result from papillary muscle coaption with the septum rather than from the mitral leaflets themselves in patients with hypertrophied papillary muscle that inserts directly into the mitral valve leaflets.[20] In these cases, mitral valve pli-cation or replacement may be the most appropriate man-agement in order to separate the papillary muscle from the mitral valve movement.[21]

The level of LV cavity narrowing can also be deter-mined by color flow Doppler, since it demonstrates non-linear (mosaic) flow on two-dimensional images at the site of narrowing. The degree of outflow tract obstruction or mid-cavity obliteration is determined by continuous-wave Doppler recordings in the form of a pressure drop. The shape of the continuous-wave velocity trace is helpful in differentiating between outflow tract obstruc-tion (that peaks in mid systole) and mid-cavity oblitera-tion (whose velocity peaks in late systole).

With symmetric hypertrophy, the LV cavity is crescentic rather than ellipsoid on the apical views. This shape change may itself contribute to the systolic anterior mitral valve movement and narrowing of the outflow tract. Complete apical obliteration may occur when asymmetric septal hypertrophy is solely apical.[22,23]

In HCM, the septum is commonly hypokinetic and contributes little to the overall systolic function of the left ventricle. To maintain the stroke volume, the ventricular free wall becomes hyperactive. Septal hypokinesis[24,25] should not be confused with that due to coronary artery disease, particularly its lengthening velocity, in early

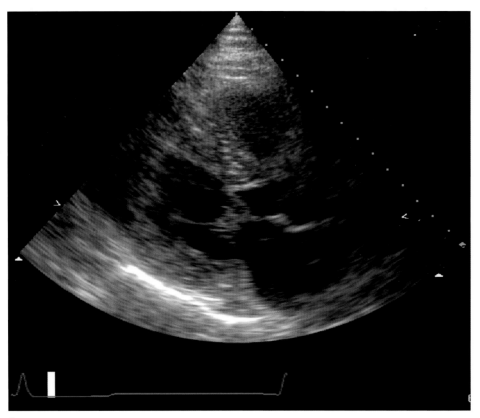

A

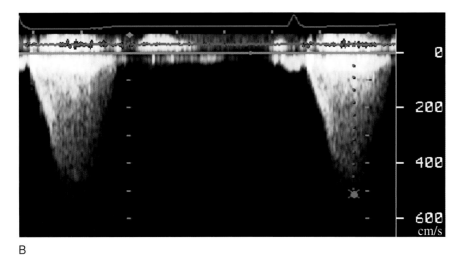

B

FIGURE 10.5. Parasternal long-axis view of the left ventricle from a patient with HCM. Note the systolic anterior movement of the mitral valve, narrowing the outflow tract in systole. (A) Two-dimensional image and (B) continuous-wave Doppler gradient.

diastole. This can be confirmed by stress echo, as it demonstrates normal increase in septal velocities of movement but less than normal increase of its amplitude. These findings suggest compromised septal distensibility rather than ischemic dysfunction. The coronary arteries in HCM are commonly large and not obstructed, although coronary velocities may be less than normal in a considerable number of patients.

Mid-systolic aortic valve closure accompanies SAM of the mitral valve and probably reflects its disturbing effect to the outflow tract jet during systole. This is a fre-

quently seen echocardiographic feature of subaortic (outflow tract) obstruction; if not present at rest, it appears with stress as SAM of the mitral valve obstructs the outflow tract in late systole.

Raised LV outflow tract velocities at rest or with stress must be distinguished from mitral regurgitation using color flow and continuous-wave Doppler.[26] Although color flow Doppler may demonstrate jet direction at rest, continuous-wave Doppler is more confirmatory, particularly during stress and fast heart rate. The main difference between the two is that the outflow tract velocity signal

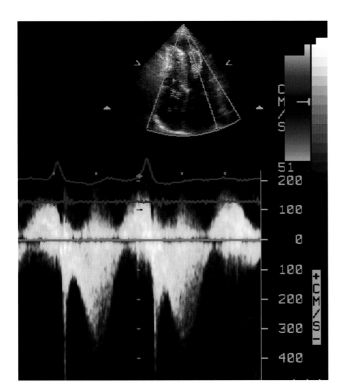

FIGURE 10.6. Continuous wave Doppler from a patient with hypertrophic cardiomyopathy and mid-cavity narrowing demonstrating late systolic pressure drop with stress, characteristic for mid-cavity obliteration.

stops at end ejection in HCM but persists beyond A2 in mitral regurgitation.

A number of observations consistent with LV hypertrophy but not specific for HCM are observed during diastole. Isovolumic relaxation time is prolonged, and early diastolic LV filling velocity is reduced with prolonged deceleration time. These findings are consistent with increased dispersion of early diastolic lengthening velocities and normal LV filling pressure.[27,28]

Patients with apical hypertrophy and mid-cavity obliteration may show intracavitary flow during the isovolumic periods, suggesting either differences in pressure within the ventricle or significant shape change of the cavity.[29] Passive stiffness of the myocardium may also be abnormal in late diastole. This results in raised ventricular end-diastolic pressure and left atrial pressure. Late stages of myocardial disease are associated with left atrial dilatation, mitral regurgitation, and atrial fibrillation.

NATURAL HISTORY

HCM may remain silent for years until it is accidentally discovered. There is no set course for the disease process. Symptoms may remain well controlled by medications for years, but once the myocardium becomes stiff and intraventricular pressure rises, patients complain of breathlessness or arrhythmia (often atrial fibrillation). Patients presenting with HCM picture later in life (sixth decade and beyond) are usually hypertensive with some degree of ventricular hypertrophy that predominantly affects the proximal septum.[30] These patients' main complaint is often exertional breathlessness rather than chest pain or arrhythmia. Symptoms can easily be provoked and cardiac function assessed using dobutamine stress. Basal septal hypertrophy, if significant, causes LV outflow tract obstruction during stress with the development of SAM

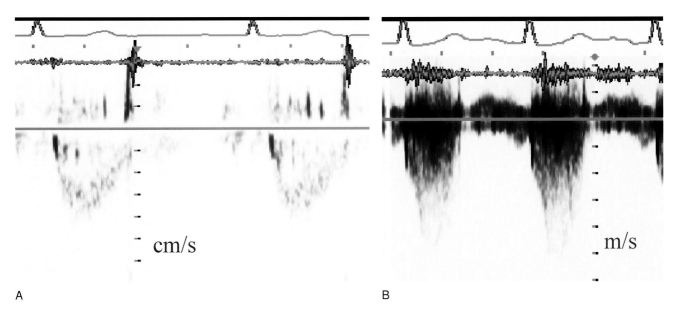

A   B

FIGURE 10.7. Left ventricular (LV) outflow tract velocity (continuous-wave Doppler) from a patient with hypertrophic cardiomyopathy, (A) at rest and (B) peak stress. Note the significant increase in LV outflow tract pressure drop (gradient) to 110 mmHg with stress, also notice the appearance of systolic murmur on the phonocardiogram.

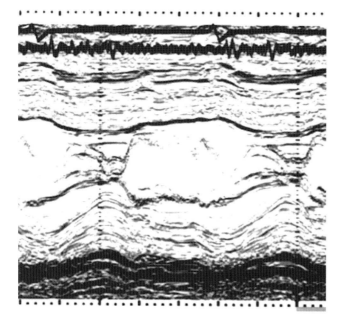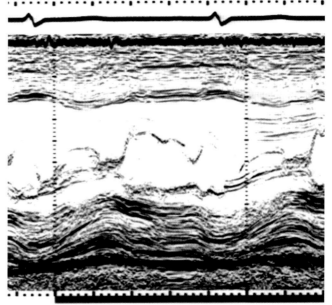

FIGURE 10.8. Mitral valve echogram from a patient with hypertrophic cardiomyopathy showing systolic anterior movement of the mitral valve (left) that disappeared after alcohol septal ablation (right).

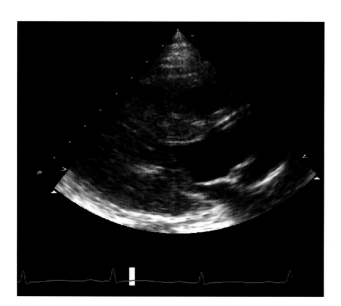

FIGURE 10.9. Parasternal long-axis view from a patient with hypertrophic cardiomyopathy involving the papillary muscles. Note the anterior displacement of the papillary muscles and their movement that narrows the outflow tract.

of the mitral valve and a modest drop in systolic blood pressure at the time of symptoms in a similar fashion to middle-age HCM.[31] This basal septal hypertrophy has a benign outcome, in contrast to HCM, and in the majority of patients symptoms can be controlled by β blockers.[32] Regardless of the echocardiographic picture, the clinical course in HCM is unpredictable. In a number of patients, the classical picture of HCM may change over the years

to that of dilated cardiomyopathy, leaving residual asymmetric segmental hypertrophy. This progression is difficult to predict.[33]

MITRAL VALVE DYSFUNCTION IN HCM

Mitral regurgitation is commonly seen in HCM. It is often mild but may become significant in advanced LV disease. A number of mechanisms may contribute to the alteration of normal function of the mitral valve and development of mitral regurgitation in HCM.

1. Hypertrophy of the posterior papillary muscle may displace the mitral valve anteriorly, resulting in apposition of the anterior mitral valve leaflet to the septum.[34]

2. The anterior mitral valve leaflet area and length are both greater than normal in HCM despite the normal diameter of the mitral valve annulus circumference. This causes the two leaflets to coapt together half way through their length, leaving the distal part redundant in the LV cavity. With the increase in LV cavity pressure during early systole the freely mobile mitral leaflet tips are forced against the proximal part of the ventricular septum, hence reducing the outflow tract diameter and causing outflow tract pressure gradient.[35,36]

3. The abnormal behavior of the mitral valve leaflets in systole results in significant deformation of its orifice area; consequently, mitral regurgitation, of varying severity, may develop.

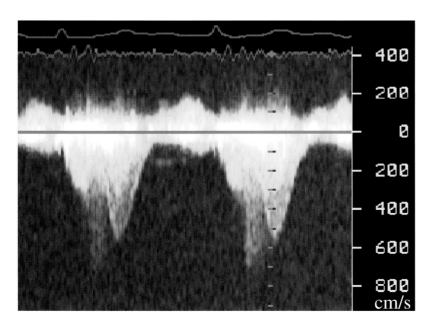

FIGURE 10.10. Continuous-wave Doppler of the left ventricular outflow tract from a patient with hypertrophic cardiomyopathy and outflow tract narrowing. Note the raised velocities that peak in mid systole in addition to another late-systolic high-velocity component due to mid-cavity obliteration.

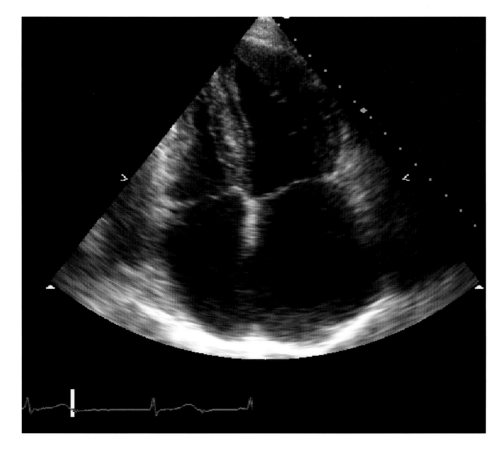

FIGURE 10.11. Apical four-chamber view from a patient with hypertrophic cardiomyopathy demonstrating obliterated apex.

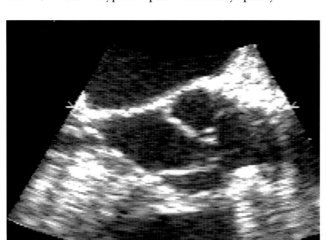

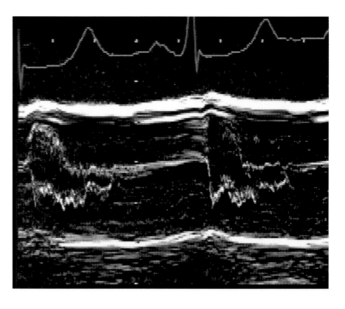

FIGURE 10.12. Transesophageal echo of the aortic valve from a patient with hypertrophic cardiomyopathy demonstrating mid-systolic valve closure on two-dimensional echo (left) and M-mode (right).

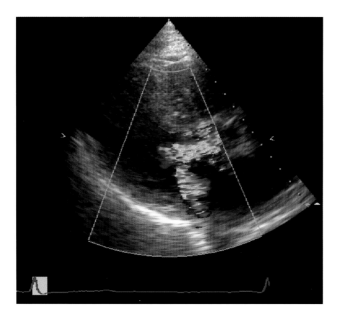

FIGURE 10.13. Color flow Doppler recordings from a patient with hypertrophic cardiomyopathy at peak dobutamine stress showing systolic anterior movement of the mitral valve and high outflow tract velocities and functional mitral regurgitation.

4, In late stages of the disease, diastolic pressure and left atrial pressure increase as the LV cavity becomes stiff and the atrium and mitral ring dilate. This may result in functional mitral regurgitation.

EXERCISE INTOLERANCE IN HYPERTROPHIC CARDIOMYOPATHY

A number of factors may contribute to exercise intolerance known in patients with HCM:

1. An increase in LV outflow tract velocities (gradient) with exercise results in a drop in systolic blood pressure at the time of symptom development.

2. High outflow tract pressure drop may aggravate mitral regurgitation, thus adding to the increase in left atrial pressures and pulmonary congestion.

3. Exercise-induced increased outflow tract pressure drop prolongs systole and shortens diastole, thus limiting ventricular filling time. This disturbed physiology is associated with raised left atrial pressure.

4. The raised left atrial pressure itself may contribute to exercise intolerance by increasing pulmonary venous pressure and causing exacerbating subendocardial ischemia.

5. Arrhythmia may be the main exercise-limiting factor in HCM. This tends to manifest at fast heart rates and during exercise/stress.

6. Right ventricular function is an important contributing factor to exercise tolerance. When involved in the disease process, its function is bound to be disturbed and hence its overall performance may influence exercise capacity.

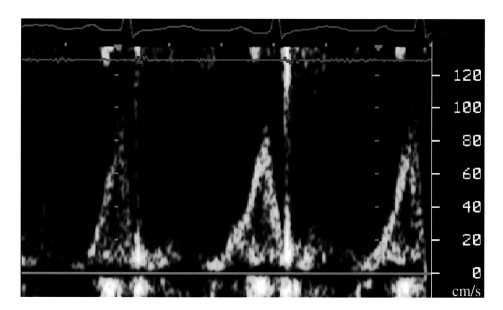

FIGURE 10.14. Left ventricular filling from a patient with hypertrophic cardiomyopathy and slow relaxation, demonstrating dominant late diastolic filling.

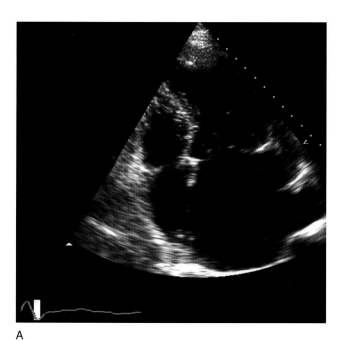

A

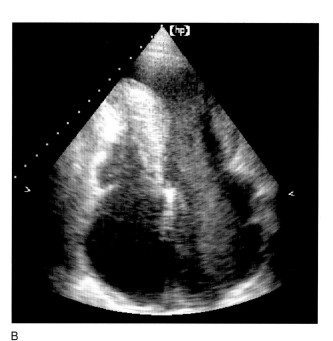

B

FIGURE 10.15. (A) Apical views from a patient with HOCM. Note the systolic anterior movement of the mitral leaflets and the dilated left atrium. (B) Apical 4 chamber view from a patient with HCM and impaired LV function. Note the spontaneous echo contrast in the cavity, a sign of slow circulation.

MANAGEMENT

Medical

No current treatment is expected to prevent or stop disease progression in HCM. The main objective of medical treatment is symptom control. β blockers and/or calcium antagonists (e.g., verapamil) have been used to control frequent arrhythmia and increases in heart rate that may be associated with syncopal attacks. Disopyramide, with its negative inotropic effect, has been used as an alternative to verapamil, mainly in patients demonstrating outflow tract obstruction at rest. Digitalis or amiodarone can be used to control the ventricular rate in patients with symptomatic atrial fibrillation along with anticoagulation to prevent thromboembolism. Reversion to sinus rhythm either medically or electrically and its maintenance is always desirable. However, patients with poor ventricular compliance and raised left atrial pressure may prefer atrial fibrillation to sinus rhythm, since the stroke volume generated by atrial contraction is pumped retrogradely into the pulmonary veins, resulting in wors-

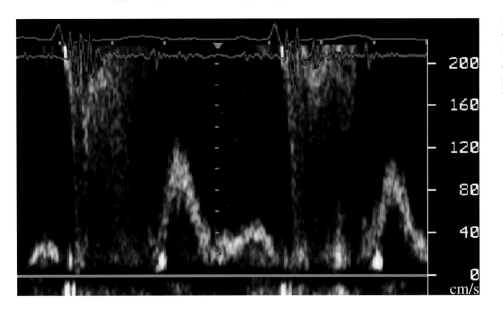

FIGURE 10.16. Left ventricular filling from a patient with hypertrophic cardiomyopathy demonstrating restrictive filling pattern and a third sound III on the phonocardiogram.

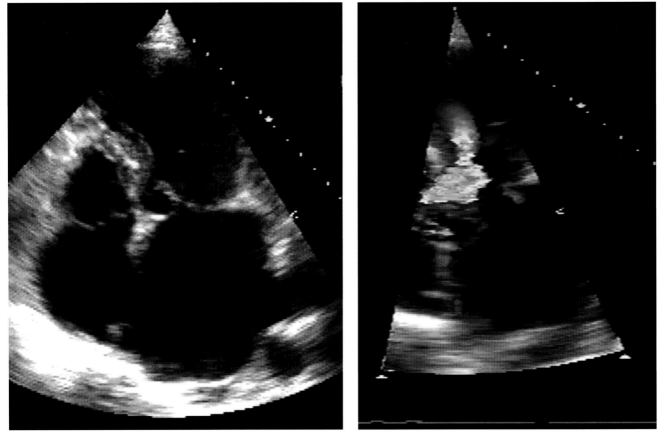

FIGURE 10.17. Apical view from an elderly patient with basal septal hypertrophy, SAM (left) and color aliasing in the outflow tract (right).

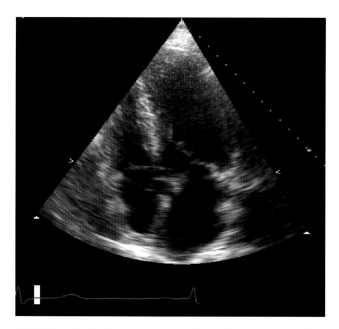

FIGURE 10.18. Apical view of the mitral valve leaflets showing mid-length coaption in mid systole and anterior movement of the leaflet tips.

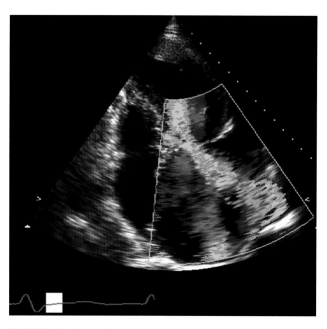

FIGURE 10.19. Apical four-chamber view from a patient with hypertrophic cardiomyopathy and severe mitral regurgitation.

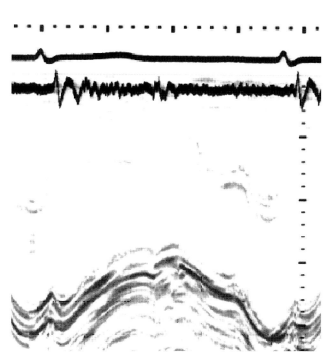

FIGURE 10.20. Left ventricular free-wall long-axis recording demonstrating gross incoordination (postejection shortening) consistent with subendocardial ischemia.

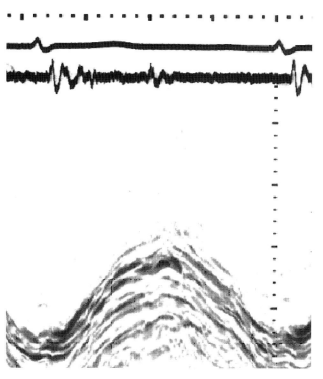

FIGURE 10.21. Right ventricular long-axis recording from a patient with hypertrophic cardiomyopathy and right ventricular involvement demonstrating reduced amplitude of movement (that corresponds to ejection fraction).

ening pulmonary congestion. When there are symptoms of congestion due to a high left atrial pressure, careful use of a diuretic or even an angiotensin-converting enzyme inhibitor may be considered.

Pacing

Dual chamber pacing has been used in patients in whom medical treatment is unsuccessful in an attempt to divert septal contraction from being left-sided to become right ventricular. The procedure rationale is widening the LV outflow tract and lowering the pressure drop (gradient) in the outflow tract and hence improvement of symptoms. Results of DDD pacing are unpredictable, and early changes in ventricular behavior have not been thoroughly documented. Pacing the right ventricular apex has produced significant reduction in LV outflow tract gradient compared with upper septal pacing. However, in some patients, symptoms do not change or even become worse with dual-chamber pacing. Long-term symptomatic improvement reflected in quality-of-life data has not been accompanied by objective assessment of exercise tolerance.[37]

Surgical

The standard surgical procedure is septal myectomy (the Morrow procedure), in which a small portion of the proximal septal myocardium is resected to widen the outflow tract and reduce the pressure drop across it.[34] Major complications of this operation are known: thromboembolism, ventricular septal defect, complete heart block, and severe aortic insufficiency. In most patients, complete left bundle branch block develops, which is always considered a criterion for success. Less commonly, a permanent pacemaker implantation may be required for complete heart block. Alternatively, patients with papillary muscles inserting into the mitral valve leaflets are considered as having variant degree of mitral valve disease. In these patients, attempts have been directed toward abolishing the outflow tract obstruction by either plicating the mitral leaflets or replacing the entire valve with a prosthesis. Overall surgical management of HCM may completely resolve the outflow tract obstruction, but patients may later complain of symptoms compatible with restrictive ventricular physiology or limiting arrhythmia.

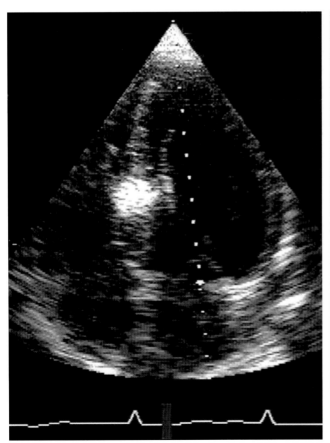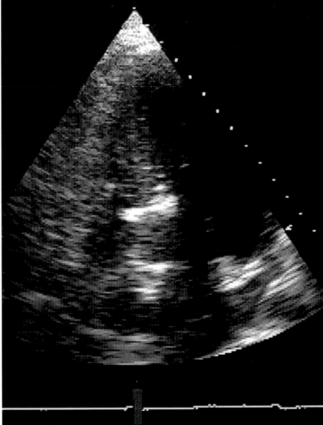

FIGURE 10.22. Echo contrast injected in the second (left) then first (right) septal branches of the left anterior descending artery. Note the localization of the opacified septal myocardium in each.

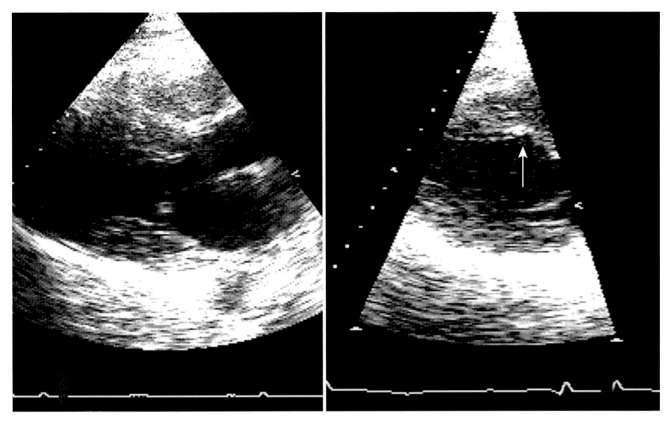

FIGURE 10.23. Left ventricular long-axis view of a patient with hypertrophic cardiomyopathy before (left) and after (right) transcatheter nonsurgical septal reduction. Note the widening of the left ventricular outflow tract (arrow) at the site of the localized septal infarction.

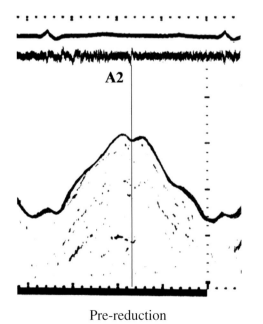

Pre-reduction

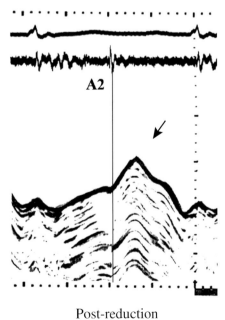

Post-reduction

FIGURE 10.24. Left ventricular septal long axis before (left) and after (right) nonsurgical septal reduction technique in a hypertrophic cardiomyopathy patient. Note the marked incoordinate septal behavior in diastole (arrow).

Nonsurgical Septal Reduction

This transcatheter procedure aims at creating a small, localized upper septal infarct by alcohol injection at the site of narrowing of the ventricular outflow tract in an attempt to widen it. A balloon is inflated in the upper septal coronary branch, usually the proximal segment of the first septal branch of the left anterior descending artery. If the outflow tract pressure drops, 1 to 3 mL of absolute alcohol is injected down the cannulated artery, distal to the inflated balloon. Outflow tract pressure drop is again assessed at rest and with stress using either dobutamine or isoprenaline. If the results are not satisfactory, as assessed by outflow tract gradient, the same steps are repeated while cannulating the second perforator of the left anterior descending artery and creating a larger area of septal akinesia.[38,39]

Echo contrast material, if available, aids in identifying the bulk of muscle supplied by each septal branch of the left anterior descending artery and hence determining the target artery.[40] A diluted myocardial echo contrast is injected distal to the inflated balloon in the cannulated septal perforator, and the location and size of the opacified myocardium is assessed.

Procedural success results in a significant rise in myocardial enzyme levels and a reduction in outflow tract velocities, along with the development of conduction disturbances (right bundle branch block or absent septal q wave) and septal incoordination.[41]

PROGNOSIS

In most patients who symptomatically improve after the procedure, mid- and long-term follow-ups demonstrate low outflow tract velocities, with a modest increase in ventricular cavity size and improved quality of life and exercise tolerance. Few may require permanent pacemakers for complete heart block.[42]

REFERENCES

1. Jarcho JA, McKenna W, Pare JA, et al. Mapping a gene for familial hypertrophic cardiomyopathy to chromosome 14q1. *N Engl J Med* 1989;321:1372–1378.
2. Solomon SD, Geisterfer-Lowrance AA, Vosberg HP, et al. A locus for familial hypertrophic cardiomyopathy is closely linked to the cardiac myosin heavy chain genes, CRI-L436, and CRI-L329 on chromosome 14 at q11-q12. *Am J Hum Genet* 1990;47:389–394.
3. Solomon SD, Jarcho JA, McKenna W, et al. Familial hypertrophic cardiomyopathy is a genetically heterogeneous disease. *J Clin Invest* 1990;86:993–999.
4. Geisterfer-Lowrance AA, Kass S, Tanigawa G, et al. A molecular basis for familial hypertrophic cardiomyopathy: a beta cardiac myosin heavy chain gene missense mutation. *Cell* 1990;62:999–1006.
5. Epstein ND, Fananapazir L, Lin HJ, et al. Evidence of genetic heterogeneity in five kindreds with familial hypertrophic cardiomyopathy. *Circulation* 1992;85:635–647.
6. Solomon SD, Wolff S, Watkins H, et al. Left ventricular hypertrophy and morphology in familial hypertrophic cardiomyopathy associated with mutations of the beta-myosin heavy chain gene. *J Am Coll Cardiol* 1993;22:498–505.
7. Goodwin JF. ?IHSS. ?HOCM. ?ASH. a plea for unity. *Am Heart J* 1975;89:269–277.
8. Maron BJ, Epstein SE. Hypertrophic cardiomyopathy: a discussion of nomenclature. *Am J Cardiol* 1979;43:1242–1244.
9. Maron BJ, Gottdiener JS, Bonow RO, et al. Hypertrophic cardiomyopathy with unusual locations of left ventricular hypertrophy undetectable by M-mode echocardiography. Identification by wide-angle two-dimensional echocardiography. *Circulation* 1981;63:409–418.
10. Shapiro LM, McKenna WJ. Distribution of left ventricular hypertrophy in hypertrophic cardiomyopathy: a two-dimensional echocardiographic study. *J Am Coll Cardiol* 1983;2: 437–444.
11. Henry WL, Clark CE, Epstein SE. Asymmetric septal hypertrophy. Echocardiographic identification of the pathognomonic anatomic abnormality of IHSS. *Circulation* 1973;47: 225–233.
12. Henry WL, Clark CE, Epstein SE. Asymmetric septal hypertrophy (ASH): the unifying link in the IHSS disease spectrum. Observations regarding its pathogenesis, pathophysiology, and course. *Circulation* 1973;47:827–832.
13. Wigle ED, Sasson Z, Henderson MA, et al. Hypertrophic cardiomyopathy. The importance of the site and the extent of hypertrophy. A review. *Prog Cardiovasc Dis* 1985;28:1–83.
14. Wigle ED, Adelman AG, Silver MD. Pathophysiological consideration in muscular subaortic stenosis. In: Wolstenholme GEW, ed. *Hypertrophic obstructive cardiomyopathy.* Ciba Foundation Study Group 47. London: Churchill, 1971.
15. Shah PM, Gramiak R, Kramer DH. Ultrasound localization of left ventricular outflow obstruction in hypertrophic obstructive cardiomyopathy. *Circulation* 1969;40:3–11.
16. Maron BJ, Gottdiener JS, Arce J, et al. Dynamic subaortic obstruction in hypertrophic cardiomyopathy: analysis by pulsed Doppler echocardiography. *J Am Coll Cardiol* 1985;6: 1–18.
17. Wigle ED, Henderson M, Rakowski H, et al. Muscular (hypertrophic) subaortic stenosis (hypertrophic obstructive cardiomyopathy): the evidence for true obstruction to left ventricular outflow. *Postgrad Med J* 1986;62:531–536.
18. Yamaguchi H, Ishimura T, Nishiyama S, et al. Hypertrophic nonobstructive cardiomyopathy with giant negative T waves (apical hypertrophy): ventriculographic and echocardiographic features in 30 patients. *Am J Cardiol* 1979;44: 401–412.
19. Pellikka PA, Oh JK, Bailey KR, et al. Dynamic intraventricular obstruction during dobutamine stress echocardiography. A new observation. *Circulation* 1992;86:1429–1432.
20. Maron BJ, Gottdiener JS, Epstein SE. Patterns and significance of distribution of left ventricular hypertrophy in hypertrophic cardiomyopathy. A wide angle, two-dimensional echocardiographic study of 125 patients. *Am J Cardiol* 1981; 48:418–428.
21. McIntosh CL, Maron BJ, Cannon RO III, et al. Initial results of combined anterior mitral leaflet plication and ventricular

septal myotomy-myectomy for relief of left ventricular outflow tract obstruction in patients with hypertrophic cardiomyopathy. *Circulation* 1992;86(5 Suppl):II60–II67.

22. Rodger JC. Motion of mitral apparatus in hypertrophic cardiomyopathy with obstruction. *Br Heart J* 1976;38:732–737.

23. Spirito P, Maron BJ, Bonow RO, et al. Severe functional limitation in patients with hypertrophic cardiomyopathy and only mild localized left ventricular hypertrophy. *J Am Coll Cardiol* 1986;8:537–544.

24. Rossen RM, Goodman DJ, Ingham RE, et al. Ventricular systolic septal thickening and excursion in idiopathic hypertrophic subaortic stenosis. *N Engl J Med* 1974;291:1317–1319.

25. Tajik AJ, Giuliani ER. Echocardiographic observations in idiopathic hypertrophic subaortic stenosis. *Mayo Clin Proc* 1974;49:89–97.

26. Kinoshita N, Nimura Y, Okamoto M, et al. Mitral regurgitation in hypertrophic cardiomyopathy. Non-invasive study by two dimensional Doppler echocardiography. *Br Heart J* 1983;49: 574–583.

27. Spirito P, Maron BJ. Relation between extent of left ventricular hypertrophy and diastolic filling abnormalities in hypertrophic cardiomyopathy. *J Am Coll Cardiol* 1990;15:808–813.

28. Nihoyannopoulos P, Karatasakis G, Frenneaux M, et al. Diastolic function in hypertrophic cardiomyopathy: relation to exercise capacity. *J Am Coll Cardiol* 1992;19:536–540.

29. Nakamura T, Matsubara K, Furukawa K, et al. Diastolic paradoxic jet flow in patients with hypertrophic cardiomyopathy: evidence of concealed apical asynergy with cavity obliteration. *J Am Coll Cardiol* 1992;19:516–524.

30. Sutton MG, Tajik AJ, Smith HC, et al. Angina in idiopathic hypertrophic subaortic stenosis. A clinical correlate of regional left ventricular dysfunction: a videometric and echocardiographic study. *Circulation* 1980;61:561–568.

31. Henein MY, O'Sullivan C, Sutton GC, et al. Stress-induced left ventricular outflow tract obstruction: a potential cause of dyspnea in the elderly. *J Am Coll Cardiol* 1997;30: 1301–1307.

32. Al Nasser F, Duncan A, Sharma R, et al. Beta-blocker therapy for dynamic left-ventricular outflow tract obstruction. *Int J Cardiol* 2002;86:199–205.

33. Spirito P, Maron BJ, Bonow RO, et al. Occurrence and significance of progressive left ventricular wall thinning and relative cavity dilatation in hypertrophic cardiomyopathy. *Am J Cardiol* 1987;60:123–129.

34. Grigg LE, Wigle ED, Williams WG, et al. Transesophageal Doppler echocardiography in obstructive hypertrophic cardiomyopathy: clarification of pathophysiology and importance in intraoperative decision making. *J Am Coll Cardiol* 1992; 20:42–52.

35. Petrone RK, Klues HG, Panza JA, et al. Coexistence of mitral valve prolapse in a consecutive group of 528 patients with hypertrophic cardiomyopathy assessed with echocardiography. *J Am Coll Cardiol* 1992;20:55–61.

36. Zhu WX, Oh JK, Kopecky SL, et al. Mitral regurgitation due to ruptured chordae tendineae in patients with hypertrophic obstructive cardiomyopathy. *J Am Coll Cardiol* 1992;20:242–247.

37. Fananapazir L, Cannon RO III, Tripodi D, et al. Impact of dual-chamber permanent pacing in patients with obstructive hypertrophic cardiomyopathy with symptoms refractory to verapamil and beta-adrenergic blocker therapy. *Circulation* 1992;85:2149–2161.

38. Sigwart U. Non-surgical myocardial reduction for hypertrophic obstructive cardiomyopathy. *Lancet* 1995;346: 211–214.

39. Knight C, Kurbaan AS, Seggewiss H, et al. Nonsurgical septal reduction for hypertrophic obstructive cardiomyopathy: outcome in the first series of patients. *Circulation* 1997;95: 2075–2081.

40. Faber L, Seggewiss H, Gleichmann U. Percutaneous transluminal septal myocardial ablation in hypertrophic obstructive cardiomyopathy: results with respect to intraprocedural myocardial contrast echocardiography. *Circulation* 1998;98: 2415–2421.

41. Henein MY, O'Sullivan CA, Ramzy IS, et al. Electromechanical left ventricular behavior after nonsurgical septal reduction in patients with hypertrophic obstructive cardiomyopathy. *J Am Coll Cardiol* 1999;34:1117–1122.

42. Faber L, Meissner A, Ziemssen P, et al. Percutaneous transluminal septal myocardial ablation for hypertrophic obstructive cardiomyopathy: long term follow up of the first series of 25 patients. *Heart* 2000;83:326–331.

11

Restrictive Cardiomyopathy

Restrictive cardiomyopathy is a condition characterized by normal left ventricular cavity size and systolic function but with increased myocardial stiffness.[1] This makes the ventricle incompliant and fills predominantly in early diastole. When atrial systolic function is maintained, the ventricle may accommodate a small volume of blood during atrial systole but at the expense of raising the end-diastolic pressure. These physiologic disturbances are associated with raised left atrial pressures, atrial dilatation, and possible arrhythmias.[2]

Restrictive cardiomyopathy is uncommon, and usually no specific cause is identified.

The most common forms of restrictive cardiomyopathies are idiopathic,[1] endomyocardial fibrosis (EMF)[3,4], associated with Löffler's syndrome, and infiltrative myocardial disease.[5] In the West, amyloid heart disease[6] remains the most common cause of restrictive cardiomyopathy. Among other diseases of the myocardium that may present with a similar picture are cardiac sarcoidosis[7] and hemochromatosis.[8]

IDIOPATHIC RESTRICTIVE CARDIOMYOPATHY

Idiopathic restrictive cardiomyopathy is a benign condition, characterized by a normal left ventricular cavity size and a dilated left atrium in the absence of mitral valve pathology. It is a slowly progressing disease when compared with other infiltrative restrictive cardiomyopathies.[2] Patients diagnosed with this condition tend to respond to diuretics and angiotensin-converting enzyme inhibitors.[9] Restrictive left ventricular filling is characterized by short isovolumic relaxation time, dominant early diastolic filling with short deceleration time, and small or absent late diastolic filling component. Pulmonary venous flow demonstrates late diastolic flow reversal

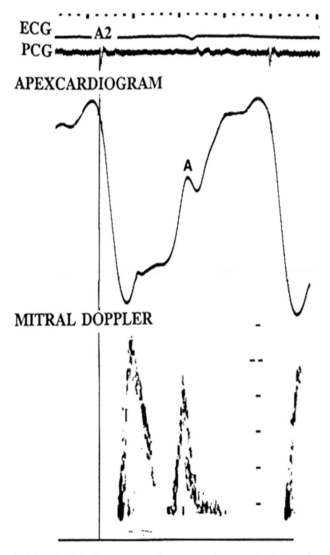

FIGURE 11.1. An apexcardiogram and transmitral Doppler velocities from a patient with restrictive cardiomyopathy, showing raised end-diastolic pressure with small filling volume.

185

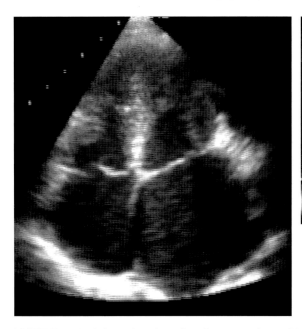

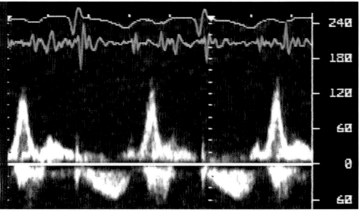

FIGURE 11.2. A four-chamber view from a patient with idiopathic restrictive cardiomyopathy showing normal left ventricular cavity size, dilated left atrium (left), and restrictive filling pattern (right).

"during atrial systole" of a longer duration than the corresponding transmitral flow.

If such patients with raised filling pressure develop atrial fibrillation D.C. cardioversion may be unsuccessful because of the large atrium.

ENDOMYOCARDIAL FIBROSIS

Endomyocardial fibrosis (EMF), a form of restrictive cardiomyopathy, is prevalent in West Africa, southern India, Thailand, and South America, among the indigenous population. Endomyocardial fibrosis is characterized by extensive fibrosis of the subendocardial layer of the myocardium involving the apices of the left and right ventricles and extending to the inflow tract. Fibrosis may be patchy or diffuse in distribution.[3,10] Endomyocardial

fibrosis results in increased chamber stiffness and hence restrictive filling. The left ventricle is normal in size but the walls are thickened with increased subendocardial myocardial echo intensity.[11–13] Ventricular function may initially be preserved but subsequently impaired. The endocardial fibrosis forms the substrate for thrombus formation that may obliterate the entire ventricular apex, particularly the right ventricle. The atria are usually dilated, not necessarily due to the resulting mitral or tricuspid regurgitation but as a consequence of the increased atrial pressure secondary to the incompliant ventricles. Severe cases may be complicated by pulmonary hypertension and tricuspid regurgitation. The disease may also involve the mitral and tricuspid valve leaflets themselves, thus adding to the severity of regurgitation. EMF may be very similar in presentation to Löffler's syndrome.[13–15]

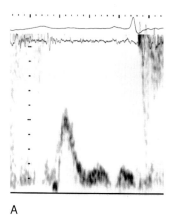

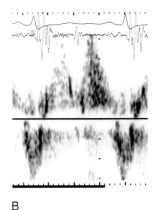

A   B

FIGURE 11.3. Transmitral forward-flow velocities from a patient with restrictive cardiomyopathy along with pulmonary venous flow. Note the classical restrictive filling pattern with late diastolic flow reversal in the pulmonary veins.

LÖFFLER'S SYNDROME

Löffler's syndrome presents with echocardiographic and physiologic signs similar to EMF, but in addition there is hypereosinophilia.[13–15] While management of EMF is directed toward subendocardial decortication with or without valve replacement, controlling the eosinophilia is the first stage in treating Löffler's syndrome.

INFILTRATIVE MYOCARDIAL DISEASE

Amyloid heart disease is the most common cause of restrictive cardiomyopathy in the West. The myocardium may be infiltrated by iron in hemochromatosis,[8,16] glycogen in Pompe's[17] and Cori's disease, or glycolipids in Fabry's disease.[18] Myocardial infiltrates disturb normal myocyte function and metabolism, resulting in fibrosis. Eventually, progressive myocardial fibrosis adds to the myocardial stiffness and increase in ventricular diastolic pressures. Amyloid deposition may be patchy or diffuse, and the ventricular walls in amyloid heart disease are usually thick, showing poor thickening fraction as well as increased myocardial echo intensity (brightness).[6,19] Amyloid deposition may involve the four cardiac chambers, and even the atrioventricular valves.

In patients with amyloid heart disease, the greater the ventricular wall thickness, the more intensive is the amyloid deposition and the poorer the clinical outcome.

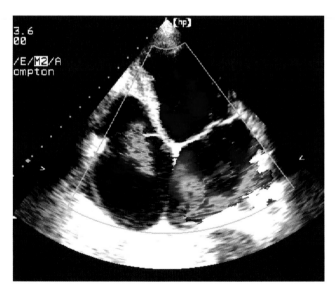

FIGURE 11.4. Apical four-chamber view from a patient with endomyocardial fibrosis. Note the large atria, the increased subendocardial echo intensity in the presence of normal ventricular size, and mitral and tricuspid regurgitation on color Doppler.

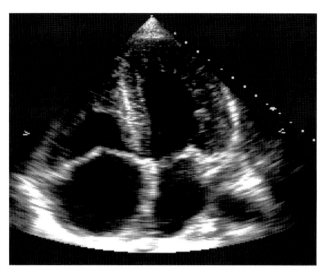

FIGURE 11.5. Apical four-chamber view from a patient with advanced amyloid disease involving the four chambers and atrioventricular valves.

Wall thickness of more than 1.5 cm is associated with mean survival of 5 months.[19] The extent of segmental dysfunction is usually out of proportion to the degree of wall thickness, showing markedly depressed segmental thickening and thinning rates.[20] By the time of clinical presentation, the echocardiographic picture of amyloid heart disease is usually severe, and ventricular filling is of the restrictive pattern.[21] Some degree of mitral and tricuspid regurgitation is commonly seen, which may be severe, particularly when the valves themselves are involved in the disease process.

In amyloid heart disease, the changes in ventricular filling pattern evolve as the disease progresses and ventricular function deteriorates. Although in early disease the E/A ratio may be less than 1.0 and isovolumic relaxation time prolonged, in later stages filling becomes restrictive and isovolumic relaxation time shortens, consistent with raised left atrial pressures. Similar abnormalities can be seen on the right side of the heart.[22,23]

The ventricular filling pattern has been shown to predict clinical outcome in amyloid heart disease. E wave deceleration time of less than 150 ms has been found to predict a life expectancy of 50% at 1 year compared with more than 90% survival at 1 year with deceleration time more than 150 ms.[24]

Amyloid left ventricular disease should be differentiated from hypertrophic cardiomyopathy.[25] While the cavity size is equally maintained in the two conditions, the overall systolic ventricular function, segmental thickening fraction, and thinning rate are preserved only in hypertrophic cardiomyopathy. The QRS voltage criteria on surface ECG may also help, demonstrating low amplitude in amyloid disease. The amyloid disease may also involve the atrial septum and may be associated with varying degrees of pericardial effusion.

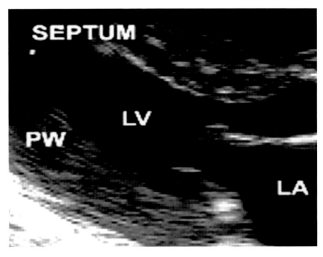
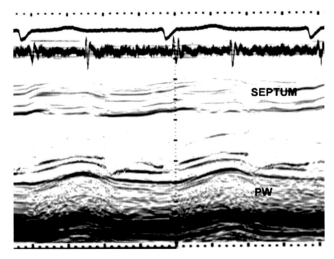

FIGURE 11.6. Parasternal long-axis view (left) and M-mode recording (right) from a patient with amyloid deposition. Note the normal left ventricular cavity size, thick walls, and poor thickening fraction.

CARDIAC SARCOIDOSIS

Cardiac involvement occurs in a minority of sarcoid cases. Cardiac involvement is manifest as patchy myocardial infiltration by granulomatous sarcoid deposits followed by fibrosis.[26] When sarcoidosis affects the posterior wall of the left ventricle, the proximal segment is usually involved, which has an echocardiographic picture similar to that of posterior wall myocardial infarction. It may also involve the lateral papillary muscle, giving rise to some degree of mitral regurgitation. Sarcoid heart disease may affect the proximal septal segment, where it may affect the conducting tissue, resulting in conduction disease and heart block. This explains the etiology of syncope in these patients. The left ventricular cavity may be slightly dilated at the basal region due to

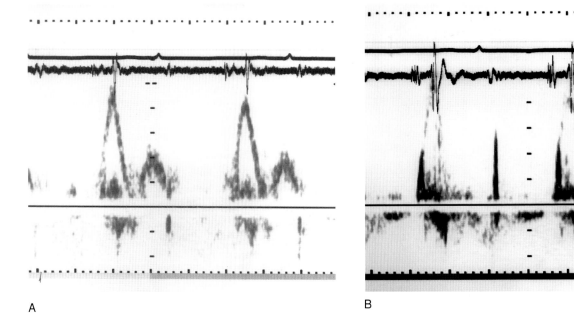

A

B

FIGURE 11.7. Left ventricular filling (restrictive) from a patient with (A) amyloid heart disease. (B) Right ventricular filling from the same patient. Note the characteristic restrictive pattern of filling on both sides of the heart and a third heart sound on the phonocardiogram.

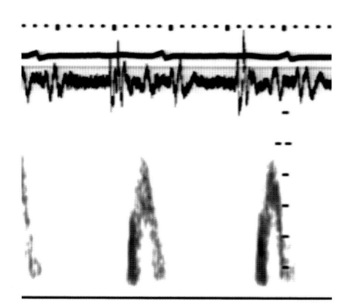

FIGURE 11.8. Left ventricular filling from a patient with late-stage amyloid disease showing restrictive pattern with very short deceleration time (100 ms).

the fibrosed segments. Ventricular filling is commonly late diastolic.

HEMOCHROMATOSIS

The ventricular myocardium may be infiltrated by iron in patients with hemochromatosis.[16] It tends to invade the outer layer of the myocardium more than the subendocardium. It is deposited in the myocytes as well as in interstitial cells, resulting in myocardial fibrosis. Although the ventricular cavity may be dilated, the clinical outcome is better than the other infiltrative diseases, since it responds well to iron chelation therapy.[27]

DIABETIC HYPERTENSIVE CARDIOMYOPATHY

Long-standing diabetes and hypertension may affect the left ventricular function in such a way as to resemble restrictive cardiomyopathy, in particular the picture associated with amyloid. The cavity size is maintained, walls are thickened, and sequential thickening fraction is significantly reduced. Most of these patients become limited by breathlessness due to raised left atrial pressures in the absence of mitral valve disease. The long-term outcome of this condition, however, is more benign than that of amyloid cardiomyopathy.

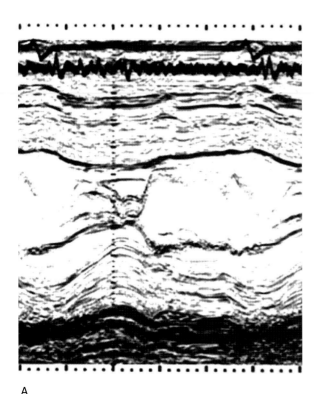

A

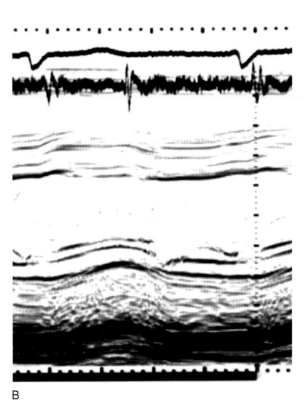

B

FIGURE 11.9. M-mode of left ventricular minor axis from two patients. (A) Hypertrophic cardiomyopathy and (B) amyloid heart disease. Note the similar extent of wall thickness but poor thickening fraction particularly of the posterior wall in the amyloid patient compared with the hypertrophic cardiomyopathy. (*Continues*)

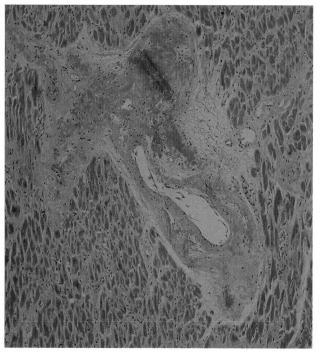

C

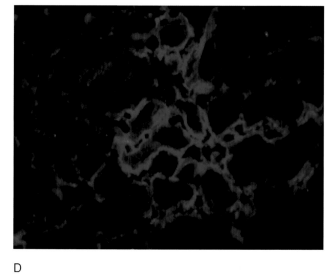

D

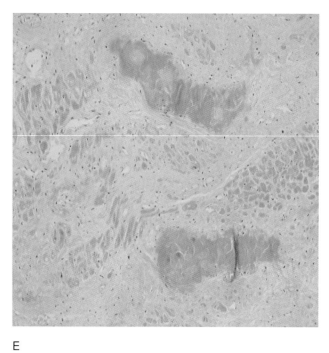

E

FIGURE 11.9. (*Continued*) (C–E) Histologic sections showing amyloid deposition in the myocardium (pink). (D) (apple green) Fluorescence staining amyloid is used in D.

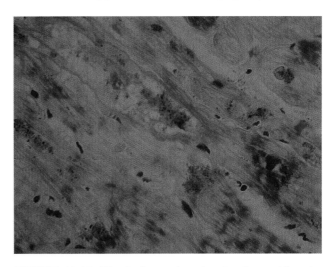

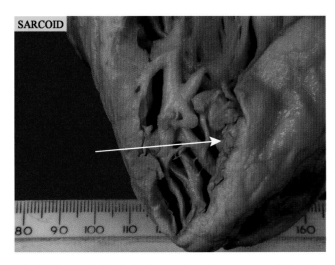

FIGURE 11.10. Pathologic section from a ventricle of a patient with sarcoid heart showing myocardial fibrosis (arrow).

FIGURE 11.12. Histologic section showing hemosiderosis, with blue purple dots of iron deposition in the myocytes.

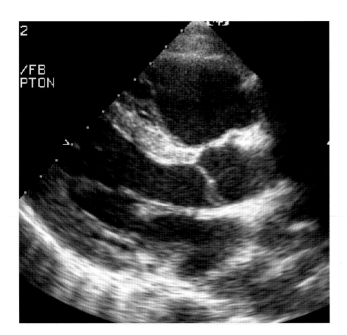

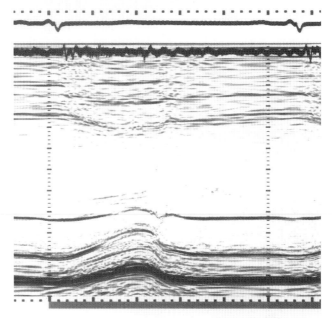

FIGURE 11.11. Parasternal long-axis view from a patient with sarcoid heart disease showing scarred proximal septum with increased echo intensity.

FIGURE 11.13. M-mode images from a patient with long-standing hypertension and diabetes. Note the modest cavity dilatation, reduced systolic function, and thickening fraction.

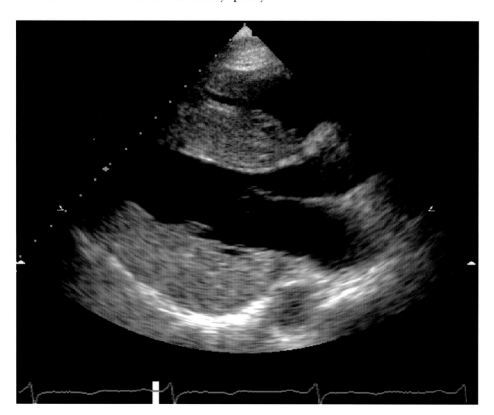

FIGURE 11.14. Parasternal long-axis view from a patient with glycogen storage disease showing thick walls with increased myocardial echo intensity.

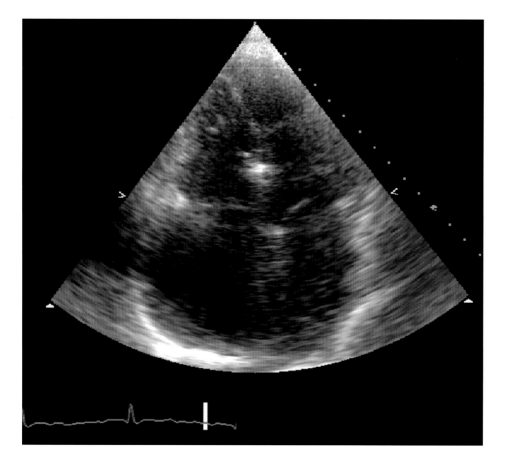

FIGURE 11.15. Apical four-chamber view from a patient with isolated right ventricular restrictive disease demonstrating large right atrium and normal-sized right ventricle.

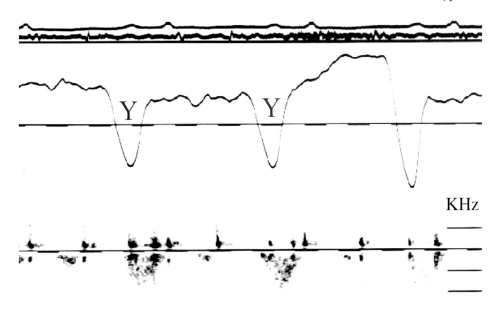

FIGURE 11.16. Jugular venous pulse and Superior vena caval flow from a patient with restrictive right ventricular disease demonstrating deep Y descent and early diastolic RA filling consistent with early diastolic drop of right atrial pressure.

KHz

Restrictive right ventricular disease: features of this condition (please refer to chapter 12).

REFERENCES

1. Siegel RJ, Shah PK, Fishbein MC. Idiopathic restrictive cardiomyopathy. *Circulation* 1984;70:165–169.
2. Benotti JR, Grossman W, Cohn PF. Clinical profile of restrictive cardiomyopathy. *Circulation* 1980;61:1206–1212.
3. Roberts WC, Liegler DG, Carbone PP. Endomyocardial disease and eosinophilia. A clinical and pathologic spectrum. *Am J Med* 1969;46:28–42.
4. Candell-Riera J, Permanyer-Miralda G, Soler-Soler J. Echocardiographic findings in endomyocardial fibrosis. *Chest* 1982;82:88–90.
5. Child JS, Levisman JA, Abbasi AS, et al. Echocardiographic manifestations of infiltrative cardiomyopathy. A report of seven cases due to amyloid. *Chest* 1976;70:726–731.
6. Cueto-Garcia L, Tajik AJ, Kyle RA, et al. Serial echocardiographic observations in patients with primary systemic amyloidosis: an introduction to the concept of early (asymptomatic) amyloid infiltration of the heart. *Mayo Clin Proc* 1984;59:589–597.
7. Silverman KJ, Hutchins GM, Bulkley BH. Cardiac sarcoid: a clinicopathologic study of 84 unselected patients with systemic sarcoidosis. *Circulation* 1978;58:1204–1211.
8. Short EM, Winkle RA, Billingham ME. Myocardial involvement in idiopathic hemochromatosis. Morphologic and clinical improvement following venesection. *Am J Med* 1981;70:1275–1279.
9. Henein MY, Gibson DG. Abnormal subendocardial function in restrictive left ventricular disease. *Br Heart J* 1994;72:237–242.
10. Hess OM, Turina M, Senning A, et al. Pre- and postoperative findings in patients with endomyocardial fibrosis. *Br Heart J* 1978;40:406–415.
11. George BO, Gaba FE, Talabi AI. M-mode echocardiographic features of endomyocardial fibrosis. *Br Heart J* 1982;48:222–228.
12. Vijayaraghavan G, Davies J, Sadanandan S, et al. Echocardiographic features of tropical endomyocardial disease in South India. *Br Heart J* 1983;50:450–459.
13. Acquatella H, Schiller NB, Puigbo JJ, et al. Value of two-dimensional echocardiography in endomyocardial disease with and without eosinophilia. A clinical and pathologic study. *Circulation* 1983;67:1219–1226.
14. Davies J, Gibson DG, Foale R, et al. Echocardiographic features of eosinophilic endomyocardial disease. *Br Heart J* 1982;48:434–440.
15. Gottdiener JS, Maron BJ, Schooley RT, et al. Two-dimensional echocardiographic assessment of the idiopathic hypereosinophilic syndrome. Anatomic basis of mitral regurgitation and peripheral embolization. *Circulation* 1983;67:572–578.
16. Olson LJ, Baldus WP, Tajik AJ. Echocardiographic features of idiopathic hemochromatosis. *Am J Cardiol* 1987;60:885–889.
17. Hwang B, Meng CC, Lin CY, et al. Clinical analysis of five infants with glycogen storage disease of the heart–Pompe's disease. *Jpn Heart J* 1986;27:25–34.
18. Bass JL, Shrivastava S, Grabowski GA, et al. The M-mode echocardiogram in Fabry's disease. *Am Heart J* 1980;100 (6 Pt 1):807–812.
19. Cueto-Garcia L, Reeder GS, Kyle RA, et al. Echocardiographic findings in systemic amyloidosis: spectrum of cardiac involvement and relation to survival. *J Am Coll Cardiol* 1985;6:737–743.
20. Siqueira-Filho AG, Cunha CL, Tajik AJ, et al. M-mode and two-dimensional echocardiographic features in cardiac amyloidosis. *Circulation* 1981;63:188–196.
21. Klein AL, Hatle LK, Burstow DJ, et al. Doppler characterization of left ventricular diastolic function in cardiac amyloidosis. *J Am Coll Cardiol* 1989;13:1017–1026.
22. Henein MY, Amadi A, O'Sullivan C, et al. ACE inhibitors unmask incoordinate diastolic wall motion in restrictive left ventricular disease. *Heart* 1996;76:326–331.
23. Child JS, Krivokapich J, Abbasi AS. Increased right ventricular wall thickness on echocardiography in amyloid infiltrative cardiomyopathy. *Am J Cardiol* 1979;44:1391–1395.
24. Klein AL, Hatle LK, Taliercio CP, et al. Prognostic significance of Doppler measures of diastolic function in cardiac amyloidosis. A Doppler echocardiography study. *Circulation* 1991;83:808–816.

25. Chandrasekaran K, Aylward PE, Fleagle SR, et al. Feasibility of identifying amyloid and hypertrophic cardiomyopathy with the use of computerized quantitative texture analysis of clinical echocardiographic data. *J Am Coll Cardiol* 1989;13: 832–840.

26. Lewin RF, Mor R, Spitzer S, et al. Echocardiographic evaluation of patients with systemic sarcoidosis. *Am Heart J* 1985;110(1 Pt 1):116–122.

27. Candell-Riera J, Lu L, Seres L, et al. Cardiac hemochromatosis: beneficial effects of iron removal therapy. An echocardiographic study. *Am J Cardiol* 1983;52:824–829.

12 Pericardial Disease

ANATOMY

The pericardium consists of two layers, a visceral layer lined by mesothelial cells and a parietal or fibrous layer lined also by mesothelial cells but with attached fat and fibrous tissue. The mesothelial layer secretes a small amount of pericardial fluid, usually 50 mL of clear fluid that allows both surfaces to slide together during the cardiac cycle. The fibrous layer is usually 1 mm in thickness, whereas the visceral layer is a transparent membrane on the surface of the heart.[1]

PHYSIOLOGY

Intrapericardial pressure normally ranges between –2 and 2 mmHg. Thus it is less than that of the right heart. It falls with the intrapleural pressure during inspiration, resulting in a fall in right-sided cardiac pressures. This causes a modest increase in right heart filling velocities with inspiration. These effects are often exaggerated in patients with clinically significant pericardial disease.

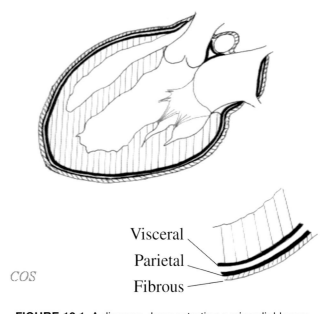

COS

Visceral
Parietal
Fibrous

FIGURE 12.1. A diagram demonstrating pericardial layers.

Pericardial Effusion

Diagnosis of pericardial effusion is only made when the volume of the fluid in the pericardial space is more than the physiologic amount of 50 mL. Two-dimensional echocardiography permits the visualization of 100 mL of fluid collection in the pericardial space.[2] Pericardial effusion can be secondary to cardiac or noncardiac etiology.[3] Acute rapid collection is usually caused by traumatic injury, iatrogenic ventricular puncture, or aortic dissection with fluid collection inside the pericardium. Chronic effusion is more common than acute effusion. The common causes of chronic fluid accumulation in the pericardial sac are viral infection, uremia, collagen vascular disease, myocardial infarction, myxoedema, and malignancy. Also, conditions associated with salt and water retention such as congestive cardiac failure, renal failure, and hepatic cirrhosis may be complicated by pericardial effusion. Most of the pericardial effusion seen in clinical practice, however, is idiopathic in origin.

A small, rapidly accumulated effusion may result in raised pericardial pressure and development of symptoms, whereas with a slowly accumulating effusion patients may remain asymptomatic even with large volumes.[4] Symptoms in pericardial effusion are not specific and may be in the form of reduced exercise tolerance or dull aching chest pain. Patients may develop symptoms of mediastinal syndrome (cough caused by bronchial compression, dyspnea due to lung compression, or hoarseness of voice caused by recurrent laryngeal

195

nerve compression). Distant heart sounds and widespread dullness to percussion may be the only physical signs until tamponade develops.

Investigations

Chest X-ray does not always confirm the presence of pericardial effusion if it is less than 250 mL. MRI and CT scanning are ideal for assessing pericardial thickness. Echocardiography is the investigation of choice for confirming the presence of pericardial effusion and for assessing its volume.[5] An echo-free space in the pericardium both on M-mode and on two-dimensional echo should be distinguished from anterior pericardial fat.[6] More than 1 cm pericardial densities that are moving with the pericardium and the epicardium suggests the presence of pericardial fat. A localized effusion should always be looked for from different views, even a small amount adjacent to the left atrium or right atrium can be visualized on two-dimensional echo images. With a large pericardial collection the entire heart may swing in the effusion, causing electrical alternans. The latter is defined as alternating small R-wave amplitudes with normal ones.[7]

Pericardial effusion should be differentiated from pleural effusion by identifying the location of the pericardial effusion with respect to the descending aorta and fibrous pericardium (from the parasternal long-axis view).[8]

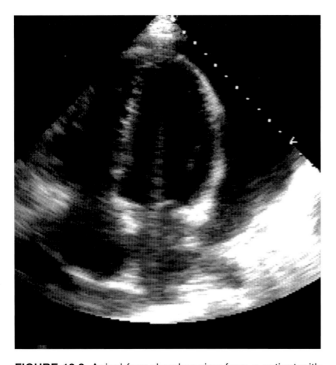

FIGURE 12.2. Apical four-chamber view from a patient with a large pericardial effusion. Note the large space between the pericardium and the epicardium.

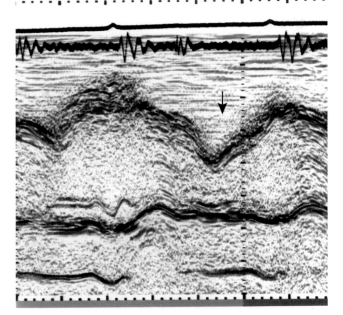

FIGURE 12.3. M-mode of the aortic valve and root demonstrating diastolic right ventricular collapse (arrow).

Quantitation of Pericardial Effusion

Semiquantitative estimation with either M-mode or two-dimensional techniques is usually adequate for clinical management. A 1-cm global collection around the heart suggests an approximate amount of 200 mL. With localized effusion a comparative assessment of the effusion size with that of the left ventricle gives a rough estimation of the collection volume. The hemodynamic effects of pericardial effusion depend on the pressure–volume relation of the pericardium, the speed of fluid collection, and the volume of the effusion. In patients with ventricular disease, ventricular compliance may also add to the hemodynamic effects of pericardial effusion.[9]

Pericardial Tamponade

Pericardial tamponade is a condition of cardiac hemodynamic instability presenting as chamber compression caused by increased intrapericardial pressure greater than the filling pressure of the right and left ventricles. The most common cause of tamponade is malignant effusion or acute fluid collection after cardiac surgery. Right ventricular collapse is a sensitive (92%) and highly specific (100%) diagnostic sign for tamponade. It reflects transient negative transmural early diastolic pressure as pericardial pressure exceeds right ventricular pressure. Right ventricular collapse is better seen from the short-axis view across the right ventricular outflow tract and should be confirmed to be diastolic in timing. Right atrial collapse has been shown to be less sensitive (82%) but equally specific (100%) for pericardial tamponade.[10]

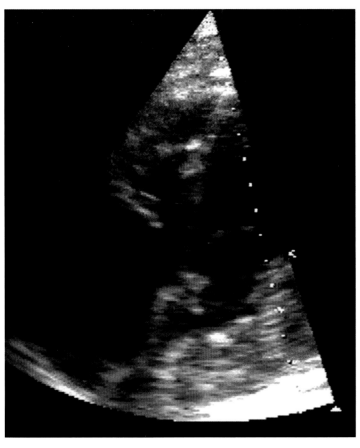

A

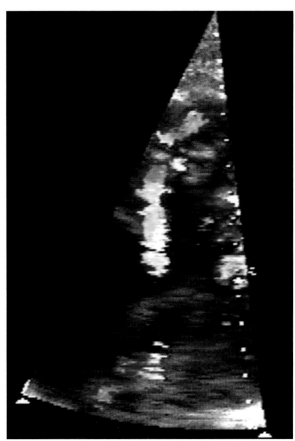

B

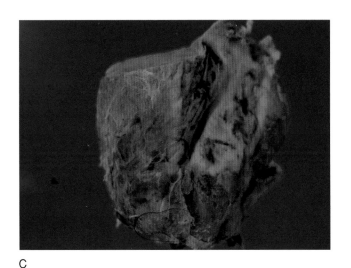

C

FIGURE 12.4. (A, B) Apical four-chamber view from a patient with a localized pericardial effusion behind the right atrium. Note the collapsed right atrial cavity that causes iatrogenic narrowing of the right ventricular inflow tract proximal to the tricuspid valve leaflets and hence functional raised filling velocities similar to tricuspid stenosis. (C) Pathologic section from a patient with pericarditis showing generalized pericardial inflammation.

Also, right atrial inversion index greater than 34% strongly suggests tamponade. In the absence of hemodynamically significant pericardial effusion, right ventricular diastolic collapse may be caused by bilateral large pleural effusion.[11] In contrast, the onset of right ventricular collapse may be delayed by myocardial hypertrophy, pulmonary hypertension, or free wall adhesions, commonly associated with malignant effusions.[11]

Pathophysiology

The pericardium is normally able to stretch to accommodate more than 2000 mL of slowly accumulated fluid without a significant increase in pressure. Rapid accumulation of as little as 200 mL increases pericardial pressure. Inability of the pericardium to distend causes its pressure to rise above right atrial pressure, which is

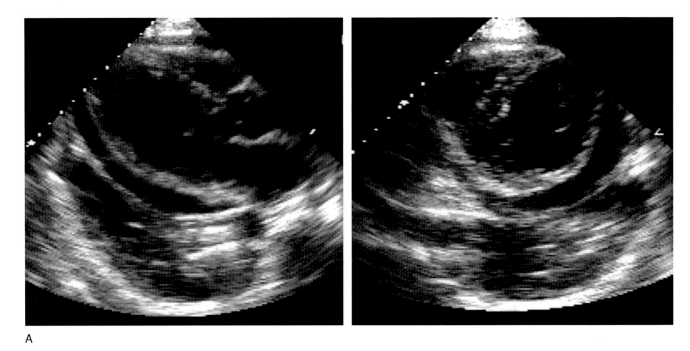

A

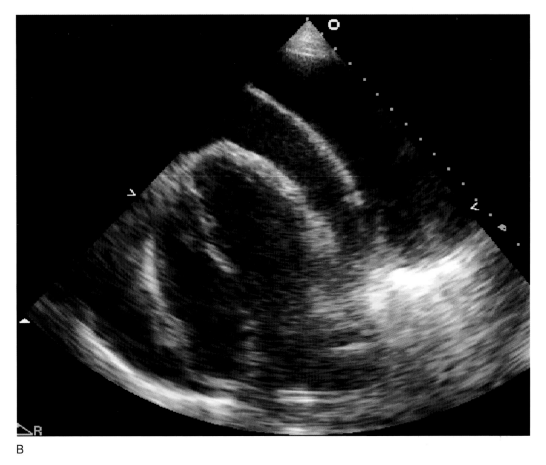

B

FIGURE 12.5. (A) Parasternal long-axis and short-axis views from a patient with pericardial and pleural effusions. Note the relationship of the latter with respect to the descending aorta and the pericardial effusion. (B) Apical 4 chamber view showing large pericardial and pleural effusions.

followed by right ventricular pressure; this eventually results in right ventricular collapse. Normally, intrapericardial and intrapleural pressures fall equally during inspiration. With tamponade intrapericardial pressure does not fall as much, resulting in less pressure gradient between intrathoracic pressure and pulmonary veins and left atrium and ventricle.[12] This results in reduced left-sided filling velocities during inspiration as well as stroke volume.[13] On the right side of the heart the increase in right ventricular dimensions during inspiration enhances right-sided filling and ejection during inspiration. Progressive increase in pericardial pressure and right ventricular pressure may affect the left heart, adding to its compromised filling during inspiration and significantly dropping the stroke volume. The combined effect of the two mechanisms may eventually compromise cardiac output.[14] Pericardial pressure greater than 10 mmHg results in right ventricular collapse and raised diastolic

pressures of both ventricles as well as increased capillary wedge pressure. This leads to inspiratory fall of aortic pressure and hence pulsus paradoxus and hypotension. Pericardial effusion to that extent is not the sole cause of arterial paradox, since its mechanisms are complex.[15] Loculated high-pressure posterior pericardial effusion may have a similar effect on left ventricular physiology in the absence of large-volume effusion. Patients with such disturbed hemodynamics often present with raised jugular venous pressure (JVP), tachycardia, and tachypnea. In the absence of pericardial effusion, right ventricular diastolic collapse may be caused by a large pleural effusion that results in disturbed physiology similar to that of pericardial effusion.

Left ventricular and left atrial collapse are much less commonly seen with tamponade. However, left ventricular invagination caused by localized collection around the free wall has been reported after open-heart surgery.[16]

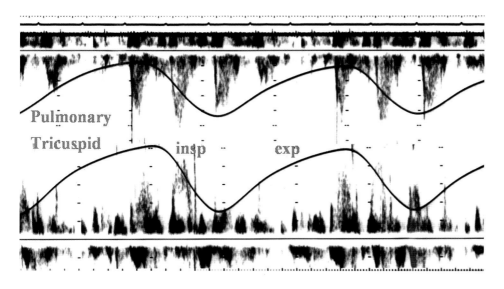

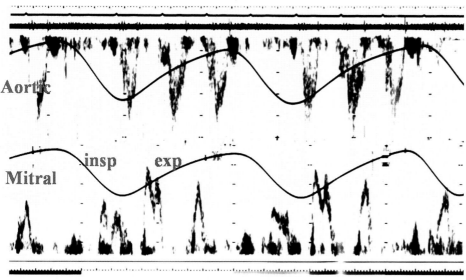

FIGURE 12.6. Transtricuspid and pulmonary pulsed Doppler velocities from a patient with large pericardial effusion and tamponade (upper) and transmitral and aortic Doppler velocities from the same patient (lower) demonstrating reciprocal significant alteration of right- and left-sided filling and ejection velocities with respiration; being predominantly inspiratory on the right side of the heart and expiratory on the left side.

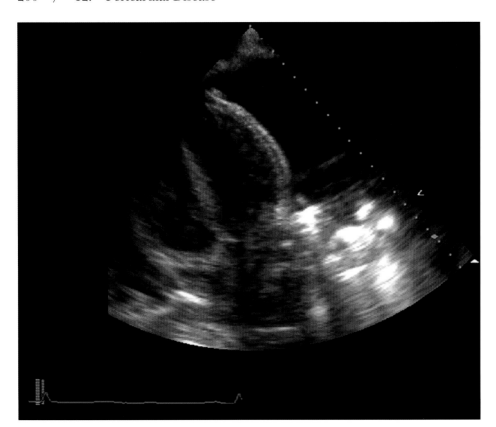

FIGURE 12.7. Large left pleural effusion from a patient with phasic right heart filling and empting. Note the insignificant amount of pericardial effusion.

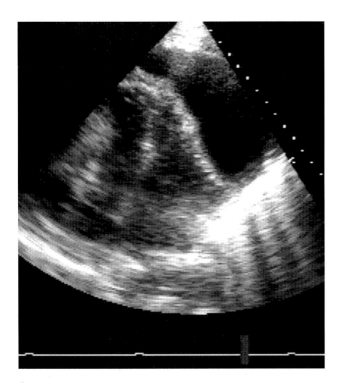

A

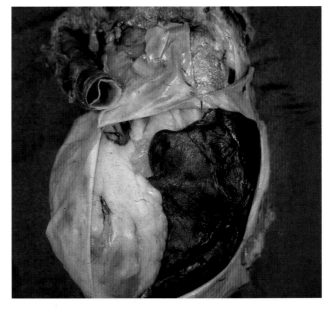

B

FIGURE 12.8. (A) Apical four-chamber view from a patient with localized pericardial effusion around the left ventricular free wall. Note the effect of the raised localized pericardial pressure compressing the ventricular free wall. (B) Pathologic section from a patient with hemopericardium.

Significant localized posterior effusion is usually caused by anterior adhesions between the right ventricle, the right atrium, and the pericardium.[17]

Intrapericardial clot formation after cardiac surgery or as a complication of an interventional procedure (e.g., trans-septal puncture) may result in signs of tamponade due to the rapid increase in intrapericardial pressure even in the absence of a significantly large fluid volume, because of fluid absorption. Diagnosis of this condition is important, since it does not usually respond to percutaneous needle aspiration. Transesophageal echo postoperatively is of great value in making the differential diagnosis.[18]

Management

Pericardiocentesis is traditionally performed under fluoroscopy, but currently available ultrasound imaging can provide enough guidance to achieve maximum drainage.[19] However, ultrasound guidance cannot provide needle aspiration guidance, since the needle tip is poorly visualized on ultrasound images. Substernal window drainage is usually recommended in patients with resistant, recurrent, or fast accumulating effusion. Although surgical in nature, the procedure allows for therapeutic symptomatic pressure relief, fluid drainage, and pericardial biopsy for cytology. It is generally successful with a large effusion and much less successful with small collections. A subcostal window is also the ideal means for dealing with localized effusion that is not accessible by needle drainage.

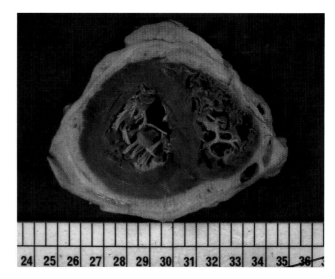

FIGURE 12.10. Specimen demonstrating thickened pericardium with complete fusion of its layers (constriction) in a patient after cardiac surgery.

Constrictive Pericarditis

Pericardial constriction is a pathologic condition characterized by pericardial thickening and fibrosis that results in adhesion of its two layers and calcium deposition.[20] Constrictive pericarditis is usually seen by the pathologist as a thickened adherent sheet on the cardiac surface that cannot be separated from the underlying myocardium. Both fibrous and visceral layers fuse together.

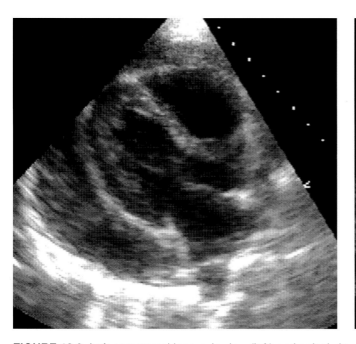 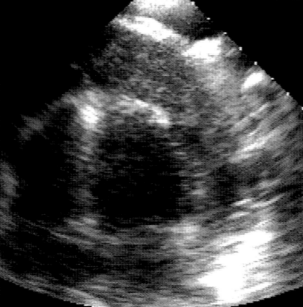

FIGURE 12.9. Left parasternal long-axis view (left) and apical view (right) from a patient with post-operative clotting in the pericardial space.

Etiology

The most common cause of constrictive pericarditis is viral infection, which can be missed for a long time until presentation. Viral etiology is frequently invoked when no cause is found.[21] Tuberculosis is currently an uncommon cause, particularly in the West. Other causes may be radiation, connective-tissue disease, chronic renal failure, neoplastic disease, and previous cardiac surgery.

Pathophysiology

The stiff pericardium loses its stretching ability to accommodate normal changes in intracardiac pressures. This is demonstrated by the equalization of end-diastolic pressures in the right and left ventricles "dip and plateau pattern," a cardinal sign for diagnosing pericardial constriction. Since this pathology is uniform it manifests itself in the form of raised venous pressure, usually seen in the jugular veins and with systemic fluid retention. This picture also complicates acute or chronic inflammatory processes that involve the pericardium. A thickened pericardium on any imaging technique is not an exclusive diagnostic criterion for constrictive physiology. Furthermore, in rare cases of rapidly increasing ventricular volumes as in dilated cardiomyopathy, the pericardium may be completely normal but demonstrates an external constricting effect, thus adding to the deterioration of the clinical condition.

A fibrosed and unstretchable pericardium being adherent to the epicardial layer of the myocardium can limit its normal movement during the cardiac cycle, particularly in systole, along the ventricular transverse axis. It cannot, however, affect shortening and lengthening of the longitudinal myocardial fibers that are located in the subendo-

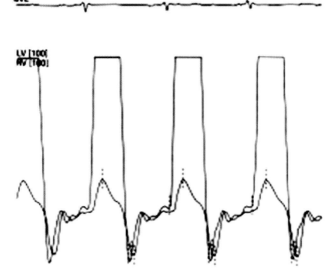

FIGURE 12.11. Combined right and left ventricular pressures from a patient with constrictive pericarditis. Note the equalization of the two ventricular pressures in late diastole.

cardium. This longitudinal myocardial function can easily be studied from the movement of the mitral and tricuspid valve annuli in systole and diastole, respectively. The downward displacement of the tricuspid ring and valve in systole results in increased right atrial surface area and volume and a fall in right atrial pressure. This allows a column of blood to fill the atrium and hence the characteristic systolic drop of venous pressure, the "X descent."[1] Similar presentation can be seen in the left heart physiology. The chronic increase in venous pressure results in systemic congestion and dilatation of hepatic veins, which demonstrate a similar pattern to that of the jugular veins.

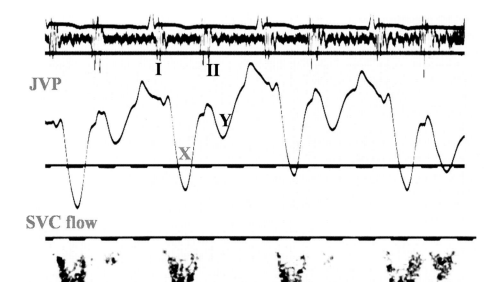

FIGURE 12.12. Jugular venous pulse from a patient with pericardial constriction. Note the dominant systolic (X) descent (top) coinciding with a systolic right atrial filling component from the superior vena cava (bottom).

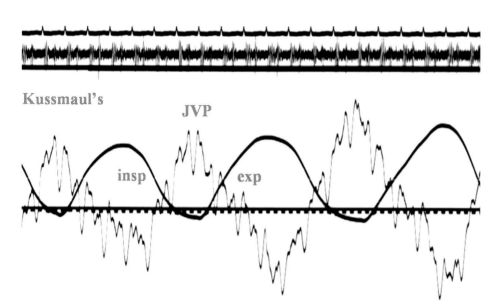

FIGURE 12.13. Jugular venous pulse with superimposed respiration recording demonstrating increased venous pressure during inspiration (Kussmal's sign).

The preceding disturbed physiology results in fluid retention due to low cardiac output and venous return, raised JVP, congested liver, and lower limb edema. Calcification of the pericardial border may be seen in the chest X-ray but is not always a diagnostic criterion. Pericardial thickening may be better demonstrated by MRI or CT scanning.

Echocardiographic Findings

A deep X descent on JVP recording from a patient with raised venous pressure along with predominant systolic flow in the superior or inferior vena cava is a very reliable finding for pericardial constriction. Thickened pericardium is a poorly sensitive marker, since it can easily be confused with small pericardium effusion with adhesions, with fibrous strands, or with pericardial fat. In constrictive pericarditis, there is less intracardiac than extracardiac respiratory variation, particularly on the right side when compared with that seen with pericardial tamponade.[22] Nonspecific signs include (a) rapid early diastolic posterior motion of the aortic root, with little additional movement in mid and late diastole caused by pressure equalization between the atrium and the ventricle in late diastole, limiting filling and ring movement[23]; (b) premature opening of the pulmonary valve occurring before the P wave of the electrocardiogram, suggesting significant increase in right ventricular pressures in mid diastole, and occasionally raised right atrial pressure during inspiration (Kussmaul's sign).

These findings can similarly be seen in other conditions, such as left bundle branch block and right ventricular disease. Although a dilated inferior vena cava is commonly seen, it is not solely a diagnostic sign for peri-

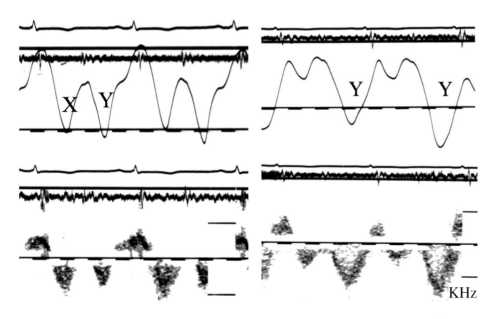

FIGURE 12.14. Jugular venous pulse from a patient with constrictive pericarditis before (left) and after (right) pericardiectomy. Note the diagnostic deep X descent and systolic right atrial filling before surgery that disappeared a few days after surgery.

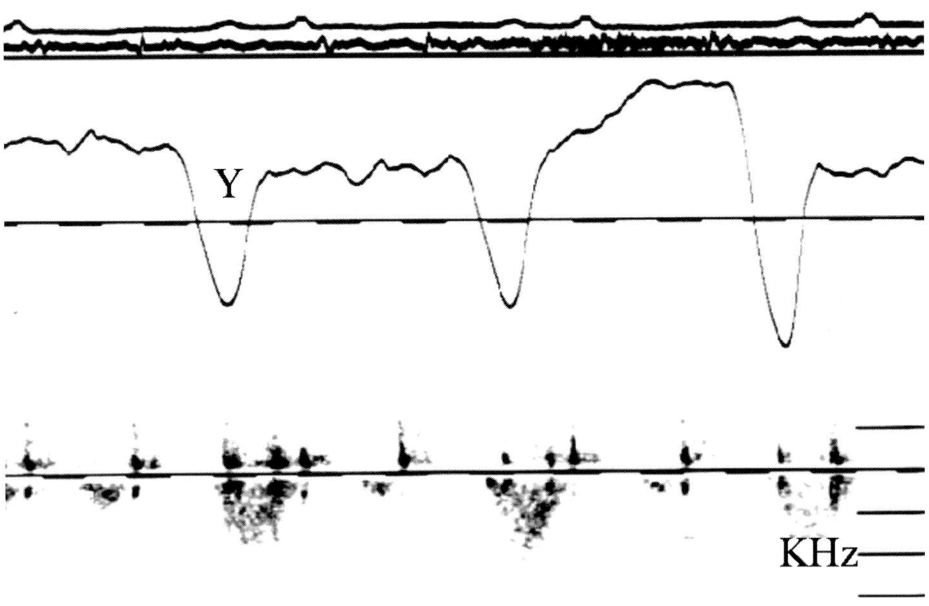

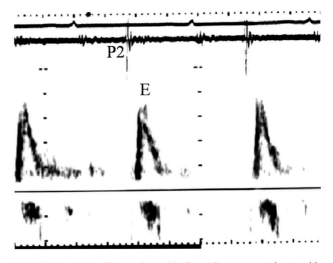

FIGURE 12.15. Jugular venous pulse from a patient with restrictive cardiomyopathy. Note the predominant early diastolic Y descent and right atrial filling (superior vena caval flow).

cardial constriction. Spontaneous contrast in the inferior vena cava, resulting from the limited venous return, may be an additional finding in favor of constrictive pericarditis.[24] In summary, therefore, the most sensitive Doppler sign for pericardial constriction in patients with persistent raised venous pressure and fluid retention is the predominant systolic atrial filling along with the X descent on the JVP.

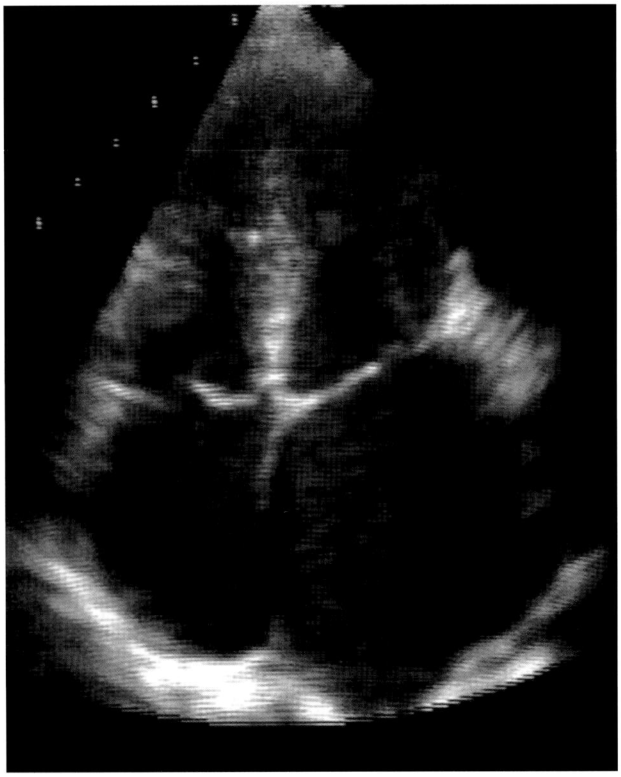

Management

Diuretics are usually given as an attempt to control the raised venous pressures. Pericardiectomy is usually recommended in patients resistant to pharmacologic therapy. After surgical removal of the pericardium the venous pressure drops and the X descent on the JVP disappears. This is not always instantaneous and may take up to a few days or even weeks to settle.

FIGURE 12.16. Apical four-chamber view from a patient with restrictive cardiomyopathy showing normal right ventricular size and dilated right atrium in the absence of tricuspid valve stenosis.

FIGURE 12.17. Transtricuspid flow from a patient with restrictive cardiomyopathy showing signs of raised right atrial pressure, fast acceleration, and short deceleration time.

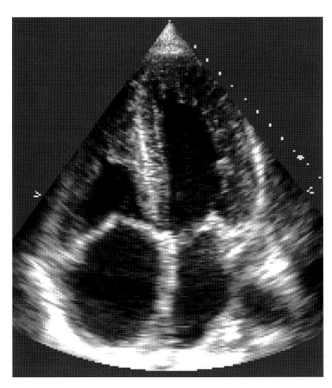

FIGURE 12.18. Apical four-chamber view from a patient with amyloid heart disease. Note the massive infiltration of the ventricles and atria judged by the increased myocardial echo intensity.

Differentiation Between Constrictive Pericarditis and Restrictive Cardiomyopathy

The clinical similarity between constrictive pericarditis and restrictive cardiomyopathy[25] makes the differential diagnosis difficult (i.e., raised venous pressure and fluid retention that is resistant to medical therapy). While con-strictive pericarditis is an extra-cardiac constraint, restrictive cardiomyopathy is an intrinsic myocardial disease of the ventricle. Restrictive cardiomyopathy is either idiopathic or infiltrative in origin (e.g., amyloid disease). The ventricular muscle may preserve its contractile function but loses its compliance, thereby becoming stiff and incompliant. This is specifically manifested in late diastole as the ventricle becomes unable to fill without a significant rise in the end-diastolic pressure. Therefore ventricular filling becomes restricted to early diastole with high acceleration and deceleration frequently associated with right-sided third heart sound. A concurrent fall in systemic venous pressure in early diastole "deep Y descent" is an additional diagnostic sign. Since restrictive cardiomyopathy is a chronic condition it results in a gradual increase in right atrial pressure and size, which in advanced stages may become the cause of arrhythmia, particularly atrial flutter.

Respiratory variation of ventricular filling and ejection velocities may be modestly present in constriction but is absent in restrictive right ventricular disease.[26] As pericardiectomy is largely a radical surgical management for constriction, empirical medical treatment remains the only available management to control patient symptoms in restrictive cardiomyopathy. Isolated right ventricular restrictive disease is rare. Right ventricular restriction is commonly seen in association with restrictive left ventricular disease, particularly amyloid infiltration and occasionally after recurrent open heart surgery or coronary artery disease. When right ventricular restriction and constriction physiology are present, even pericardiectomy does not provide radical treatment of the venous congestion because it only alleviates the extracardiac effect of constriction, being unable to alter the restrictive behavior of the right ventricle.

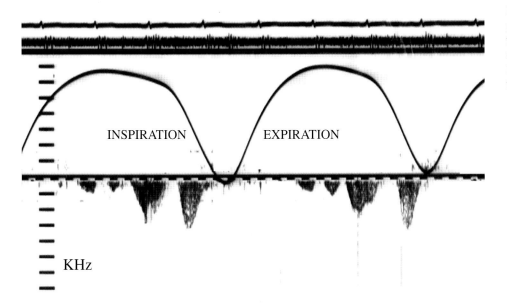

INSPIRATION   EXPIRATION

KHz

FIGURE 12.19. Jugular venous pulse and superior vena caval flow from a patient with postoperative tight pericardium. Note predominantly right-sided filling during inspiration.

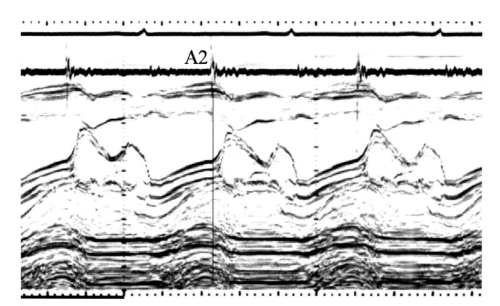

A

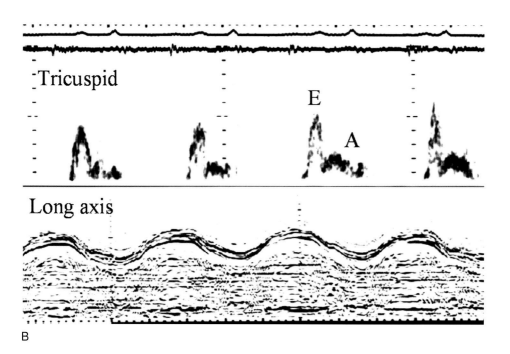

B

FIGURE 12.20. (A) Mitral echogram from a patient with restrictive pericarditis. Note the short isovolumic relaxation time consistent with raised left atrial pressure. (B) Right ventricular long-axis recording from the same patient showing markedly depressed amplitude and systolic function along with restrictive filling.

PERICARDIAL COMPLICATIONS POST OPEN HEART SURGERY

Apart from the commonly seen pericardial effusion, other complications, although rare, may occur:

1. Pericardial clot: Clot collection in the pericardial space with or without pericardial effusion is often associated with delayed postoperative clinical recovery. Irrespective of the amount present, it may have an important physiologic effect on the overall cardiac function. With time, the clot results in increased intrapericardial pressure and hence disturbed hemodynamics. Surgical removal of the clot is the ideal management of this condition through reopening and emptying the pericardial space. Early detection and management secures complete recovery.[18]

2. "Tight" pericardium: In the absence of postoperative pericardial effusion or detectable clotting, intrapericardial pressure may be raised to the extent that it affects right-sided physiology, making it phasic with respect to respiration. This condition is uncommon but may be seen after open heart surgery with signs of raised venous pressure. JVP is raised and right-sided physiology, filling and ejection, is predominantly inspiratory. On two-dimensional images there is no evidence for right atrial or ventricular collapse. The exact underlying etiology of this condition is not clear, although a potential element of pericardial tightness that is self-limited may be involved. Although these signs may resolve with time, delayed sternal closure has proved beneficial in some of the patients presenting with this phenomenon. The condition tends to settle within days of, if not a few weeks after, surgery, with complete normalization of venous pressure. This self-limited course supports the idea of it being iatrogenic pericardial inflammation that resolves with time.

3. Restrictive pericarditis: This is a rare clinical presentation that usually occurs following open heart surgery.[25] It presents with resistant fluid retention and raised venous pressure. Two-dimensional echocardiographic images may not show any specific abnormality, although MRI may demonstrate a thickened pericardium. The underlying pathology seems to be chronic combined pericardial and epicardial inflammation that consequently results in massive fibrosis and adhesions between the two layers. Patients with restrictive pericarditis are usually

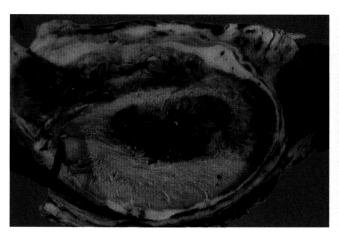
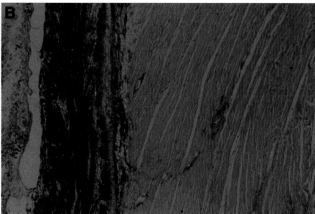

FIGURE 12.21. Section of the heart and pericardium from a case of restrictive pericarditis showing pericardial fibrosis invading the epicardium.

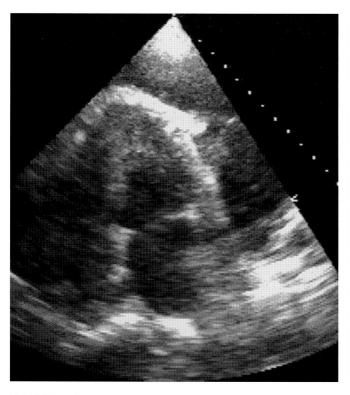
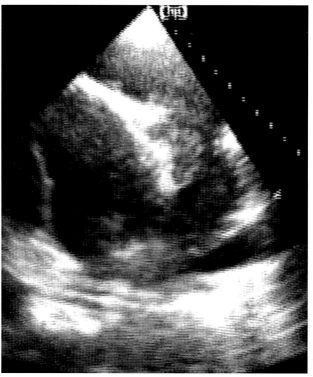

FIGURE 12.22. Apical four-chamber view from a patient with pleural carcinoma invading the pericardium and the apical free wall of the left ventricle.

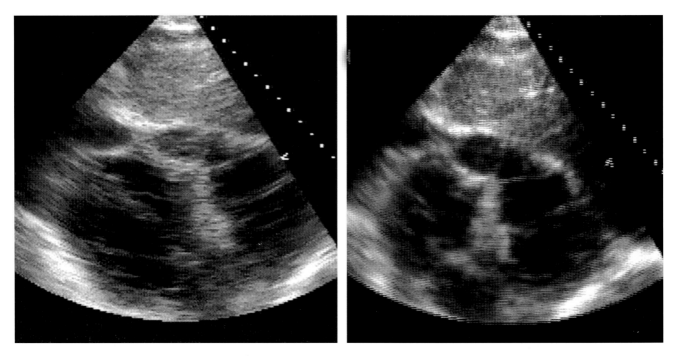

FIGURE 12.23. Subcostal view from a patient with small cell carcinoma that invaded the pericardium, causing effusion and adhesions to right ventricular free wall.

resistant to medical therapy and demonstrate signs of restrictive physiology on both sides of the heart, with a dominant early diastolic filling component and short deceleration time. Atrial pressures are usually raised as shown by the extraordinarily short isovolumic relaxation time. Atrial filling is predominantly early diastolic due to the raised ventricular end-diastolic pressure. The jugular venous pulse demonstrates a deep Y descent. Although left ventricular minor-axis dimensions and systolic function may be preserved, ventricular long-axis amplitude is consistently depressed in keeping with myocardial dysfunction.

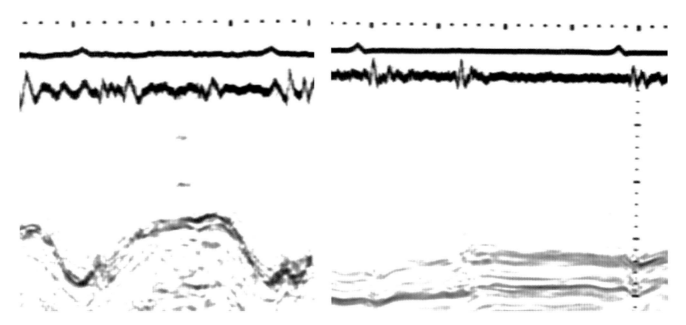

FIGURE 12.24. Right ventricular free-wall long axis before (left) and after (right) pericardial invasion showing significantly reduced free wall amplitude caused by adhesion.

Management

Cases that resist medical therapy may respond to surgical decortication of the pericardium. This does not always secure complete recovery, since the epicardial layer of the myocardium is usually involved in the pathology with fibrosis extending into the underlying myocardium.

PERICARDIAL TUMORS

The most common tumors of the pericardium are secondaries. The most frequent primary sources are carcinoma of the breast and lung, malignant melanoma, lymphoma, and leukemia.[27] They invade the pericardium either directly or via lymphatics or hematogenous dissemination. Primary tumors are rare but usually include malignant mesothelioma and sarcomas. While carcinomas metastasize in the pericardium in the form of localized masses, lymphomas and leukemia present in the form of uniform pericardial infiltration and thickening that may cause tumor incarceration of the heart and hence the clinical syndrome of "constrictive physiology." A mild degree of pericardial thickening may easily be missed on two-dimensional images. Magnetic resonance or CT scanning may offer a more conclusive diagnostic picture for pericardial thickening. Recurrent pericardial effusion of unknown etiology should suggest malignancy until otherwise proved. In addition, pericardial effusion in the presence of intracardiac mass suggests malignancy.

REFERENCES

1. Lorell BH, Braunwald E. Pericardial disease. In: Braunwald E, ed. *Heart disease.* Philadelphia: WB Saunders, 1992: 1465–1516.
2. Hagan AD. Evaluation of pericardial diseases by M-mode and two-dimensional echocardiography. In: Mason DT, ed. *Advances in heart disease.* New York: Grune & Stratton, 1980:699–702.
3. Guberman BA, Fowler NO, Engel PJ, et al. Cardiac tamponade in medical patients. *Circulation* 1981;64:633–640.
4. Chandraratna PA. Echocardiography and Doppler ultrasound in the evaluation of pericardial disease. *Circulation* 1991;84(3 Suppl):I303–I310.
5. Horowitz MS, Schultz CS, Stinson EB, et al. Sensitivity and specificity of echocardiographic diagnosis of pericardial effusion. *Circulation* 1974;50:239–247.
6. Isner JM, Carter BL, Roberts WC, et al. Subepicardial adipose tissue producing echocardiographic appearance of pericardial effusion. Documentation by computed tomography and necropsy. *Am J Cardiol* 1983;51:565–569.
7. Nanda NC, Gramiak R, Gross CM. Echocardiography of cardiac valves in pericardial effusion. *Circulation* 1976;54: 500–504.
8. Come PC, Riley MF, Fortuin NJ. Echocardiographic mimicry of pericardial effusion. *Am J Cardiol* 1981;47:365–370.
9. D'Cruz IA, Hoffman PK. A new cross-sectional echocardiographic method for estimating the volume of large pericardial effusions. *Br Heart J* 1991;66:448–451.
10. Singh S, Wann LS, Schuchard GH, et al. Right ventricular and right atrial collapse in patients with cardiac tamponade–a combined echocardiographic and hemodynamic study. *Circulation* 1984;70:966–971.
11. Gillam LD, Guyer DE, Gibson TC, et al. Hydrodynamic compression of the right atrium: a new echocardiographic sign of cardiac tamponade. *Circulation* 1983;68:294–301.
12. Katz LN, Gauchat HW. Observations on pulsus paradoxus (with special reference to pericardial effusions): II. Experimental. *Arch Intern Med* 1924;33:371–393.
13. Appleton CP, Hatle LK, Popp RL. Cardiac tamponade and pericardial effusion: respiratory variation in transvalvular flow velocities studied by Doppler echocardiography. *J Am Coll Cardiol* 1988;11:1020–1030.
14. Shabetai R, Fowler NO, Fenton JC, et al. Pulsus paradoxus. *J Clin Invest* 1965;44:1882–1898.
15. Reddy PS, Curtiss EI, O'Toole JD, et al. Cardiac tamponade: hemodynamic observations in man. *Circulation* 1978;58: 265–272.
16. Chuttani K, Pandian NG, Mohanty PK, et al. Left ventricular diastolic collapse. An echocardiographic sign of regional cardiac tamponade. *Circulation* 1991;83:1999–2006.
17. Kronzon I, Cohen ML, Winer HE. Diastolic atrial compression: a sensitive echocardiographic sign of cardiac tamponade. *J Am Coll Cardiol* 1983;2:770–775.
18. Kochar GS, Jacobs LE, Kotler MN. Right atrial compression in postoperative cardiac patients: detection by transesophageal echocardiography. *J Am Coll Cardiol* 1990;16:511–516.
19. Callahan JA, Seward JB, Nishimura RA, et al. Two-dimensional echocardiographically guided pericardiocentesis: experience in 117 consecutive patients. *Am J Cardiol* 1985;55: 476–479.
20. Nishimura RA, Kazmier FJ, Smith HC, et al. Right ventricular outflow obstruction caused by constrictive pericardial disease. *Am J Cardiol* 1985;55:1447–1448.
21. Cameron J, Oesterle SN, Baldwin JC, et al. The etiologic spectrum of constrictive pericarditis. *Am Heart J* 1987;113(2 Pt 1): 354–360.
22. Shabetai R, Fowler NO, Guntheroth WG. The hemodynamics of cardiac tamponade and constrictive pericarditis. *Am J Cardiol* 1970;26:480–489.
23. Voelkel AG, Pietro DA, Folland ED, et al. Echocardiographic features of constrictive pericarditis. *Circulation* 1978;58: 871–875.
24. Himelman RB, Lee E, Schiller NB. Septal bounce, vena cava plethora, and pericardial adhesion: informative two-dimensional echocardiographic signs in the diagnosis of pericardial constriction. *J Am Soc Echocardiogr* 1988; 1:333–340.
25. Henein MY, Rakhit RD, Sheppard MN, et al. Restrictive pericarditis. *Heart* 1999;82:389–392.
26. Hatle LK, Appleton CP, Popp RL. Differentiation of constrictive pericarditis and restrictive cardiomyopathy by Doppler echocardiography. *Circulation* 1989;79:357–370.
27. Kutalek SP, Panidis IP, Kotler MN, et al. Metastatic tumors of the heart detected by two-dimensional echocardiography. *Am Heart J* 1985;109:343–349.

13 Cardiac Tumors

BENIGN TUMORS

Cardiac tumors are rarely suspected clinically but usually appear as unexpected findings when patients are investigated for syncope, breathlessness, thromboembolism, or constitutional manifestations such as congestive heart failure or pulmonary hypertension.[1] Echocardiography provides a great opportunity to identify tumors that are clinically silent,[2] although extension to extra cardiac structures should be further investigated by transesophageal echocardiography,[3] CT scanning, or MRI. Benign tumors form approximately 80% of all cardiac tumors, 70% of which are myxomas.[4]

Myxoma

Myxomas affect adults in the third to the sixth decades of life with 3:1 female predominance.[5;6] They may remain completely silent until either accidentally discovered or become large enough to interfere with cardiac function and give symptoms.[7] Myxomas may occur anywhere in the heart, but in more than 80% of patients the left atrium is involved.[8] They rarely occur concurrently in more than one chamber.[9] Left atrial myxomas originate from the inter-atrial septum. They may increase in size and eventually occupy nearly all the atrium. Being redundant, they may obstruct the left ventricular inlet and prolapse into the left ventricle in diastole, so-called tumor plop. Large tumors may thus cause mitral stenosis, secondary pulmonary hypertension, and tricuspid regurgitation.[10]

Right atrial myxoma is much less common.[11] It may obstruct the right ventricular inlet, damage the tricuspid valve leaflets, and cause tricuspid valve obstruction.[12] Papillary fragments on the tumor surface may break off and cause systemic thromboemboli.[13;14]

The most important differential diagnosis of atrial myxoma is atrial thrombus. In contrast to atrial myxoma, a thrombus is commonly attached to the atrial wall by a

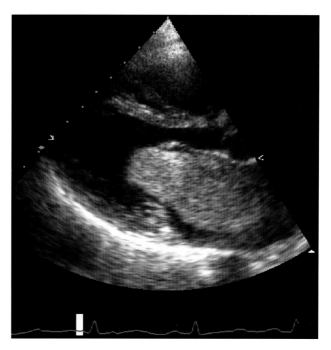

FIGURE 13.1. Parasternal long-axis view from a patient with left atrial myxoma. Note the size of the tumor and its relationship to anterior mitral valve leaflet.

large base and at any segment. The atrial thrombus is not pedunculated and is immobile.[15] The thrombus usually does not have a rounded contour, as does the myxoma. Atrial thrombus is also commonly associated with other pathologies (e.g., mitral valve disease, dilated atrium, atrial fibrillation, and raised atrial pressures secondary to left ventricular disease).

Surgical excision is the only management for large tumors and results in normalization of atrial size and function. Atrial myxoma may recur after excision either in the same area or in adjacent segments if its origin in the left atrium is not completely removed.

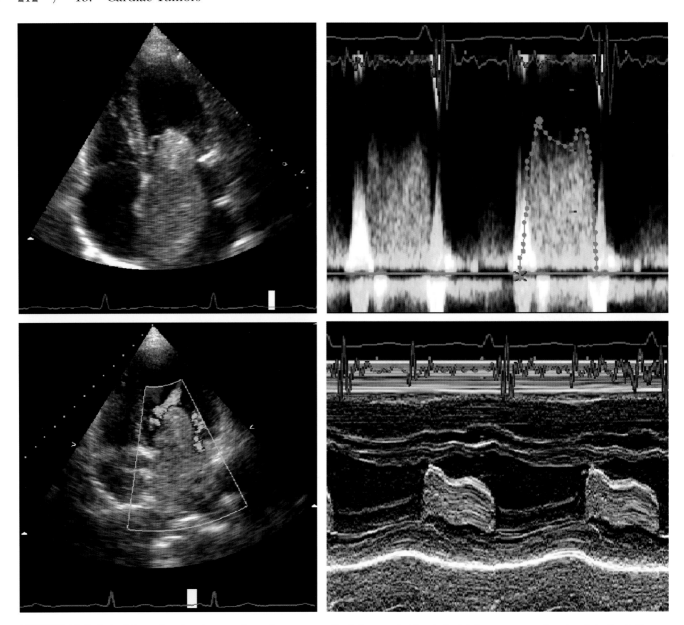

FIGURE 13.2. Apical four-chamber images from the same patient demonstrating left atrial myxoma prolapsing into the left ventricular cavity. Note the aliasing of the color flow Doppler, the raised inflow velocities consistent with narrowed ventricular inflow tract, and the classical mitral valve M-mode of prolapsing myxoma.

Fibroelastoma

Fibroelastoma is a benign mass that appears as a small, frond-like tumor, is usually solitary, but is rarely multiple.[16;17] Although it can be found anywhere in the heart, it is commonly attached to the valves or ventricular outflow tract. A fibroelastoma is not usually associated with any symptoms but is accidentally found during either routine scanning or surgery for other pathology.

Lipoma

Lipomas are rare benign tumors that are found attached to the endocardium or epicardium. Demonstrating that

they are encapsulated and sessile may help in differentiating them from fat deposition inside and outside the heart.[18;19] Lipomas are rarely associated with symptoms or clinical manifestations. Although lipomas attached to the interatrial septum may be difficult to differentiate from benign septal hypertrophy, their localization and encapsulation may support the diagnosis of lipoma.

Rhabdomyoma

Rhabdomyoma[20] is a congenital tumor that may grow large enough to obstruct valves and cause sudden death. Characteristically, it is associated with tuberous

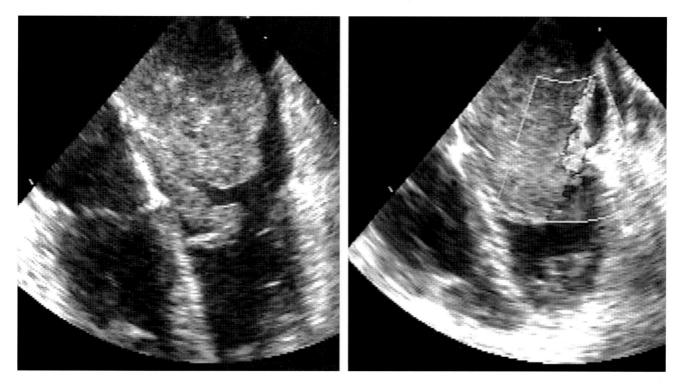

FIGURE 13.3. Transesophageal echo from a patient with left atrial myxoma demonstrating the prolapsing tumor in diastole that narrows ventricular inlet and causing raised filling velocities.

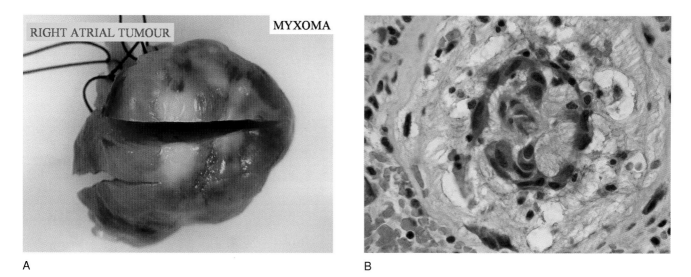

A   B

FIGURE 13.4. (a) Pathologic specimen of left atrial myxoma b) shows myxoid cells in histologic section.

sclerosis, and multiple tumors are usually found. After birth the size of the tumors tends to regress.

Fibroma

Cardiac fibroma is usually solitary, occurring either at the ventricular free wall or at the septum when involving the septal myocardium. Large fibromas are often inoperable.

They are benign and can regress with increasing age in childhood.

Teratoma

Often detected antenatally, teratomas are evident in infancy.

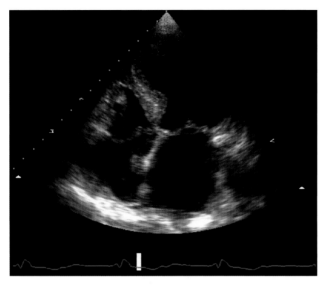

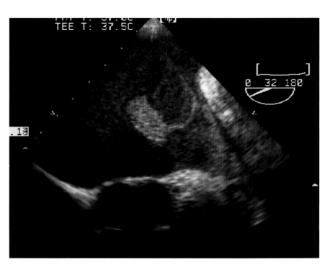

FIGURE 13.6. Transesophageal echo demonstrating large left atrium, spontaneous contrast, and a free-wall thrombus.

FIGURE 13.5. Apical four-chamber view from a patient with small right atrial myxoma.

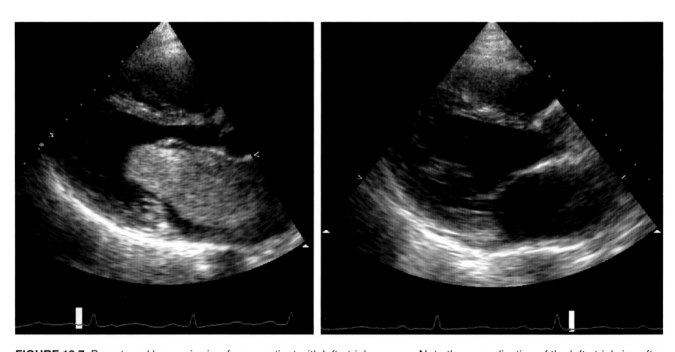

FIGURE 13.7. Parasternal long-axis view from a patient with left atrial myxoma. Note the normalization of the left atrial size after excision of the tumor (right).

MALIGNANT TUMORS

Primary Malignant Tumors

While benign tumors favor the left atrium, malignant ones tend to occur more commonly in the right heart.[21] More than 80% of primary malignant tumors are sarcomas, the most common one being angiosarcoma.[22] In more than 70% of cases it occurs in the right atrium, invading the myocardium, epicardium, and pericardium and frequently metastasizes to the lungs. Other sarcomas may also occur but are extremely rare. Osteosarcoma may occur in the left atrium as well.

Mesothelioma

Mesothelioma is the second most common primary malignant tumor that grows from the visceral or parietal layer of the pericardium.[23] It rarely invades the myocardium. It is rarely intracardiac and may mimic a myxoma.

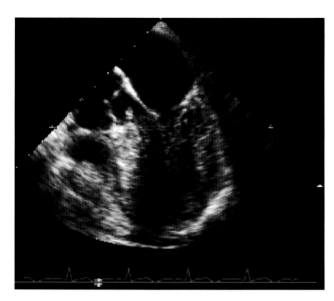

FIGURE 13.8. Apical four-chamber view demonstrating a small fibroelastoma attached to left ventricular outflow tract.

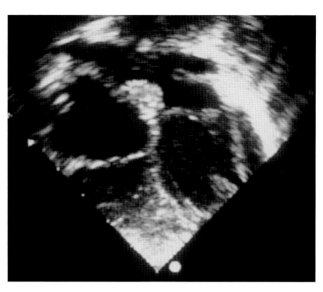

FIGURE 13.10. Subcostal views from a patient with atrial septal lipomas.

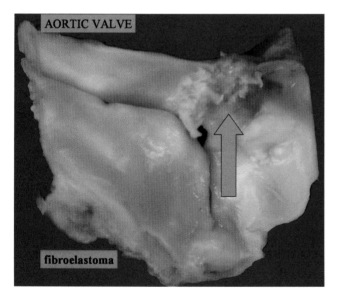

AORTIC VALVE

fibroelastoma

FIGURE 13.9. Pathologic section showing a small fibroelastoma attached to the aortic valve.

Secondary Malignant Tumors

Secondary malignant tumors are commonly found in autopsies. However, their incidence in the heart is much less than that in other organs, possibly due to frequent obliteration of the malignant cells by myocardial contraction, sliding of its layers, and poor lymphatic cardiac flow. Secondary tumors may complicate carcinoma of the lung and breast and are less frequently seen with melanoma,[24] leukemia, and lymphoma.[25] When blood-borne secondaries invade the heart, the right heart is most commonly affected, particularly with malignant melanoma and renal cell carcinoma. Direct invasion of the heart via lung or breast carcinoma is usually associated with large pericardial effusions. Lymphatic spread as in breast carcinoma and lymphoma may invade the pericardium without any obvious intracardiac secondary growth. Melanoma and leukemia commonly involve the heart without pericardial effusion.

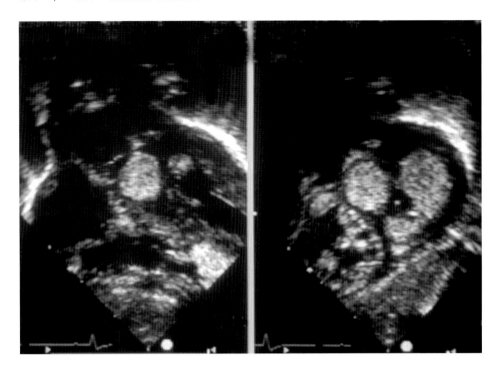

FIGURE 13.11. Subcostal views from a patient with multiple rhabdomyomata.

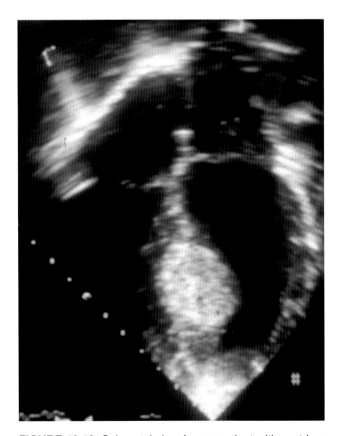

FIGURE 13.12. Subcostal view from a patient with ventricular septal fibroma. Notice the tumor size and its distant relationship to the left ventricular inlet.

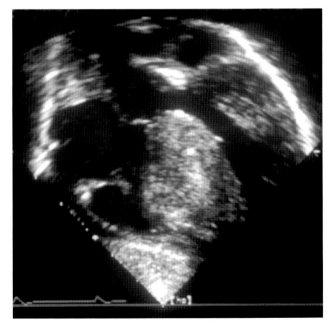

FIGURE 13.13. Subcostal view from a patient with teratoma invading the distal septum and right ventricular apex.

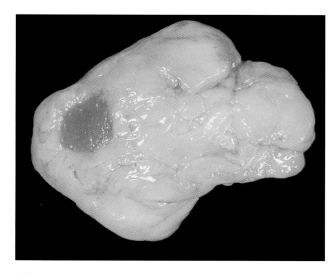

FIGURE 13.14. Pathologic section demonstrating malignant tumour excised from the right atrium.

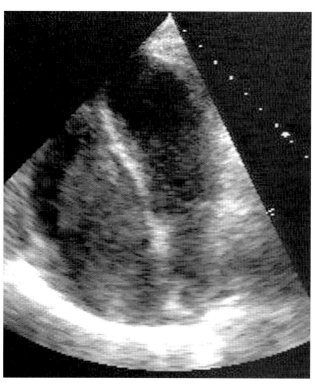

FIGURE 13.15. Apical four-chamber view showing right atrial angiosarcoma invading the atrial wall and disturbing atrial blood flow.

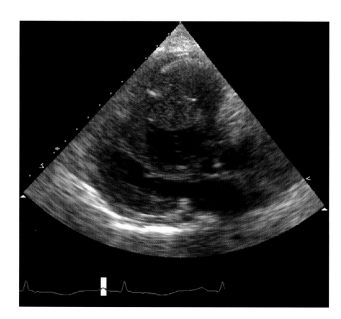

FIGURE 13.16. Parasternal long axis showing melanoma invading right ventricular free wall.

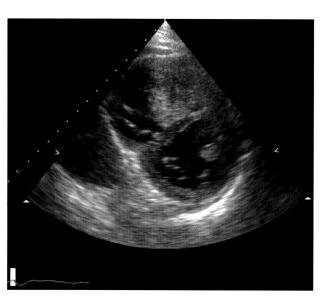

FIGURE 13.17. Short-axis view showing malignant melanoma invading the right ventricular free wall.

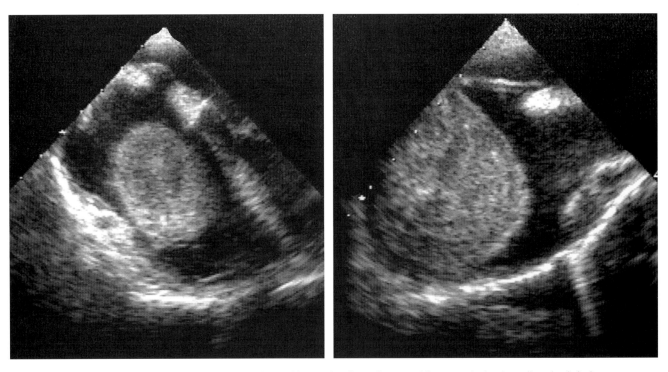

FIGURE 13.18. Transesophageal echo from a patient with renal cell carcinoma with secondaries invading the inferior vena cava and the right atrium.

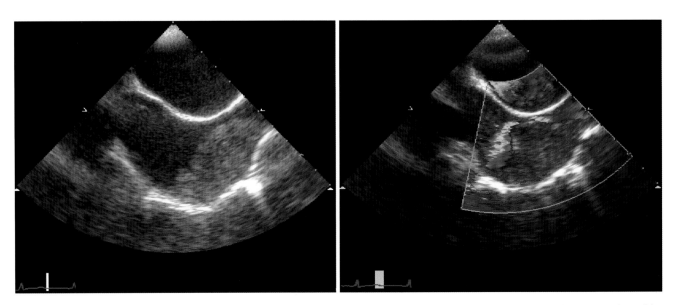

FIGURE 13.19. Transesophageal echo showing osteosarcoma invading the right atrial free wall and causing narrowing of its inflow.

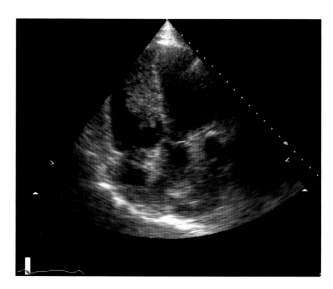

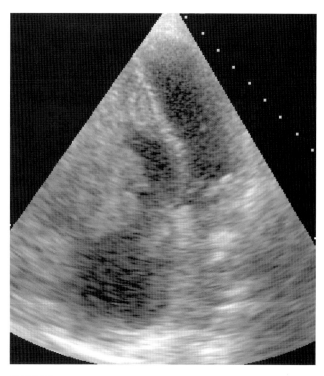

FIGURE 13.20. Apical view showing malignant melanoma invading right ventricular septal region near the apex.

FIGURE 13.21. Apical view showing renal cell carcinoma invading right ventricular free wall.

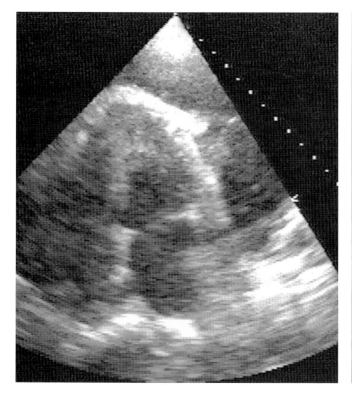

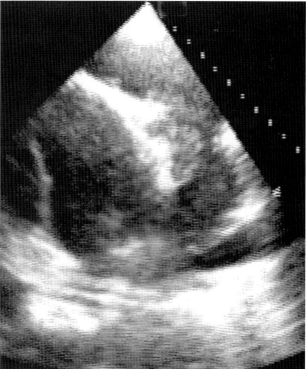

FIGURE 13.22. Apical views demonstrating left pleural carcinoma invading and eroding the pericardium and the epicardium of the left ventricular free wall.

REFERENCES

1. Bloor CM, O'Rourke RA. Cardiac tumors: clinical presentation and pathologic correlations. *Curr Probl Cardiol* 1984;9: 7–48.

2. Fyke FE III, Seqard JB, Edwards WD, et al. Primary cardiac tumors: experience with 30 consecutive patients since the introduction of two-dimensional echocardiography. *J Am Coll Cardiol* 1985;5:1465–1473.

3. Reeder GS, Khandheria BK, Seward JB, et al. Transesophageal echocardiography and cardiac masses. *Mayo Clin Proc* 1991;66:1101–1109.

4. Goodwin JF. The spectrum of cardiac tumors. *Am J Cardiol* 1968;21:307–314.

5. Prichard RW. Tumors of the heart: review of the subject and report of one hundred and fifty cases. *Arch Pathol* 1951;51:98–128.

6. Nasser WK, Davis RH, Dillon JC, et al. Atrial myxoma. I. Clinical and pathologic features in nine cases. *Am Heart J* 1972;83:694–704.

7. McAllister HA, Fenoglio JJ. *Tumors of the cardiovascular system. Atlas of tumor pathology.* Washington, DC: Armed Forces Institute of Pathology, 1978.

8. Salcedo EE, Adams KV, Lever HM, et al. Echocardiographic findings in 25 patients with left atrial myxoma. *J Am Coll Cardiol* 1983;1:1162–1166.

9. Vargas-Barron J, Romero-Cardenas A, Villegas M, et al. Transthoracic and transesophageal echocardiographic diagnosis of myxomas in the four cardiac cavities. *Am Heart J* 1991;121(3 Pt 1):931–933.

10. Gorcsan J III, Blanc MS, Reddy PS, et al. Hemodynamic diagnosis of mitral valve obstruction by left atrial myxoma with transesophageal continuous wave Doppler. *Am Heart J* 1992;124:1109–1112.

11. Dashkoff N, Boersma RB, Nanda NC, et al. Bilateral atrial myxomas. Echocardiographic considerations. *Am J Med* 1978; 65:361–366.

12. Turlapati RV, Jacobs LE, Kotler MN. Right atrial myxoma causing total destruction of the tricuspid valve leaflets. *Am Heart J* 1990;120:1227–1231.

13. Bryhn M, Gustafson A, Stubbe I. Two-dimensional echocardiography in the diagnosis of hemorrhages in a left atrial myxoma. *Acta Med Scand* 1982;212:433–435.

14. Rahilly GT Jr., Nanda NC. Two-dimensional echographic identification of tumor hemorrhages in atrial myxomas. *Am Heart J* 1981;101:237–239.

15. Reeder GS, Tajik AJ, Seward JB. Left ventricular mural thrombus: two-dimensional echocardiographic diagnosis. *Mayo Clin Proc* 1981;56:82–86.

16. Lee KS, Topol EJ, Stewart WJ. Atypical presentation of papillary fibroelastoma mimicking multiple vegetations in suspected subacute bacterial endocarditis. *Am Heart J* 1993; 125(5 Pt 1):1443–1445.

17. Richard J, Castello R, Dressler FA, et al. Diagnosis of papillary fibroelastoma of the mitral valve complicated by non–Q-wave infarction with apical thrombus: transesophageal and transthoracic echocardiographic study. *Am Heart J* 1993; 126(3 Pt 1): 710–712.

18. Shirani J, Roberts WC. Clinical, electrocardiographic and morphologic features of massive fatty deposits ("lipomatous hypertrophy") in the atrial septum. *J Am Coll Cardiol* 1993; 22:226–238.

19. Kamiya H, Ohno M, Iwata H, et al. Cardiac lipoma in the interventricular septum: evaluation by computed tomography and magnetic resonance imaging. *Am Heart J* 1990;119: 1215–1217.

20. Smythe JF, Dyck JD, Smallhorn JF, et al. Natural history of cardiac rhabdomyoma in infancy and childhood. *Am J Cardiol* 1990;66:1247–1249.

21. Burke AP, Cowan D, Virmani R. Primary sarcomas of the heart. *Cancer* 1992;69:387–395.

22. Glancy DL, Morales JB Jr, Roberts WC. Angiosarcoma of the heart. *Am J Cardiol* 1968;21:413–419.

23. Skhvatsabaja LV. Secondary malignant lesions of the heart and pericardium in neoplastic disease. *Oncology* 1986;43:103–106.

24. Glancy DL, Roberts WC. The heart in malignant melanoma. A study of 70 autopsy cases. *Am J Cardiol* 1968;21:555–571.

25. Roberts WC, Glancy DL, DeVita VT Jr. Heart in malignant lymphoma (Hodgkin's disease, lymphosarcoma, reticulum cell sarcoma and mycosis fungoides). A study of 196 autopsy cases. *Am J Cardiol* 1968;22:85–107.

Diseases of the Aorta

CONGENITALLY SMALL AORTIC ROOT

For a discussion of congenitally small aortic root please refer to the aortic valve disease chapter 2.

AORTIC DISSECTION

Aortic dissection is a surgical emergency that requires accurate diagnosis and prompt management. Aortic dissection is classified into two types: type A, which involves all forms that include the ascending aorta, and type B, which does not involve the ascending aorta. Although type A is usually an emergency diagnosis and management, type B can be managed medically or conservatively. Mortality from type A dissection may be 60% within the first 24 hours, 80% over the first 2 weeks, and 90% within 3 months of acute attack. Dissection of the proximal ascending aorta can often be seen on transthoracic echo imaging, and even those involving the distal ascending aorta may occasionally be detected. However, transthoracic echo cannot always exclude type A dissection. Instead transesophageal echocardiography is the investigation of choice.[1-3]

The diagnostic marker of dissection is the luminal flap that can take different shapes and forms during the cardiac cycle according to its size.

1. Freely mobile flap with detached edges that prolapse back into the left ventricle in diastole. This tends to hold the leaflets apart and the valve open during diastole, resulting in severe aortic regurgitation.

2. Mobile flap that is distal to the aortic leaflets. Blood fills the false lumen at the entry point, which may

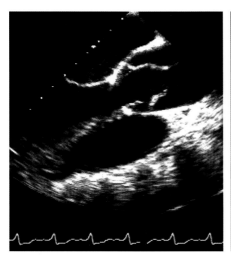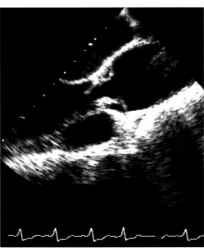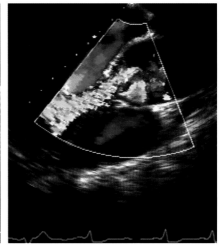

FIGURE 14.1. Transesophageal echo from a patient with aortic dissection. Note the freely mobile flap in the ascending aorta in systole (left) that prolapses into the left ventricle in diastole (middle), resulting in severe aortic regurgitation on color flow Doppler (right).

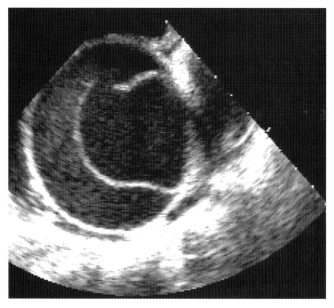

A

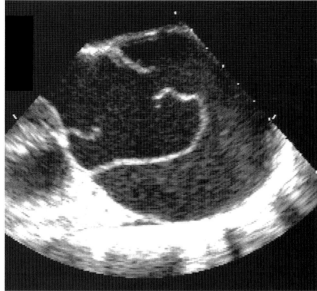

B

C

FIGURE 14.2. (A, B) Transesophageal echo of the aorta showing dilated ascending aorta with a dissection flap in the middle separating the true from the false lumen. (C) M-mode of the proximal ascending aorta showing the true aortic lumen and a clotted dissection (*arrow*).

thrombose if left untreated. This results in dilatation of the ascending aorta and distal root and, consequently, significant aortic regurgitation. Identifying the true and false aortic lumens depends on the position of the dissection flap in the aortic lumen and its relationship to the image planes and flow patterns.

3. Coincidental chronic dissection that has settled spontaneously and is thrombosed (organized) in the distal ascending aorta. Such cases may be followed up clinically without the need for intervention.

An apparent dissection flap may be mimicked on transthoracic echo by other conditions, such as calcified

aortic valve, pacing leads, aortic calcification, or pericardial effusion. However, an independently moving flaplike layer in a dilated ascending aorta is suggestive of dissection until proven otherwise.

Transesophageal echo provides clear images of the aortic root and ascending aorta in the majority of patients with suspected aortic dissection. The entry site is usually identified, the flap is clearly seen, and the extent of dissection, to the arch or even to the descending aorta, can be followed. Associated coronary artery or carotid artery dissection can often be confirmed, although it occurs in a very small percentage of patients.[4–6]

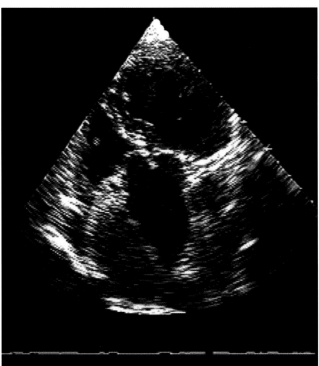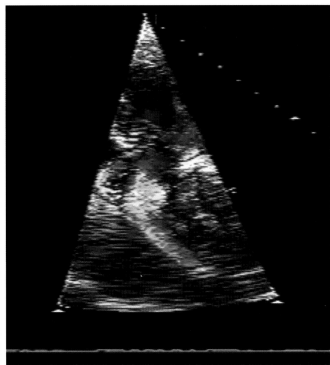

FIGURE 14.3. Apical four-chamber view from an elderly patient with distal dissection in the ascending aorta. Note the organized thrombus in the false lumen (left) and the blood flow in the true lumen parallel to the flap edge (right).

Color flow Doppler with transthoracic and transesophageal echo imaging helps in identifying the entry site of the false lumen and in assessing the severity of aortic regurgitation. Transesophageal echo has similar sensitivity to MRI and CT scanning for diagnosing aortic dissection but lower specificity, particularly for the ascending aorta. This has been attributed to the extent of aortic calcification, plaque formation, debris, and echo reverberations. It has the advantage, though, of being performed at bedside and on ventilated patients in the intensive care unit.[7,8]

Management

The classification of dissection of the aorta is closely related to the current optimal initial treatment. Thus type A dissection involving either the ascending aorta or the ascending arch and descending aorta is an indication for urgent operation. A type B dissection that classically originates in the proximal third of the descending aorta immediately distal to the origin of the left subclavian artery is initially treated by medical therapy with surgery reserved for selected patients 8 to 12 weeks later. The objective in surgery for acute type A ascending dissection is to relieve pericardial tamponade, restore the integrity of the aortic valve, and stabilize the ascending aorta. These operations are done using cardiopulmonary bypass, and frequently the distal aortic anastomosis is done during a period of circulatory arrest involving core cooling of the patient to between 15°C and 18°C for a period of approximately 20 to 25 minutes. The principle of the operation is to remove the area of aorta where the entry site or tear exists and to reconstitute the layers of the aorta, both proximal and distal to this point. In the vast majority of patients it is possible to resuspend the commissures of the aortic valve, thus saving the aortic valve, the leaflets of which are usually quite normal. An interposition graft of collagen-impregnated Dacron is then placed between the two reconstructed areas of aorta. Frequently it is necessary to extend the distal anastomosis into the proximal part of the aortic arch. The risk of this surgery is of the order of 8% to 10% mortality with a 1% to 2% incidence of stroke.

By comparison, acute operations on the descending aorta that are not routinely performed carry a similar mortality risk and a small risk of paraplegia.

It is vital that these patients remain under surveillance, preferably by a surgeon interested in surgery of the aorta, and that they undergo MRI scans annually or CT scans if MRI is inappropriate. In the majority of these cases the distal part of the aorta heals and the false lumen thromboses, but in a small minority this does not occur, and further dilatation of the descending aorta may take place, requiring intervention at a later date.

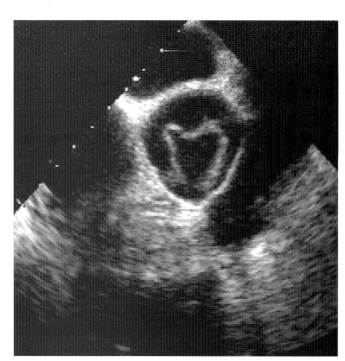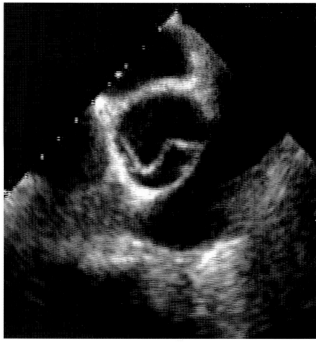

FIGURE 14.4. Short axis of the ascending aorta from a patient with dissection showing freely mobile flap, changing its shape during the cardiac cycle.

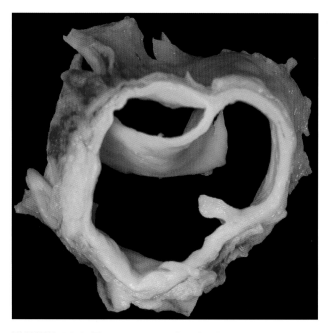

FIGURE 14.5. Transverse section in the ascending aorta demonstrating a dissection flap dividing the aorta into two lumens.

AORTIC ATHEROSCLEROTIC DEBRIS

Aortic atherosclerotic debris are small, localized, atherosclerotic plaques in the aortic wall that protrude into the aortic lumen and can be identified by transesophageal echo. Different grades of debris may be recognized, varying from thickened intima, atherosclerotic plaques, and mobile atheromata greater than 5 mm in diameter. An atherosclerotic aortic wall can be the source of strokes in a number of conditions[9,10]:

1. Patients undergoing aortic clamping as part of cardiopulmonary bypass.

2. High-risk patients with carotid or peripheral vascular disease.

3. Patients with recurrent embolization.

AORTIC ANEURYSM

A dilated ascending aorta can be readily diagnosed by transthoracic echo and the diameter measured from M-mode recordings. Aneurysms involving the arch or the descending thoracic aorta are better studied by transesophageal echocardiography or MRI. A true aneurysm may be differentiated from a dissecting aneurysm.[11,12] A common cause of aortic aneurysm is Marfan's syndrome, but the lesion may occur in the absence of external stigmata of the disease.[13] According to Laplace's law, wall tension increases directly with diameter, so that a dilated aorta is inherently unstable, particularly if medial necrosis is present. Such patients should therefore be regularly monitored for changes in aortic diameter. Patients with an aortic root exceeding 5 cm are likely to be taking prophylactic β blocker therapy to prevent progressive aortic dilatation.[12] Aortic replacement with resuspension or replacement of the aortic valve is a commonly applied surgical management for aortic aneurysm, when the aortic diameter exceeds 5.5 to 6 cm.[14] Such patients are at high risk from dissection, and ideally the operation should be performed before this occurs. Whether or not prophylactic aortic root replacement should be considered in patients with normal-diameter aorta but strong family history of dissection, particularly at a young age, remains controversial.

AORTIC SINUS OF VALSALVA ANEURYSM

Aneurysm of the aortic sinuses has been reported with Marfan's syndrome. The congenital form of aneurysmal sinuses is rare but has been reported with the sinus diameter exceeding 2.5 cm. Intact dilated sinuses carry the risk of blood clots inside them, hence the need for prophylactic anticoagulants. Coronary sinus rupture into the right heart establishes a fistulous connection between the aorta and the right atrium or right ventricle. Color flow Doppler helps to establish the exact relationship between the aortic sinuses and right heart chambers.[14–16]

AORTIC ROOT ABSCESS

Aortic root abscess is a form of infective endocarditis that can involve the paravalvular tissue of the aortic root. It is commonly associated with prolongation of the PR interval and conduction disturbances. Transthoracic echo often confirms the presence of paravalvular space lesions. A well-defined abscess enlarges during systole due to the blood flowing in and out of it. Aortic root abscess may consist of one or more small cavities either in isolation or connected together. Transesophageal echo, particularly the short-axis view, is ideal for demonstrating an aortic root abscess, and color flow Doppler may confirm space continuity between the compartments and the aortic root. If the latter is found it is usually demonstrated as a fistula between the cavity and the aortic root with the hemodynamics of aortic regurgitation. Aortic root abscess is a strong indication for early surgery. Small cavities may be sterilized, repaired, or grafted by pericardial tissue during surgery, followed by aortic valve replacement. Large and widely spread cavities may require entire aortic root replacement.[17,18]

INTRAOPERATIVE ECHOCARDIOGRAPHY

Intraoperative transesophageal echocardiography provides an invaluable tool for assessing early results of aortic surgery. In patients with aortic dissection, the inlet site of the dissection as well as its extent can be confirmed. The flap morphology and lumens can all be clearly visualized, and hence the right surgical plan can be made. Early results of dissection repair (with homograft or Dacron) can be evaluated and the aortic valve function (suspended native valve or substitute) can be assessed. The same benefits apply to surgical procedure for aortic aneurysm. Additional information on left ventricular size and function is provided, and any pericardial collection that may delay early postoperative recovery can also be quantified.

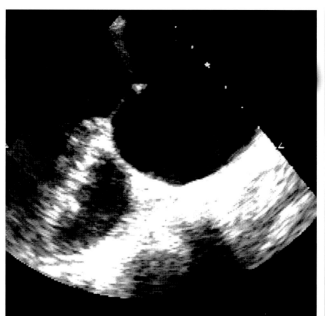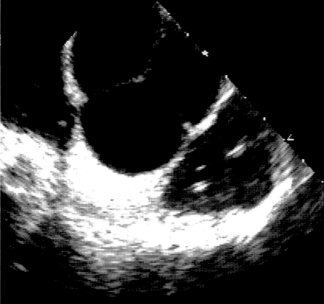

FIGURE 14.6. Transesophageal echo from a patient with aortic root aneurysm (localized).

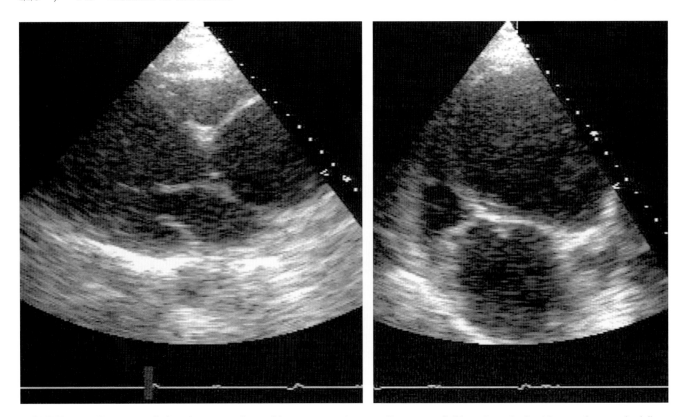

FIGURE 14.7. Parasternal view from a patient with aneurysmal ascending aorta (left) and equivalent image from apical five-chamber views (right) demonstrating aneurysm diameter of 7 cm.

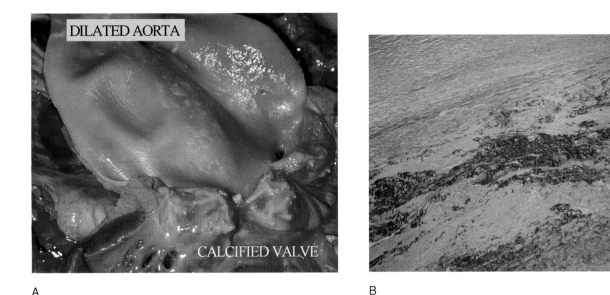

A

B

FIGURE 14.8. (A) Section demonstrating dilated and aneurysmal ascending aorta. (B) Histologic section from the aorta showing cystic medial necrosis characteristic of aortic aneurysm.

COARCTATION OF THE AORTA

Coarctation is a localized aortic stricture that commonly affects the descending aorta distal to the origin of the left subclavian artery with significant aortic narrowing.

Coarctation of the aorta results in collateral development between the proximal and distal aortic segments to the coarctation in order to secure the peripheral circulation. Coarctation of the aorta may present as a single congenital anomaly or may be associated with bicuspid aortic

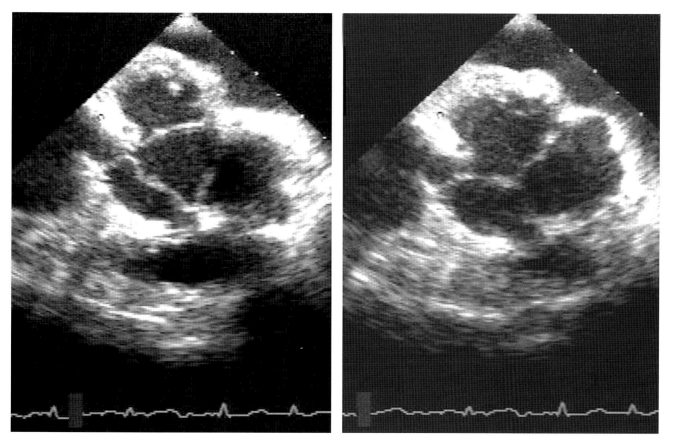

FIGURE 14.9. Parasternal short-axis views from a patient with aneurysmal aortic sinuses. Note the large sinus diameter and the retained clot behind the leaflet.

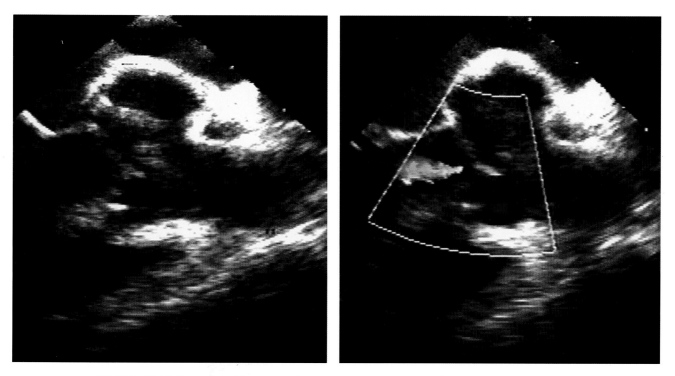

FIGURE 14.10. Parasternal long-axis view from the same patient showing aortic regurgitation.

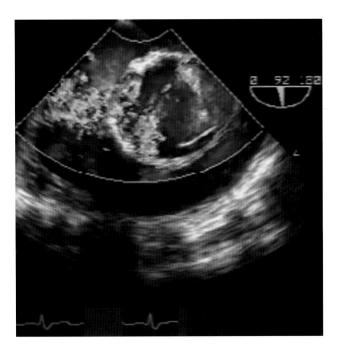

FIGURE 14.11. Transesophageal echo images of the aortic root from a patient with infective endocarditis showing ruptured sinus of Valsalva aneurysm into the right atrium demonstrating continuous flow.

valve, atrial septal defect, ventricular septal defect, or patent ductus arteriosus. Most patients with coarctation survive until adulthood. Coarctation is best visualized from the suprasternal notch with leftward angulation of the imaging probe. Post-stenotic dilatation is commonly seen as well as prestenotic dilatation of the descending thoracic aorta. Color flow Doppler helps in localizing the segment involved, but continuous-wave Doppler is the diagnostic technique to confirm the presence and severity of coarctation. With mild degree of aortic lumen narrowing, the velocity across the coarctation is low and its deceleration limb stops at end ejection. With significant stenosis the systolic velocities are increased and the pressure decline continues through diastole, so-called diastolic tail. This is a diagnostic Doppler criterion for significant coarctation.[19,20]

From continuous wave Doppler recordings, peak pressure drop across the coarctation can be calculated from the peak velocity using the modified Bernoulli equation. This may overestimate the pressure drop across the coarctation. Therefore applying the equation $4 (V_2^2 - V_1^2)$ as a measure of pressure drop, where V_2 is distal velocity and V_1 is proximal velocity provides a closer value to that from catheterization.[21] Patients who demonstrate a modest systolic pressure drop and raised diastolic pressure drop across the coarctation greater than 16 mmHg should be considered as having significant coarctation. Combined significant aortic stenosis and coarctation may exist, and decision making for managing such patients may be difficult, since severe aortic stenosis can underestimate the degree of coarctation narrowing and vice versa. The situation may be even more complex when there is additional significant left ventricular disease and low cardiac output state. Stress echo may have an important role in confirming severity of aortic stenosis and coarctation based on changes in

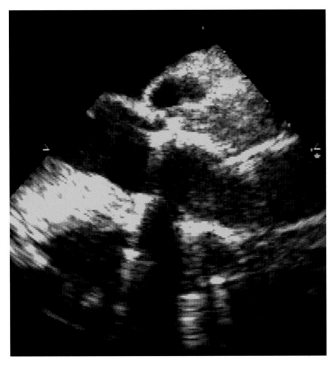

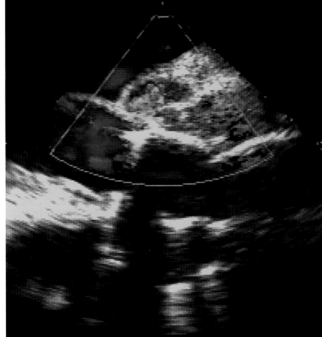

FIGURE 14.12. Parasternal long-axis view from a patient with localized abscess cavity.

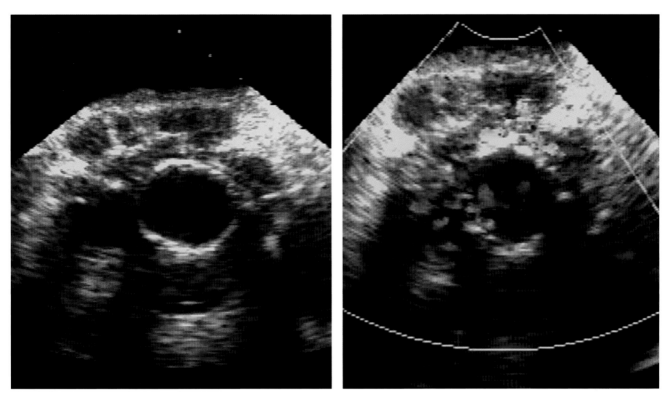

FIGURE 14.13. Short axis of the aortic root showing paravalvular abscess cavities with color flow inside them.

effective valve area and lumen diameter, respectively, with stress.

Management

Significant coarctation can be treated by balloon angioplasty (particularly in the young) or surgical resection with end-to-end anastomosis in adults who are not suitable for the nonsurgical procedure. Transesophageal echo monitoring during surgery provides excellent imaging of the site of stricture and anastomosis. In patients with coexisting aortic stenosis and coarctation, current surgical policy recommends managing the coarctation first, preferably by percutaneous balloon intervention, followed by aortic valve replacement.

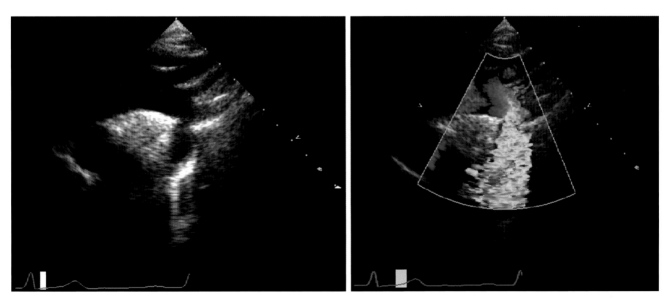

FIGURE 14.14. Suprasternal images of the aortic arch and proximal descending aorta from a patient with coarctation of the aorta. Note the color aliasing at the site of aortic narrowing.

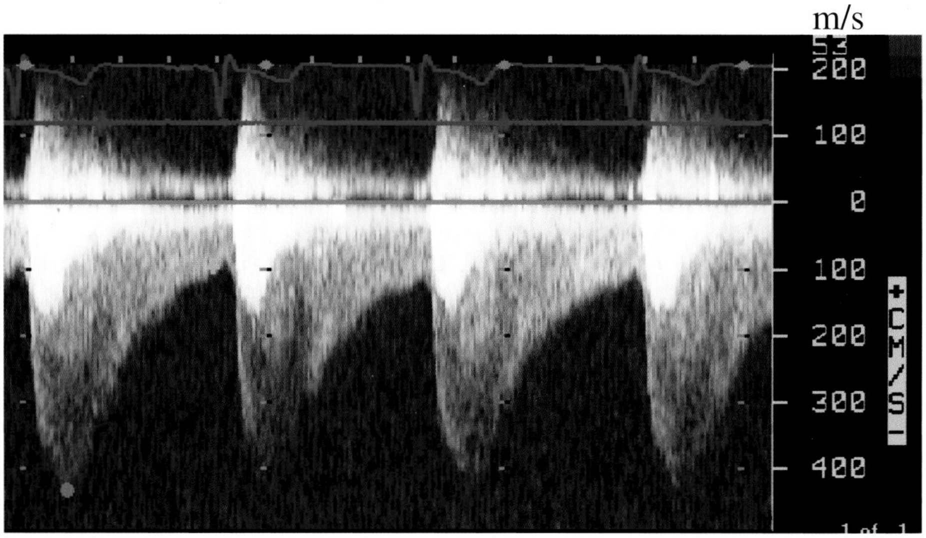

FIGURE 14.15. Continuous-wave Doppler recording from a patient with severe coarctation of the aorta showing velocity of 3.5 m/s equivalent to a pressure drop of 50 mmHg and a diastolic tail.

Surgery for coarctation in children is an operation that is usually carried out before the child attends school. An end-to-end anastomosis is the primary aim following resection of the coarct segment. Interrupted sutures are used over the anterior third of the anastomosis to allow for subsequent growth. In situations where the aorta is hypoplastic, particularly in the neonate, more complex methods of repair are required, and one of the commonest approaches is the use of the subclavian flap. By this operation the left subclavian artery is sacrificed and the proximal part of this artery is used as a flap to augment the area adjacent to the coarctation. Flow to the arm in the majority of instances is maintained due to the collateral circulation from the suprascapular arteries.

In adult patients coarctation of the aorta is a more complex operation, as there is commonly calcification at the site of the duct, and if collaterals are not well developed it is vital to ensure that the lower half of the body is well perfused during the clamping period. It is in this group of patients that there is an incidence of paraplegia of approximately 3% to 5%, which can be reduced by techniques to ensure adequate perfusion to the lower half of the body and in some instances a drainage of the cerebrospinal fluid via a lumbar catheter. The overall mortality for a coarctation in childhood is of the order of 1% to 2%, and in adult life it is around 2% to 3%. These patients need to be followed up for life, as there are significant complications that can arise from coarctation, particularly if Dacron grafts are employed for the intervening segment when a direct end-to-end anastomosis cannot be affected. Between one-half and two-thirds of patients still require medical treatment for hypertension lifelong.

AORTITIS

Takayasu's Disease

Takayasu's disease is a form of aortitis that affects people in the second to fifth decade of life. It is characterized by intimal proliferation and fibrosis along with fibrous scarring of the arterial media. Takayasu's disease affects mainly the aorta and its major branches, more markedly at the arterial origin. Clinically, the disease is manifested by weak or absent pulses along the arterial course. Takayasu aortitis rarely affects the aortic root, but when it does occur, it results in aortic regurgitation and poststenotic dilatation. An echocardiogram may be inconclusive, but in some cases, significant diffusely thickened aortic wall may be demonstrated by two-dimensional echo imaging. This picture should be differentiated from an aortic root abscess where the site of infection is always localized to one segment of the root. Once the diagnosis is made, conservative management is usually recommended, but pacemaker insertion may be required if the condition is complicated by heart block.[22]

Aortitis of Rheumatic Disease

As in rheumatoid arthritis and ankylosing spondylitis, arteritis is the result of complex immune disturbances. When the aorta is involved, the inflammatory process results in panaortitis affecting the three arterial layers. The only echocardiographic finding may be mild aortic regurgitation, which rarely progresses. This is probably because of the early disease recognition, the arthritis, and commencement of therapy that limits further progression.

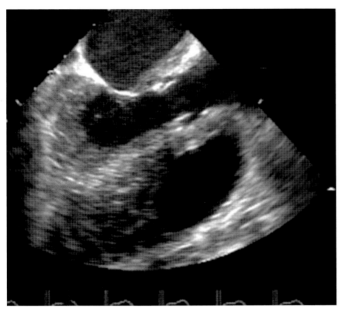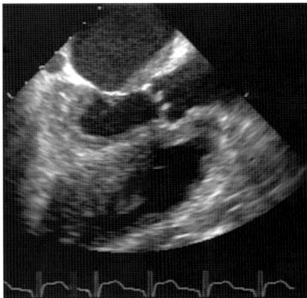

FIGURE 14.16. Parasternal long-axis view from a patient with Takayasu disease showing significantly thickened aortic root wall (10 mm).

However, extensive involvement with severe aortic regurgitation may occur.[23]

Syphilitic Aortitis

Syphilitic aortitis is a rare condition that results in scarring of the media and adventitia. It is manifested late after the onset of infection (10 to 30 years). The ascending aorta is the commonly affected site that becomes dilated. In severe disease a large aneurysm is formed that may cause mediastinal syndrome by pressing on adjacent structures: bronchi, esophagus, and recurrent laryngeal nerve. Surgery is the only means for managing complications of syphilitic aortic aneurysm.[24,25,26,27]

REFERENCES

1. Erbel R, Engberding R, Daniel W, et al. Echocardiography in diagnosis of aortic dissection. *Lancet* 1989;1:457–461.
2. Harris PD, Bowman FO Jr, Malm JR. The management of acute dissections of the thoracic aorta. *Am Heart J* 1969; 78:419–422.
3. Nienaber CA, von Kodolitsch Y, Nicolas V, et al. The diagnosis of thoracic aortic dissection by noninvasive imaging procedures. *N Engl J Med* 1993;328:1–9.
4. Bansal RC, Chandrasekaran K, Ayala K, Smith DC. Frequency and explanation of false negative diagnosis of aortic dissection using aortography and transesophageal echocardiography. *J Am Cell Cardiol.* 1995;25:1393–401.
5. Khandheria BK, Tajik AJ, Taylor CL, et al. Aortic dissection: review of value and limitations of two-dimensional echocardiography in a six-year experience. *J Am Soc Echocardiogr* 1989;2:17–24.
6. Kotler MN. Is transesophageal echocardiography the new standard for diagnosing dissecting aortic aneurysms? *J Am Coll Cardiol* 1989;14:1263–1265.
7. Chia BL, Yan PC, Ee BK,et al. Two-dimensional echocardiography and Doppler color flow abnormalities in aortic root dissection. *Am Heart J* 1988;116(1 Pt 1):192–194.
8. Iliceto S, Nanda NC, Rizzon P, et al. Color Doppler evaluation of aortic dissection. *Circulation* 1987;75:748–755.
9. Karalis DG, Chandrasekaran K, Victor MF, et al. Recognition and embolic potential of intraaortic atherosclerotic debris. *J Am Coll Cardiol* 1991;17:73–78.
10. Tobler HG, Edwards JE. Frequency and location of atherosclerotic plaques in the ascending aorta. *J Thorac Cardiovasc Surg* 1988;96:304–306.
11. Fox R, Ren JF, Panidis IP, et al. Anuloaortic ectasia: a clinical and echocardiographic study. *Am J Cardiol* 1984;54:177–181.
12. Pyeritz RE. Propranolol retards aortic root dilatation in the Marfan syndrome, abstracted. *Circulation* 1983;68 (Suppl III): 365.
13. el Habbal MH. Cardiovascular manifestations of Marfan's syndrome in the young. *Am Heart J* 1992;123:752–757.
14. Rothbaum DA, Dillon JC, Chang S, et al. Echocardiographic manifestation of right sinus of Valsalva aneurysm. *Circulation* 1974;49:768–771.
15. Haaz WS, Kotler MN, Mintz GS, et al. Ruptured sinus of Valsalva aneurysm: diagnosis by echocardiography. *Chest* 1980;78:781–784.
16. Nishimura K, Hibi N, Kato T, et al. Real-time observation of ruptured right sinus of Valsalva aneurysm by high speed ultrasono-cardiotomography. Report of a case. *Circulation* 1976; 53:732–735.
17. Ellis SG, Goldstein J, Popp RL. Detection of endocarditis-associated perivalvular abscesses by two-dimensional echocardiography. *J Am Coll Cardiol* 1985;5:647–653.
18. Shively BK, Gurule FT, Roldan CA, et al. Diagnostic value of transesophageal compared with transthoracic echocardiogra-

phy in infective endocarditis. *J Am Coll Cardiol* 1991;18: 391–397.

19. Carvalho JS, Redington AN, Shinebourne EA, et al. Continuous wave Doppler echocardiography and coarctation of the aorta: gradients and flow patterns in the assessment of severity. *Br Heart J* 1990;64:133–137.

20. Houston AB, Simpson IA, Pollock JC, et al. Doppler ultrasound in the assessment of severity of coarctation of the aorta and interruption of the aortic arch. *Br Heart J* 1987;57:38–43.

21. Marx GR, Allen HD. Accuracy and pitfalls of Doppler evaluation of the pressure gradient in aortic coarctation. *J Am Coll Cardiol* 1986;7:1379–1385.

22. Choe YH, Kim DK, Koh EM, et al. Takayasu arteritis: diagnosis with MR imaging and MR angiography in acute and chronic active stages. *J Magn Reson Imaging* 1999;10: 751–757.

23. Townend JN, Emery P, Davies MK, et al. Acute aortitis and aortic incompetence due to systemic rheumatological disorders. *Int J Cardiol* 1991;33:253–258.

24. Frank MW, Mehlman DJ, Tsai F, et al. Syphilitic aortitis. *Circulation* 1999;100:1582–1583.

25. Pugh PJ, Grech ED. Images in clinical medicine. Syphilitic aortitis. *N Engl J Med* 2002;346:676.

26. Fagan, A, Yacoub M, Pillai R, Radley-Smith R. Dacon replacement of the ascending aorta and sinuses with re-suspension of the aortic valve and re-implantation of the coronary arteries: a new method for treatment of aneurysmal or acute dissection of the aortic root. Proc. Joint Inter. CV and Thoracic Surgical Conference Stockholm. *Scan J. Cardiothoracic Surg.* 1982.

27. Yacoub M, Fagan A, Stauono P, Radley-Smith R. Results of valve conserving operations for aortic regurgitation. *Circulation* 1983;68:311–21.

Index